Materia Medica for Nurses
A Textbook of Drugs and Therapeutics

W Gordon Sears
MD (Lond.), MRCP (Lond.)
Honorary Consultant Physician, Mile End Hospital, London

R S Winwood
MB, FRCP
Consultant Physician, Whipps Cross Hospital, London

Ninth Edition

Edward Arnold

© W. Gordon Sears 1980

First Published 1943
by Edward Arnold (Publishers) Ltd,
41 Bedford Square, London WC1B 3DQ

Reprinted 1943, 1944 (twice), 1945
Second Edition 1947
Reprinted 1948
Third Edition 1955
Reprinted 1958
Fourth Edition 1959
Fifth Edition 1962
Reprinted 1964
Sixth Edition 1966
Reprinted 1968
Seventh Edition 1971
Reprinted 1974
Eighth Edition 1976
Ninth Edition 1980

British Library Cataloguing in Publication Data

Sears, William Gordon
  Materia medica for nurses. – 9th ed.
  1. Drugs
  I. Title   II. Winwood, Robert Sidney
  615′.1′024613   RM125
  ISBN 0-7131-4385-4

Printed in Great Britain by
Butler & Tanner Ltd, Frome and London

Preface to the ninth edition

Materia Medica and Therapeutics are subjects of rapid and excit-
ing advances. Therapy is increasingly more specific and frequently
provides a fascinating insight into the normal biochemical work-
ings of the body. The treatment of patients has become progressively more logical and in many cases there are useful therapeutic
alternatives which act by differing mechanisms. Thus a patient
with a peptic ulcer may be treated by directly counteracting gastric acidity with an antacid, by inhibiting gastric acid secretion
with a histamine H_2-receptor antagonist, or by prescribing a product such as carbenoxolone which provides a protective coat over
the ulcer and diminishes its exposure to gastric acid.

Therapeutics goes beyond the use of drugs, however, and in
some cases it may be of equal or greater importance that the patient
gives up smoking, moderates alcohol consumption, or reduces
weight. It is the responsibility of doctors and nurses to inform
patients when this is so and to try to persuade them to forsake
their undesirable habits.

Similarly, patients may need education and persuasion if their
co-operation is to be obtained in taking whichever drugs are prescribed. This matter of *compliance* with the demands of treatment
is an important one in which the persuasiveness of the nurse can
help. The likelihood of compliance by patients falls progressively
as the frequency of prescribed dosage increases. There has therefore been a growth in the number of sustained-release formulations and other long-acting medications which need be taken only
once or twice daily.

Many patients need concurrent therapy for several different
diseases. Clearly, caution must be exercised in administering a
drug for one disease if it may cause unacceptable effects in relation
to any other disease from which the patient suffers. Thus anti-
anginal therapy with a 'beta-blocker' may not be feasible if the
patient also has asthma, in which beta-adrenergic-receptor-block-
ade could increase the bronchospasm, or peripheral vascular
disease, in which it could cause arterial constriction and an increase in ischaemia of the extremities.

It must be borne in mind that when a patient is required to take two or more drugs, there is a possibility of *interactions* between them. These may be hazardous or may reduce the effectiveness of one of the treatments.

The doctor or nurse should never ignore the possibility of *side-effects* when a patient undergoing treatment complains of new symptoms. Sometimes, these will necessitate stopping a drug while at other times a reduction in dosage or simple reassurance will suffice.

The nurse is not required, in the UK, to sit a finals examination specifically in Materia Medica and Therapeutics. Clearly, however, these are vitally important subjects of which the nurse is rightly expected to have a good working knowledge. It is hoped that this book will go a long way towards providing this. In revising the text, the authors were again grateful for the help of Miss P. Stone, B.Pharm, MPS, in revising 'The Legal Control of Drugs' and in helping to exclude obsolete drugs from the text. Thanks are also due to our Publishers for their consistent helpfulness.

WGS
RSW

Contents

1 Introduction

The subject of drugs and their uses is a very large one and has many branches. It is constantly expanding and, while new drugs are being discovered, others are falling into disuse.

The release of a drug for general clinical use in Britain has to be approved by the Committee on Safety of Medicines (CSM). The Committee issues a Clinical Trial Certificate for a new drug if a variety of conditions are fulfilled. This enables clinical trials to be carried out and if the results indicate an acceptable level of efficacy and safety, a Product Licence is granted for the drug. It is then made generally available to the medical profession.

The CSM has expert subcommittees, one of which is concerned with the 'early warning' of adverse reactions to drugs. It relies on reports of suspected adverse reactions from doctors, dentists and pharmaceutical companies.

It must be emphasized that, from time to time, accidents and tragedies have occurred as a result of misreading the dosage of drugs. In former days the symbols for ounces and drachms were confused; likewise grains and grams. With metrication, attention is drawn to the terms micrograms (sometimes abbreviated to μg) and milligrams (mg).

The abbreviation 'μg' is used for 'micrograms' in laboratory practice but is not recommended for prescribing because it may be confused with 'mg', resulting in a patient receiving one thousand times the intended dose. The word 'micrograms' is best written out in full but the nurse may occasionally see the abbreviation 'mcg' used in prescriptions. Many doctors continue to write small doses in mg. This is 'unscientific' but has the advantage that it immediately alerts the nurse to the fact that only a very small quantity (e.g. digoxin 0·0625 mg) of a potentially toxic drug is being prescribed.

Definitions

(1) The term **Materia Medica** may be used to include the whole subject.

(2) A **drug** is any substance taken into the body or applied to its surface for the prevention or treatment of disease or symptoms.

(3) **Pharmacy** is the science concerned with the presentation of drugs in a form suitable for administration to a patient. This includes studies of formulation, design of a suitable manufacturing process, quality control and tests to determine stability. One aspect of pharmacy is **dispensing**, which involves the production of mixtures, ointments and sterile preparations, etc., from their various constituents. Pharmacists are also trained in, and have a legal duty to enforce, the various laws governing the production, distribution, storage and dispensing of medicines.

(4) **Pharmacology** deals with the mode of action of various drugs. It endeavours to explain on which organs of the body a drug acts and exactly how it operates. It is, therefore, closely united with physiology. For example, pharmacology explains how digitalis acts on the conducting tissue in the heart, slows the rate of the ventricle in atrial fibrillation, and improves the strength of cardiac contraction.

Drugs given in excessive amounts are liable to act as poisons, the study of which is called **toxicology.**

(5) **Therapeutics** is the art of using remedies in the treatment of disease. It embraces all the methods employed in the management and care of a patient whereby we endeavour to aid Nature in restoring the individual to health. Included also are the efforts made to relieve the patient's symptoms even if the disease cannot be cured, i.e. remedies may be (*a*) symptomatic, (*b*) palliative, or (*c*) curative.

Patients vary in their response to drugs. This variability is due to three principal factors:

(*a*) **the disease,** its severity and complications;
(*b*) **the responsiveness of the tissues** to the drug;
(*c*) **the concentration of the drug** at its site of action.

The latter factor is reflected by the plasma concentration of the drug. The effectiveness of treatment and the early recognition of toxicity can sometimes be improved by measurement of the plasma concentration of drugs, as with digoxin, phenytoin and nortriptyline.

Sources of reference

The British Pharmacopoeia (BP) is a list of 'official' drugs and their doses published by HM Stationery Office on behalf of the Health Ministers on the recommendations of the Medicines Commission in accordance with the Medicines Act, 1968. It lays down the chemical standard which must be maintained in the manufacture of all drugs labelled BP. The Medicines Commission appoints the British Pharmacopoeia Commission which actually undertakes the work of preparing the BP.

The British Pharmaceutical Codex (BPC) is an 'unofficial' work published by the Pharmaceutical Society of Great Britain which acts as a supplement to the BP and contains a number of other drugs and useful preparations.

The British National Formulary (BNF) is a handbook which includes those drugs and preparations in common use, and is widely employed both in hospital and general practice as a basis for prescribing. There are also many useful notes on drugs which a nurse may well study. The BNF is published jointly by the BMA and the Pharmaceutical Society.

Proprietary preparations. In addition to the official preparations, there are an enormous number of drugs prepared and sold by firms of manufacturing chemists all over the world. Some of them are very valuable, others are more or less useless, but it is only fair to say that many advances in therapeutics and the introduction of useful new drugs are due to the research and enterprise of these commercial undertakings. A number of these preparations ultimately become **'official'** and are included in the BP, usually under a different name.

Most of the proprietary preparations in use are listed in such publications as MIMS and the Data Sheet Compendium. In addition to the **proprietary name** (e.g. Inderal) chosen by the manufacturer, drugs are allotted an **approved name** (e.g. propranolol) by the British Pharmacopoeia Commission. If the drug is later described in the British Pharmacopoeia, its approved name becomes its **official title.**

(**NB.** Proprietary names are given in brackets or starting with a capital letter in the present text.)

Terminology

One of the most difficult and confusing aspects of the subject to the beginner is the terminology used in the naming of drugs. In the first place it must be understood that therapeutic substances are of very varied origin.

1. Vegetable

Drugs may be obtained from various parts of many plants such as their leaves, roots, seeds, flowers, fruit or bark. Resins and some oils are also obtained from vegetable sources.

The modern practice has been to extract the active principles from medicinal plants rather than to use the actual plants.

The two most important types of active principles extracted are:

(*a*) alkaloids;
(*b*) glycosides.

Alkaloids

These are usually highly active substances which are only used in very small doses. They contain nitrogen and their names generally terminate in -INE (*in Latin -ina*) thus:

morphine is an alkaloid of opium;
strychnine   „   „   „ nux vomica;
atropine   „   „   „ belladonna;
nicotine   „   „   „ tobacco.

Glycosides or glucosides

These are very potent vegetable substances in the formation of which glucose, or some other sugar, takes part.

Digoxin is a glycoside of digitalis.

The names of the glycosides terminate in -IN, although not every substance ending in this way is a glycoside, e.g. liquid paraffin is a mineral oil.

2. Mineral

This group includes salts of sodium, potassium, calcium, magnesium and iron. Examples are sodium chloride (common salt), magnesium sulphate (Epsom salts) and ferrous gluconate.

3. Animal

This term applies in particular to vaccines, sera, gland extracts, hormones and similar preparations.

4. Synthetic

The term 'synthetic' is used to describe a large number of compounds (e.g. the sulphonamides) which are synthesized (built up from simpler components) in chemical laboratories. The composition of many natural substances is known, and some of these can be synthesized in the laboratory and factory as well as being obtained from their natural sources. For example, adrenaline can be obtained from the suprarenal gland, but is more economically manufactured by ordinary chemical processes.

5. Antibiotics

These drugs play a very important part in the modern treatment of infections and consist of antibacterial substances derived from various moulds. They may be defined as chemical substances produced by micro-organisms, which prevent the growth of other micro-organisms. Many of these can now be made synthetically or semi-synthetically. Well-known antibiotics are penicillin, streptomycin, the tetracyclines and the cephalosporins (p. 273).

Classification of drugs

It is convenient in a textbook to consider drugs acting on the various systems of the body together. It is also useful to classify them in general terms which indicate their main action. Although individual drugs will be dealt with in appropriate chapters the following definitions in common use may be found helpful.

Analgesics are used to relieve pain.
Antacids neutralize hydrochloric acid in the stomach.
Anthelmintics are used in the treatment of parasitic worms.
Antibiotics (see above) and other antibacterial drugs.
Anticancer drugs (carcino-chemotherapeutic agents).
Anticoagulants such as heparin and Dindevan diminish the clotting power of the blood.

Anticonvulsants such as phenytoin are used in the treatment of epilepsy.

Antidepressants such as nortriptyline stimulate the higher centres of the brain.

Antidiabetic drugs. In addition to insulin, oral hypoglycaemic agents (e.g. chlorpropamide and glibenclamide) lower the blood sugar in diabetes.

Antihistamines counteract the action of histamine, a substance liberated in the tissues in a number of allergic conditions such as hay fever and urticaria.

Antipruritics are drugs which relieve itching.

Antiviral agents, such as idoxuridine, prevent or check the replication (multiplication) of viruses.

Diuretics increase the secretion of urine.

Haematinics contain iron and/or other factors necessary for the formation of haemoglobin and mature red blood cells.

Haemopoietic drugs stimulate the formation of red cells, e.g. vitamin B_{12} in the treatment of pernicious anaemia.

Haemostatics stop bleeding and help in the clotting of blood.

Hypnotics help in the production of sleep.

Sedatives and tranquillizers help to calm the nervous system.

Thymoleptic drugs help to change the mood of the patient in states of depression and anxiety (see p. 168).

In Great Britain the use of Latin names for drugs is no longer recommended and their English titles should be used in prescribing. Likewise, the Metric System has replaced the Apothecary's and the Imperial measures.

Many of the synthetic drugs are extremely complicated chemical compounds with very long names, the meaning of which is only appreciated by a chemist. In such instances, simpler names are usually given. As a rule the approved name differs from the proprietary name as the latter is protected by law and may only be used by the manufacturer. Aspirin was the trade name (originally owned by Bayer) for acetylsalicylic acid but is now the official name of the drug in the UK. Chloromycetin is a trade name for chloramphenicol, Epanutin is the trade name of phenytoin.

The legal control of drugs

Because many drugs are powerful poisons if employed in the wrong dose, and others have dangerous habit-forming properties (see p. 164), the manufacture, distribution and care of drugs are carefully protected by law. For many years the two main Acts dealing with drugs were the Dangerous Drugs Act, 1965 (DDA), and the Pharmacy and Poisons Act, 1933. These Acts were supplemented by the Dangerous Drugs Regulations, by the Poisons Regulations, and also by the Poisons List, 1970, and the Poisons Rules, 1970. The Dangerous Drugs Act has now been superseded by the Misuse of Drugs Act, 1971, and the sections of the Pharmacy and Poisons Act relating to medicines were superseded by Part III of the Medicines Act in February 1978. Non-medicinal poisons are now controlled by the Poisons Act, 1972.

Medicines Act, 1968
Part III—Legal classification of medicines

There are now three main classes of medicines:

General Sale (GSL)
Items on the General Sale List may be sold by any type of retail shop. There are some restrictions on pack sizes and labelling.

Pharmacy (P)
These medicines may be sold only from a pharmacy under the personal supervision of a pharmacist.

Prescription Only Medicines (POM)
Medicines so designated may be sold or supplied by a pharmacy to a patient only on the prescription of a doctor. The title 'Prescription Only Medicines' could be a little confusing when applied to hospital practice, since in hospitals no drugs are administered to patients without a doctor's prescription.

Application of the Medicines Act to hospitals

Although the law described above is already in force, and the Pharmacy and Poisons Act has been repealed, in hospitals there has been delay in implementation. The detailed application of the new regulations to the ordering and storage of medicines in wards has not yet (October 1979) been finalized, and the Department of Health and Social Security has directed that existing arrangements should be continued until further guidance is issued. Thus hospitals will continue for the time being to apply the provisions of the Pharmacy and Poisons Act, described below.

The Pharmacy and Poisons Act and the Poisons Rules

The provisions of this Act and Rules governed the storage and issue of poisons in hospitals. There can be no standard definition of a poison because the poisonous effect may depend on the dose given. However, for legal purposes, an arbitrary standard has been applied and the term poison means a substance included in the Poisons List made under the provisions of the Act. Medicines containing poisons can be supplied to wards from the pharmacy department only on the receipt of a signed order written by the sister, nurse in charge or by a doctor. Certain substances are subject to extra restrictions under the Rules and these are listed in the Schedules to the Poisons Rules.

Schedule 1

In hospital wards these drugs must be kept in a special cupboard reserved for the storage of Schedule 1 poisons and other poisonous substances. The pharmacist will indicate on the label the drugs to which this applies. (There is a British Standard design of cupboard for this purpose which also incorporates a special interior cupboard for Controlled Drugs.) All poison cupboards must be inspected by a pharmacist at intervals not exceeding three months.

Some examples of Schedule 1 poisons are:

carbachol	dihydrocodeine (DF 118)
physostigmine (eserine)	morphine
digoxin	barbiturates.

Schedule 4A and 4B

Poisons listed in this Schedule were subject to extra control in that they could not be sold to the general public without a doctor's prescription. All those listed in Schedule 4A are also in Schedule 1 and will be so labelled in hospitals.

Some examples of Schedule 4 poisons are:

barbiturates
some cytotoxic agents such as busulphan (Myleran)
gallamine (Flaxedil).

Supply of poisons to out-patients

Medicines containing poisons can be supplied to out-patients only on a doctor's prescription. In the case of Schedule 1 poisons, a record of the prescription must be kept for 2 years after the date on which it was written, in such a way that it can be traced readily. This is usually done by filing in the patient's case notes the prescription sheet bearing his details such as the address or alternatively the hospital registration number.

The Misuse of Drugs Act

The supply and prescription of habit-forming drugs are controlled by the Misuse of Drugs Regulations, 1973, under this Act. In these Regulations there are 4 Schedules and the drugs listed in them are subject to varying degrees of control according to their potential for abuse, and are known as Controlled Drugs (CD). Note that these Schedules are not the same ones previously described under the Poisons Rules, although some drugs are 'Scheduled' under both Acts.

Schedule 1

This Schedule contains preparations of certain Controlled Drugs, for example, codeine, pholcodine, cocaine and morphine, combined with other substances in such small amounts or in such ways that they are not liable to produce dependence or cause harm if misused.

Examples are:

codeine linctus BPC
squill opiate linctus BPC (Gee's Linctus) which contains 800 micrograms (0·8 mg) of morphine in 5 ml
kaolin and morphine mixture BPC which contains 700 micrograms (0·7 mg) of morphine in 10 ml
dihydrocodeine tablets BP.

Such preparations may be sold to the public without a prescription or supplied to a hospital ward without any formalities other than those required by the Poisons Rules. They do not have to be kept in the Controlled Drugs cupboard.

Schedule 2

A person can obtain these drugs from a retail pharmacy only on a doctor's prescription, and the way in which this must be written is fully specified by law. It is important to remember that the following parts of the prescription must be written by the doctor in his own handwriting: the name and address of the patient, the dose, and the quantity of the drug or preparation ordered (in both words and figures). He must also sign it and date it himself.

In a hospital, the sister in charge of a ward is entitled to keep a stock of these drugs in her ward which she may, of course, administer only to a patient who has been prescribed them by a doctor. She obtains her stock from the pharmacy by writing a signed and dated order in duplicate which must specify the name of the drug and the amount required. The pharmacist must sign and date the order when he dispenses it, and he must keep his copy for 2 years. The sister must also retain her copy for 2 years. In the ward the Controlled Drugs, which will bear an identifying label, must be kept in a special locked cupboard used for storing nothing else. (See note above about British Standard cupboard.)

Some examples of drugs included in this Schedule are:

the opiates (diamorphine or heroin, morphine, etc.) and related drugs such as pethidine, methadone, etc.
major CNS stimulants such as dexamphetamine and amphetamine
methaqualone, an ingredient of Mandrax
dihydrocodeine injection (DF 118), cf. tablets in Schedule 1 above.

Schedule 3

This consists of a few minor stimulant drugs which are now rarely prescribed. They are not subject to such stringent controls as the drugs in Schedule 2.

Schedule 4

These are the hallucinogenic drugs like lysergic acid diethylamide (LSD) and cannabis which have virtually no therapeutic uses. It is an offence to possess these drugs either inside or outside a hospital unless the person has a special licence granted by the Home Office.

Control of dangerous drugs and poisons in hospitals (The Aitken Report)

This report, which was published in 1958 by the Central Health Services Council of the Ministry of Health, made a number of recommendations which supplement the laws dealt with above and which have become standard practice in hospitals throughout the United Kingdom. Some important recommendations relevant to the laws already described are as follows:

(1) Ward sisters should keep a stock record book for Controlled Drugs in which they record the receipts of all such drugs and should record all the details of drugs administered so that a stock balance can be kept. It surprises most people to learn that this is not a requirement of the Misuse of Drugs Regulations—a ward sister is the one person entitled to possess Controlled Drugs by law who is not legally obliged to account for their subsequent use, apart from a patient using them in his own home. A procedure for the administration of all drugs is recommended in the report and this involves checking by a second person.

(2) Although the pharmacist checks the Poison and Controlled Drugs cupboards, he should not be responsible for checking the numerical stock of Controlled Drugs since this should be the responsibility of the sister who is in possession of them. Any discrepancies should be reported to, and investigated by, the senior nursing staff, although the pharmacist must be kept informed.

(3) Special arrangements must be made for delivering Controlled Drugs to the wards. A receipt should be signed when they are taken from the pharmacy and again on arrival at the ward if a messenger is employed.

(4) The keys of the Controlled Drug and Schedule Poison cupboards should always be in the personal possession of the nurse at that time in charge of these cupboards. No other person at all should have access to the cupboards except in her presence.

2 Pharmaceutical preparations

There are a number of preparations in use some of which are only occasionally encountered. Those commonly employed are listed in the BNF.

Aerosols

Salbutamol (Ventolin) aerosol for asthma is an example of these.

Applications

There are various preparations which are applied to the surface of the body, e.g.:

benzyl benzoate applications
dicophane (DDT) application.

Capsules

These are containers usually made of gelatin. Cachets and capsules are generally used for unpleasant drugs and are intended to be swallowed like pills, e.g.:

vitamin capsules
ampicillin capsules.

Collodions or collodia

These are substances dissolved in a volatile and highly inflammable solvent which evaporates when applied to the surface of the body, leaving a film-like skin or protective covering, e.g.:

flexible collodion
salicylic acid collodion.

Creams

Creams are similar to ointments but contain water and an emulsifying agent. Their ingredients are more penetrating and more easily absorbed than from greasy ointments, e.g.:

calamine cream
zinc oxide cream.

Dusting-powders

These are applied locally to the skin especially where there are areas of friction, eg.:

talc dusting-powder
dicophane (DDT) dusting-powder.

Ear-drops (*auristillae*)

Examples of these are:

phenol ear-drops (p. 44)
sodium bicarbonate ear-drops.

Elixirs

Elixirs are sweet liquid preparations containing syrup, glycerin and, sometimes, alcohol to which various drugs are added. They are very pleasant but rather expensive. An example is:

triclofos elixir (Tricloryl Syrup).

Emulsions

There are many substances which will not normally mix together, such as oil and water, but which may be combined by the addition of a third substance called an emulsifying agent. In an emulsion the globules of fat or oil, instead of running together, remain separate. In some cases the oil and water tend to separate into layers on standing, in spite of the presence of an emulsifying agent, but will re-form an emulsion on shaking. Acacia gum and tragacanth are common emulsifying agents. Milk is an excellent example of a natural emulsion. An example is:

liquid paraffin emulsion.

Enemas (p. 79)

Strictly speaking, an enema consists of the rectal injection of a small quantity of fluid and does not include the administration of large infusions of saline or glucose. Enemas may be classified in the following way:

(1) *Those to be returned*
   aperient or evacuant: warm water, arachis oil, and Phosphates Enema BPC (disposable).
(2) *Those to be retained*
   sedative: starch, starch and opium
   anti-inflammatory: prednisolone.

Eye-drops (p. 249)

The drops which are applied to the eye are also called **guttae**, e.g.:

atropine sulphate eye-drops
sulphacetamide eye–drops
chloramphenicol eye-drops
hypromellose eye-drops (artificial tears).

Eye lotions

Include sodium chloride eye lotion.

Any lotion remaining unused after opening the container should be discarded immediately because of the risk of bacterial contamination.

Eye ointments (*oculenta*)

Eye ointments have a greasy base (yellow soft paraffin) and are sterile when supplied. They should be applied to the conjunctiva of the lower lid from special tubes or on a sterile glass rod, and include:

atropine eye ointment
mercuric oxide eye ointment (Golden eye ointment)
sulphacetamide eye ointment

Gargles

These are fluid preparations used for gargling and are generally similar to or identical with mouth washes, e.g.:

phenol gargle (which has a mild local anaesthetic effect)
Betadine gargle.

Granules

methylcellulose (Celevac)
Senokot.

Inhalations (vapours)

These are solutions of antiseptic or aromatic drugs or drugs themselves which are volatile or become volatile when poured into hot water, e.g.:

pine oil, menthol, menthol and eucalyptus, and Friar's balsam (*Tinctura benzoini composita*).

Anaesthetics such as chloroform, ether and nitrous oxide gas and drugs like amyl nitrite are also given by inhalation.

Injections

These are sterile solutions of drugs, generally in water but sometimes in oil or other media. They are intended for subcutaneous, intramuscular and, sometimes, intravenous administration, e.g.:

adrenaline injection, subcutaneous
morphine sulphate injection, subcutaneous or intramuscular.

In its wide sense the term injection includes:

(1) intradermal (into the skin);
(2) subcutaneous or hypodermic;
(3) intramuscular;
(4) intravenous;
(5) intraperitoneal;
(6) intrathecal (into the subarachnoid space);
(7) also rectal, vaginal and urethral injections.

NB.—Almost all subcutaneous injections may also be given intramuscularly but not vice versa.

Insufflations

These are fine powders blown by a special insufflator directly on to the skin, the mucous membrane of the nose (e.g. pituitary, posterior lobe, insufflation) or throat, or on to a wound.

Linctuses or lincti (p. 131)

A linctus is a syrupy or viscous preparation used to allay coughing. The usual dose is 5 ml.

    codeine linctus
    pholcodine linctus.

Liniments

The term embrocation is also used to describe the oily soapy or spirituous preparations which are applied to or rubbed into the skin and have a counter-irritant action. They must be labelled 'For external use only' and are supplied in fluted bottles so that the risk of giving them internally by mistake is reduced. Examples are:
    camphor liniment (known also as camphorated oil)
    turpentine liniment
    methyl salicylate liniment.

Lotions

Lotions are watery or alcoholic solutions of drugs for external application to the skin or mucous membranes. They are generally applied on gauze or similar fabric (see also Eye lotions, p. 247, and Mouth washes, p. 64. Examples are:

    calamine lotion
    aluminium acetate lotion.

Lozenges

These are solid flat tablets containing drugs incorporated in a gum or sugar basis. They dissolve slowly and are intended to be sucked. They usually have an astringent or antiseptic action on the mucous membrane of the mouth and throat. Examples are:

    amphotericin lozenges
    benzocaine compound lozenges.

Mixtures (*misturae*)

The mixture is a common method of administering medicines by mouth. Mixtures are liquid preparations of one or more drugs, generally flavoured and made up with water to a standard dose of 10 ml or 5 ml for children. The actual composition of standard mixtures varies somewhat in different hospitals and may be altered at will by the doctor to contain the desired dose of the component drugs. The constituents are not fully dissolved in every case and, therefore, **the bottle must always be carefully shaken before administration.** Examples are:

> magnesium trisilicate mixture
> potassium citrate mixture
> compound senna mixture.

Mouth washes

Examples are:

> compound thymol glycerin
> hexetidine (Oraldene)
> povidone iodine (Betadine).

Nasal drops

Examples include:

> ephedrine nasal drops
> Otrivine Nasal Drops.

Ointments (*unguenta*)

Ointments are semi-solid preparations containing drugs mixed with materials such as soft paraffin (Vaseline), wool fat or Lanette wax. They are intended to be spread on or rubbed into the skin, e.g.:

> zinc ointment
> hydrocortisone ointment.

Paints

These are liquid preparations applied to the skin or mucous membranes by means of a brush. They are often antiseptic in action, e.g.:

iodine compound paint (Mandl's paint)
crystal violet paint.

Others are caustic, e.g.:

chromic acid paint.

Some are used as adhesive varnishes, e.g.:

iodoform compound paint (*Whitehead's varnish*).

Pastes

These are preparations similar to ointments but often having a starchy or glycerin basis. They are generally stiffer and more solid than ointments and their ingredients are, therefore, less easily absorbed. They help to absorb secretions and are not easily rubbed off. Examples:

starch paste
zinc and gelatin paste (Unna's paste)
coal-tar paste (*Pasta picis carbonis*).

Pessaries

A pessary is a cone-shaped mass containing a medicament for introduction into the vagina. It is usually made of cacao butter (oil of theobroma) or gelatin base, which remains solid at atmospheric temperature but is melted by the heat of the body. Examples:

lactic acid pessaries
nystatin pessaries.

Poultices

These are soft, pasty external applications used to provide heat and moisture to an inflamed or painful part, e.g.:

kaolin poultice.

Powders

These are mixtures of finely powdered drugs for internal use when they are usually dispensed in folded paper or capsules. A very small dose of a drug is difficult to handle in powder form and in such cases the bulk of the powder is made up of some other inert substance, e.g.:

magnesium trisilicate compound powder
pancreatin powder, strong.

Special-purpose sterile solutions

Sterile solutions are available in 500-ml and 1-litre bottles for special purposes:
(1) *Intravenous infusion*
normal saline (sodium chloride injection), 5 per cent dextrose (dextrose injection);
dextrose–saline (sodium chloride and dextrose injection), and dextran injections.
(2) *Peritoneal dialysis*
Dialaflex solutions, numbers 61 (normal), 62 (hypertonic) and 63, Difusor and Dianeal solutions.
(3) *Bladder irrigation.*

Spirits

Spirits are alcoholic solutions of oils or volatile substances which are only slightly soluble in water, e.g.:

aromatic spirit of ammonia (sal volatile)
surgical spirit.

Spray solutions (*nebulae*)

These are solutions of drugs intended to be sprayed on the skin or mucous membranes by means of an atomizer or aerosol. Examples:

(1) *For the skin*
oxytetracycline-hydrocortisone (Terra-Cortril) spray.
(2) *For the nose*
ephedrine spray
xylometazoline (Otrivine) spray.

(3) *For the bronchi*
   adrenaline and atropine compound spray
   isoprenaline spray
   salbutamol (Ventolin) aerosol.

Suppositories

These are conical solid bodies, not unlike pessaries, containing drugs in a basis of cacao butter (oil of theobroma) or gelatin for insertion into the rectum, e.g.:

   glycerin suppository
   bisacodyl suppository (Dulcolax)
   aminophylline suppository.

Syrups or syrupi

These are fluid preparations of drugs in solutions of sugar, e.g.:

   compound syrup of figs (*Syrupus ficorum compositus*)
   Ventolin (salbutamol) syrup.

Tablets

Tablets consist of drugs compressed in a mould. As a general rule tablets to be taken by mouth should be given with a draught of water. Some tablets, e.g. trinitrin (p. 289) are allowed to dissolve under the tongue.

Vaccines

See p. 289.

Vitrellae

Glass capsules to be crushed and the vapour inhaled, e.g.:

   amyl nitrite vitrellae.

Extracts

By the concentration of various vegetable or animal materials either a solid (*Extractum siccum*) or a liquid extract (*Extractum liquidum*) can be made. The liquid extracts are used in the preparation of medicines given in mixture form, while solid extracts are used for pills and tablets, e.g.:

   extract of belladonna
   extract of cascara sagrada.

Medicated waters (*Aquae*)

These usually contain some volatile substance or oil in solution. A number of them are used as flavouring agents, e.g.

chloroform water (*Aqua chloroformi*)
peppermint water (*Aqua menthae piperitae*).

Oils

With the exception of liquid paraffin, which is a mineral oil, and the fish-liver oils, the oils are obtained by distillation or expression from vegetable substances, e.g.:

almond oil
peanut oil
oil of clove
linseed oil
olive oil
castor oil.

Pastilles

These are sweet-like preparations which should be dissolved slowly in the mouth.

Tinctures

These are solutions of crude drugs in alcohol and resemble spirits but differ from them in their mode of preparation. Their individual doses differ considerably. Examples:

tincture of belladonna
compound tincture of benzoin (Friar's balsam).

3 The administration of drugs

Therapeutic substances are administered or applied in a number of different ways.

(1) Via the alimentary tract

(a) By the mouth (*per os*)

Capsules	Mixtures containing:
Draughts	extracts
Elixirs	mucilages
Linctuses	oils
Lozenges	solid drugs
Pastilles	solutions (*liquores*)
Powders	tinctures
Tablets	waters (*aquae*)

(b) Sublingual tablets (under the tongue).

(c) By the rectum (*per rectum*)

Enemas   Suppositories

(2) Via the respiratory tract

Inhalations including anaesthetics

Sprays   Aerosols   Vapours

(3) Via the uro-genital tract

(a) By the urethra (*per urethram*)

Injections

(b) By the vagina (*per vaginam*)

Douches   Pessaries

(4) Drugs applied to the skin

(*a*) Local applications:

Collodions	Glycerins	Ointments
Creams	Liniments	Paints
Dusting-powders	Lotions	Pastes

(*b*) Baths

(*c*) Ionization

(5) Drugs applied to mucous membranes

Many of the above may also be applied to mucous membranes. In addition:

(*a*) Mucous membrane of the mouth:

Gargles	Mouth washes
Lozenges	Pastilles
Adhesive gels	

(*b*) Mucous membrane of the nose:

Inhalations	Nasal douches
Insufflations	Sprays

(*c*) The eye:

Eye discs (*lamellae*)	Eye ointments (*oculenta*)
Eye-drops (*guttae*)	Eye washes (*collyria*)

(*d*) The ear:

Ear-drops (*auristillae*)	Insufflations

(6) Drugs given by injection

(*a*) Intradermal (into the skin).
     e.g. BCG vaccine
     Tuberculin tests, e.g. Mantoux
     TAB vaccine

(*b*) Subcutaneous or hypodermic. (Into the loose tissue spaces just beneath the skin.)
     e.g. narcotic drugs such as morphine
          insulin

(*c*) Intramuscular or into a muscle, e.g. paraldehyde.

(*d*) Intravenous or into a vein, e.g. hydrocortisone.

(*e*) Intrathecal or into the spinal canal.
     e.g. penicillin, streptomycin. (NB.—Small doses)
          spinal anaesthetics

The term 'parenteral' means 'not through the alimentary canal' and is used to imply some type of injection.

Injections are customarily given with a syringe and needle, both of which may be disposable. However, mass inoculation programmes can be more rapidly completed with a pressure injector, e.g. the Porton Jet Injector. This delivers drugs in a high-velocity jet which painlessly penetrates unbroken skin and deposits the drugs intradermally, subcutaneously or intramuscularly. Up to 800 inoculations per hour are possible with this instrument.

Factors affecting the absorption of drugs given intramuscularly

(1) If for any reason the *local circulation* is poor in the region of the injection, absorption will be delayed.
(2) *Peripheral circulatory failure* resulting from shock or heart failure, will delay the absorption of drugs injected intramuscularly.
(3) *Oedema* of tissues delays the absorption of drugs injected into them.

Technique of administration
Rules for the administration of drugs

The administration of drugs is a matter of great importance to the nurse and is one of the routine duties which carries with it great responsibility.

Many drugs are powerful poisons and doses are carefully calculated in order to produce the desired effect.

Absolute accuracy of measurement in every case is essential and is an important part of a nurse's training. Familiarity should never lead to carelessness. In the event of any doubt entering the nurse's mind about the correctness of a dose of the drug which is about to be given, there must be no hesitation in referring the matter to a senior officer.

Points to remember about administering medicines are:

(1) Punctuality, with special regard to the instructions before and after meals and special directions, e.g. 'with water'.
   (Medicines so ordered should be given 20 minutes before meals or immediately after meals as prescribed.)
(2) Read the label on the bottle and check the drug and dose with the patient's treatment card.

(3) Make a habit of shaking the bottle in each case, irrespective of whether the medicine is clear or containing a sediment. This should be done by inverting the bottle several times.

(4) Measure the dose carefully into a suitable medicine measure. Modern mixtures are made up to doses of 10 ml (5 ml for children). The measure should, if possible, be read while it is standing on a flat surface. If not, it must be held at eye level, taking care not to tilt the measure either backwards or forwards, a movement which will obviously produce an inaccurate reading.

(5) Give the medicine or tablet to the patient and watch him take it.

It is the proud boast of some patients that they pour all their medicines down the sink. Do not leave drugs lying about or permit unauthorized persons to handle them. In a private house circumstances may, of course, modify this procedure.

(6) Observe and report any signs of over-dose, reaction or intolerance. In this connection, if any mistake should unfortunately be made in the administration of a drug either by giving the wrong drug or dose, the nurse must immediately report the fact, irrespective of any personal consequences which might ensue. An error reported at once can sometimes be rectified without serious effects on the patient.

(7) Have all injections and dangerous drugs checked by a second person and enter the dose given in the Controlled Drugs register or the poison register when this is required.

(8) Try to make the administration of unpleasant drugs as agreeable as possible, e.g. give iron mixtures with a straw to prevent blackening of the teeth, and give the patient an opportunity of brushing the teeth without delay. Sweets, fruit juice, a mouth wash or a piece of bread may help to remove a disagreeable taste.

(9) Keep medicine bottle clean by wiping after use and always pour out of the side away from the label, i.e. keep the label uppermost.

(10) Remember that tablets and capsules are supplied in various strengths and, therefore, the labelled dose must be carefully checked with the treatment card.

Notes on the administration of drugs

Linctus: should be sipped slowly.

Lozenge and *pastille:* should be sucked slowly.

Mixture: See that the patient takes any sediment which tends to collect in the medicine glass.

Tablet, capsule: should be given with a drink of water and swallowed whole.

Oil: occasionally two or three drops of a volatile oil, such as oil of peppermint, are ordered for flatulence and are best given on a cube of sugar.

Olive oil, arachis oil and liquid paraffin are given by spoon.

Suppository: this should be inserted into the rectum with the patient in the lateral position. It may be dipped in warm water (the purpose being to melt the surface of the suppository) to facilitate introduction, which should be carried out slowly with the gloved finger, taking care to pass the suppository through the anal sphincter into the rectum.

Pessary: slight moistening may be necessary before insertion into the vagina, but usually there is sufficient mucous secretion present to make introduction easy.

Powder: (i) a powder (e.g. antacid) should be stirred into a little water or milk before being taken, as there have been fatalities through inhalation of insoluble powders;

(ii) mix with jam in a sandwich for children;

(iii) effervescent powders should be stirred in half a tumbler of water and taken at once, e.g. Seidlitz powder.

Tablet: As a rule a tablet should be swallowed whole. Some may be crushed, placed on the back of the tongue and swallowed with a draught of water, but this should generally be discouraged because many tablets have special coatings or are specially designed for slow-release of their active constituents.

Tablets of glyceryl trinitrate and isoprenaline should be allowed to dissolve under the tongue, i.e. sublingually.

Some antacid tablets (e.g. Gelusil) are allowed to dissolve slowly in the mouth.

The intravenous administration of drugs

The intravenous route is used for the administration of drugs when a rapid effect is required, when other routes cannot be relied upon to achieve and maintain therapeutic serum concentrations (e.g. because of poor absorption from the gastrointestinal tract in the case of some drugs or from subcutaneous or intramuscular sites in cases of shock), when intramuscular injection would be excessively painful or would cause severe tissue damage, or when the volume of fluid to be injected is large.

The nurse may be responsible for the intravenous administration of drugs via an intravenous infusion. Intravenous infusion therapy can be used to replace abnormal losses of body fluids, to restore and maintain electrolyte balance and to administer drugs, especially those such as potassium chloride and fucidin which must be well diluted before injection.

Guide to intravenous infusion therapy

(1) A fluid-balance chart must be carefully kept so that the patient is not overloaded with fluid and sent into heart failure, which is particularly likely to occur in elderly people. When bottles are changed, the time must be recorded on the fluid balance chart.

(2) Containers must be checked for leaks or cracks immediately before use. The infusion fluid should be clear (usually) and free from visible particles. Any containers which do not pass these inspections must be discarded.

(3) The label on the container should be checked for its contents and expiry date.

(4) The closure of the container needs to be cleaned with a suitable disinfectant (e.g. 70% isopropyl alcohol) before the sterile cannula of the giving-set is inserted into it.

(5) No drug or other substance must be added to blood or blood products. Other infusion fluids which are generally unsuitable for the addition of drugs are amino-acid solutions, fat emulsions, mannitol, and sodium bicarbonate solutions. Constituents of these fluids may react with the drug or the drug may be inactivated or precipitated if the pH is unfavourable.

(6) Drugs may be incompatible with an infusion fluid and, for this reason, the fluid should be examined for cloudiness, change of colour, or formation of a precipitate after a drug has been added and evenly mixed.

(7) The infusion container must be labelled with details of whatever is added.

(8) If only a small volume of infusion fluid is required for a drug, a giving-set with a measuring chamber may be used and the drug is injected into the latter and mixed.

(9) A strict aseptic technique must always be observed in adding drugs to intravenous infusions. Ideally, additives are added in the pharmacy in an isolated area free from air-borne contamination.

(10) Some drugs may be lethal if infused too rapidly. Such an accident can occur if the drip-regulating clamp is dislodged by violent movements of the patient's arms. The ordinary giving-set is therefore insufficiently safe for the administration of potentially lethal drugs; an electric infusion pump or a giving-set with a small graduated chamber, which needs frequent refilling, should be used.

The action of drugs

It will be clear from consideration of the enormous number of drugs at our disposal and the divers conditions for which they may be employed, that no very precise summary can be given of their mode of action. However, among the ways in which drugs can act are:

(1) The direct action on micro-organisms and parasites on the surface of the body or on other objects, e.g.:

The use of antiseptics for sterilizing instruments or as lotions applied externally, for instance benzyl benzoate emulsion applied for scabies.

(2) A direct lethal effect on organisms within the tissues of the body, e.g.:

    (a) The use of chemotherapy (sulphonamides, etc.) and antibiotics, such as penicillin, against bacteria which are sensitive to their action;

    (b) Chloroquine and similar drugs for malaria.

(3) A direct and obvious chemical effect, e.g.:

    (a) neutralizing the hydrochloric acid in the gastric juice by giving antacids such as magnesium trisilicate or aluminium hydroxide;

    (b) turning an acid urine alkaline by giving potassium citrate; or an alkaline urine acid with acid sodium phosphate.

(4) Producing the desired effect by some known physiological action.

Thus atropine paralyses the nerve endings to the muscle of the pupil of the eye and its administration results in dilatation of the pupil. On the other hand, physostigmine (eserine) stimulates the nerve endings and its action is opposite to that of atropine, for it causes the pupil to contract.

The action of digitalis on the conducting tissues of the heart in the bundle of His, whereby it blocks a number of the frequent and irregular impulses coming from the atrium in atrial fibrillation, is also a good example.

(5) Drugs may be given to replace some missing factor which should normally be supplied by the body. Such drugs are usually chemically identical with the missing substance and are either made in the laboratory or obtained from some suitable animal, e.g.:

    (a) Thyroxine to replace the missing hormone in myxoedema.

(b) Vitamin B_{12} by injection to replace that which cannot be absorbed from the diet in pernicious anaemia.

(6) Vitamins, and drugs like iron and calcium given to compensate for dietetic deficiencies or defective absorption.

(7) Many other examples might be given, but they will become apparent as individual drugs are considered.

A **placebo** is a medicine given to please or satisfy a patient without having any special pharmacological effect. It is really, therefore, a form of psychotherapy.

Idiosyncrasy (drug hypersensitivity)

Idiosyncrasy may be defined as an abnormal or unusual response to a normal dose of a drug. (The word is derived from the Greek: *idios* = one's own, *syncrasis* = blending.) It is a form of over-sensitivity which is sometimes due to allergy and the term 'drug allergy' is often used.

It is only met with in isolated cases, but, in such instances, an ordinary dose may produce symptoms which are unpleasant, alarming or even dangerous. Sometimes the symptoms are similar to those seen when an over-dose of the drug has been taken by a normal person.

The symptoms may appear immediately, particularly after injections, but may be delayed for some hours or even days.

Since the nurse may administer the drug or the patient will be under the nurse's observation after it has been given, the subject is clearly one of great importance to the nurse. Any unusual symptoms occurring after a drug has been given should, therefore, be reported without delay. The condition may develop after a drug has been given internally, but not infrequently external applications to the skin produce severe local reactions. Sometimes a patient is aware of the sensitivity and gives notice of it; such a warning should not be ignored.

The most common types of reaction which occur are:

(1) Rashes and skin eruptions.

(2) General symptoms including collapse, nausea, vomiting and giddiness. Adrenaline is the drug of choice for the treatment of anaphylactic reactions in adults. Lesser symptoms may respond to an antihistimine.

(3) Aplastic anaemia and agranulocytosis, due to an unexpected toxic action of the drug in the bone marrow. These are serious conditions which may prove fatal (see p. 112).

While it is difficult to exclude any particular drugs, the following are important:

(1) *Quinine*, causing deafness, giddiness, headache, nausea, shivering, noises in the head, disturbance of vision and transient rashes such as urticaria or erythema.

(2) *Aspirin*, causing noises in the head (tinnitus), deafness, malaise, nausea, rapid pulse or an erythematous rash.

   NB.—Aspirin occasionally causes haematemesis or melaena, and may also produce serious reactions in asthmatics.

(3) *Potassium iodide* causes increased secretion from the respiratory tract resembling a severe cold in the head, laryngitis and skin eruptions similar to acne. Iodine given internally in other forms may produce the same effects (iodism).

(4) *Cocaine* (including procaine, Novocain, etc.). Malaise, vomiting, pyrexia; collapse with pallor, rapid pulse and slow respirations, and sometimes convulsions or fits, may all occur. Death occasionally follows from respiratory paralysis.

(5) *Sulphonamides*. Drugs of this group may produce serious reactions in some individuals, e.g. changes in the white cells of the blood (agranulocytosis), haematuria, pyrexia after the initial lesion for which the drug has been given has subsided (drug fever), and skin rashes (see p. 285).

(6) *Penicillin* and *ampicillin* may cause rashes or even severe collapse in sensitive persons, and streptomycin sometimes gives rise to troublesome eruptions in those who handle it.

Tolerance

This may be of two types: (i) *natural* tolerance, which is really the direct opposite of idiosyncrasy and implies that the individual resists the action of a certain drug and can tolerate much larger doses than a normal person; (ii) *acquired*, which means a state induced in the normal person by the prolonged use of a drug whereby he can gradually tolerate increasing doses which would, if administered in the first place, have produced toxic symptoms.

Tolerance is a common phenomenon and is exhibited by a number of drugs. Tobacco and alcohol are obvious examples. The first cigarette may produce nausea, vomiting and a greenish pallor of the skin, while a seasoned smoker may consume up to 60 cigarettes a day without any immediately obvious symptoms, except perhaps a well-deserved 'smoker's cough'. The difference in effect between two persons consuming the same amount of alcohol is also well known. Tolerance of the pharmacological effects does not, however, protect the smoker from lung cancer or the drinker from cirrhosis of the liver.

Among the important drugs used in therapeutics for which tolerance may be acquired are: opium and morphine, barbiturates, atropine and belladonna (p. 164).

It must always be remembered, however, that when a drug is discontinued the acquired tolerance is usually lost and, if the drug is recommenced at a later date, ordinary doses must be used.

The mechanism of acquired tolerance varies. In some cases excretion may be more rapid, in others the drug is more quickly destroyed or converted into some inert substance.

Drug addiction

The World Health Organisation prefers the more comprehensive term *'drug dependence'* to 'addiction' and 'habit'. Dependence may be *emotional* (psychic) or *physical* or both. If there is physical dependence the patient becomes physically ill on withdrawal of the drug (withdrawal syndrome) since some of the metabolic processes of the body come to depend on the drug. Continuing drug dependence may lead, however, to suffering, degradation and early death. The *types of drug dependence* (WHO) are as follows:

morphine-type (includes heroin and opium)
barbiturate- or alcohol-type
amphetamine-type
cocaine-type
hallucinogen-type (e.g. LSD)
cannabis-type (marijuana) (p. 167).

In all of these there is a degree of emotional dependence but only in the first two types is there physical dependence. The opiates cause an emotional detachment which makes them attractive to people who are intolerably anxious or despondent. An intravenous injection of heroin immediately produces an intense feeling of well being which is known as a 'rush' or a 'high'.

Opiate withdrawal symptoms include anxiety, restlessness, insomnia and yawning, aches, cramps, shivers, runny nose, vomiting, diarrhoea, anorexia, and loss of weight. In the case of heroin, withdrawal symptoms start about 6 to 8 hours after the last dose and reach a peak between 18 and 24 hours.

Heroin addicts often suffer from personal neglect, malnutrition (partly because of anorexia), and the results of using infected syringes, viz. hepatitis, abscesses and septicaemia. Gangrene sometimes results from the clumsy or unsterile intravenous injection of barbiturates ('main-lining').

Patients are sometimes dependent on a mixture of drugs, e.g. barbiturate–amphetamine or heroin–cocaine mixtures. Any substances on the Controlled Drugs list may induce dependence. This is a state in which the individual acquires a craving for a particular drug, often to such an extent that life becomes unbearable without it.

Treatment is notoriously difficult and involves the gradual withdrawal of the drug. In the case of heroin dependence, methadone may be substituted; methadone dependence is less objectionable. When cure of drug dependency is impossible the drugs may be supplied under supervision. Only doctors working in **special drug-treatment centres** may prescribe heroin or cocaine for addiction; for the treatment of organic disease any doctor may, of course, prescribe these drugs.

Cumulative effect

When a drug is taken one of two things may happen.

(*a*) It may be destroyed or converted into some inert or inactive substance by the tissues, especially the liver.

(*b*) It may be excreted unchanged by the kidneys, bowel, lungs or skin.

Clearly there will be a definite relationship for each drug, between the rate at which it is taken in and the rate of its destruction or excretion, and, as a rule, the dosage and intervals at which any drug is administered are adjusted to meet this situation. It follows that if the rate of administration is greater than the rate of destruction or excretion, the drug will accumulate in the tissues and increase in amount with each dose taken.

Some drugs and poisons are especially liable to show this phenomenon and will produce the symptoms of over-dosage or poisoning.

Digitalis is an important example. Mercury, arsenic and lead are others. In lead poisoning, small quantities of lead may be absorbed into the body over a long period and, finally, when a certain concentration exists in the tissues the typical symptoms appear, e.g. colic and various types of paralysis.

Drug interaction

Sometimes one drug will increase the effects of another if taken at the same time (potentiation) and the results may be dangerous:

(i) Alcohol increases the effect of barbiturates, tranquillizers and antihistamines, an important factor when driving a car.

(ii) The action of digitalis is enhanced by thiazide diuretics which increase potassium excretion.

(iii) Dangerous results may occur if a patient taking a monoamine oxidase inhibitor (MAOI), e.g. phenelzine (see p. 170), eats cheese or certain other foods.

(iv) Aspirin and phenylbutazone increase the activity of anticoagulant drugs.

(v) Sulphonamides should be avoided in diabetics taking tolbutamide, which is a sulphonamide derivative.

Dosage of drugs in childhood

In this book, the recommended doses are for adults unless otherwise stated.

Drugs are prescribed for children on the basis of their weight or body surface area (BSA). Sometimes one basis is preferable, sometimes the other. For example, atropine is best prescribed for an infant by reference to weight since dosage based on surface area may be excessive. Except for under-weight children, drugs are often prescribed on an age basis. No method of prescribing drugs for children is perfect and a nurse should always be on the lookout for possible adverse effects.

Many medicines are available in liquid form (suspensions or elixirs). It cannot be too strongly emphasized that liquids should be thoroughly shaken before a dose is measured out from the bottle. All BNF liquid medicines (linctuses, elixirs and paediatric mixtures) should be made up by the dispenser for individual patients so that the correct dose is contained in a 5 ml teaspoonful.

The nurse may encounter various formulae used in the calculation of dosage of drugs for children. They include *Young's formula* in which the dose for children less than 12 years of age may be obtained by dividing the age by age + 12. Thus for a child of 6:

$$6 \div (6 + 12) = \tfrac{1}{3}$$

therefore one-third of the usual adult dose would be given.

Catzel's formula

$$\frac{\text{BSA of child}}{\text{BSA of adult}} \times 100 = \% \text{ of adult dose.}$$

The weight-percentage method is another way of calculating the dose for a child.

Table 3.1

Age	Weight (kg)	(lb)	% of adult dose
Birth	3·2	7	12·5
2 months	4·5	10	15
4 ,,	6·5	14	20
12 ,,	10	22	25
18 ,,	11	24	30
5 years	18	40	40
7 ,,	23	50	50
10 ,,	30	66	60
11 ,,	36	80	70
12 ,,	40	88	75
14 ,,	45	100	80
16 ,,	54	120	90
Adult	65	145	100

Some drugs are prescribed for adults on the basis of mg/kg of body weight. The appropriate dose for a child may be calculated by taking age into account. For a child under 1 year, the dose calculated on a weight basis should be multiplied by 2. It should be multiplied by 1·5 for a child between 1 and 7 years and by 1·25 for a child of 12 years.

Weight and body surface area are not the only factors on which suitable dosage depends. Children tolerate the following drugs well and larger doses can be given than would be suggested by application of the formulae:

aperients   hyoscyamus   sulphonamides.

On the other hand, some drugs are badly tolerated and smaller doses are necessary. Morphine, opium and other narcotics fall into this category.

In **old age,** too, it is usually advisable to reduce the average dose somewhat. Doses of digitalis preparations which would be therapeutic in younger adults may be seriously toxic in elderly people. A special low-dosage form of digoxin, containing only 0·0625 mg in each tablet, has therefore been marketed under the name of Lanoxin PG, PG meaning paediatric-geriatric. Some drugs may be unsuitable for elderly patients. For example, barbiturates tend to cause mental confusion in the elderly.

In the first trimester of **pregnancy,** drugs are generally best avoided, especially if they are new ones. Some chemical compounds (and some viruses) have a malforming (teratogenic) influence on the developing embryo. This was emphasized by the thalidomide tragedy.

Drugs which should, if possible, be particularly avoided in early pregnancy are aminopterin, methotrexate, cotrimoxazole, nicotinamide, salicylates including aspirin, barbiturates, phenytoin, antacids, and hormones which may cause masculinization of the female fetus (oestrogens, progestogens and androgens). If phenytoin is essential for the control of her epilepsy, the pregnant woman should have her serum concentration of the drug monitored so as to avoid toxic concentrations.

It is also possible for drugs to adversely affect the fetus in the second and third trimesters of pregnancy. Among those which are best avoided are sulphonamides, tetracyclines, chloramphenicol, streptomycin, chloroquine, salicylates, phenothiazines, barbiturates, reserpine, thiazides, live viral vaccines, anticoagulants, and sex hormones.

4 Disinfectants and antiseptics

Only a section of the large subject of sterilization falls within the province of Materia Medica, namely, the killing of bacteria, viruses, fungi, etc. by chemical methods. This presents three problems:

(1) The killing of organisms away from the human body, viz. the sterilization of instruments, utensils, linen, dressings, excreta, etc.

(2) The killing of organisms on the surface of the body and in wounds.

(3) The killing of organisms within the tissues of the body by drugs given by internal administration, e.g. sulphonamides and antibiotics (see Chapter 18).

Methods of sterilization

The following methods of killing or removing organisms may be employed:

I. Physical methods

(*a*) *Heat*

   (i) Ordinary boiling for periods up to 20 minutes depending on the nature of the article. Two minutes boiling kills most bacteria, but spores are not necessarily destroyed by the most prolonged boiling. The addition of 2 per cent washing soda to the water is more lethal to the bacteria and spores.

   (ii) Steam under pressure, as produced in the autoclave.

   (iii) Dry heat which is not so effective as moist heat and, in comparison, requires to be of a higher temperature and to act for longer periods.

(*b*) *Radiation.* Direct exposure to sunlight or ultraviolet rays is effective in destroying a number of organisms. Gamma-irradiation is now frequently used for sterilizing surgical materials (e.g. sutures).

(*c*) *Filtration.* It is possible to remove bacteria from water and other fluids by passing them through a special very fine filter of the Berkefeld and Pasteur–Chamberland type. Viruses are smaller than ordinary bacteria and will pass through such filters, hence the term 'filter-passing virus' is sometimes used.

II. Chemical methods

The majority of these drugs owe their germicidal or antiseptic action to one of the following properties:
(1) the power to extract water from the bodies of bacteria;
(2) the power of coagulating proteins;
(3) a general poisonous action on protein;
(4) the liberation of oxygen.

The value of soap and detergents as aids to disinfection should not be overlooked. Most of them have no germicidal power in themselves but, when used on the hands or other articles, very efficiently remove the superficial layer of grease in which bacteria are lodged, and so facilitate the subsequent application of germicides. Very few disinfectant substances can be combined with toilet soap and the majority of the 'carbolic soaps' are useless from a germicidal point of view. The detergent cetrimide (Cetavlon) has mild antiseptic properties. For washing the hands before performing surgical procedures, hexachlorophane (Phiso-MED), chlorhexidine (Hibiscrub), or povidone–iodine (Betadine) may be used instead of plain soap. The patient's skin may be swabbed with cetrimide, surgical spirit, tincture of iodine or povidone–iodine prior to operation.

Whenever possible, sterilization of instruments and utensils by boiling is to be preferred to chemical methods, while the autoclave is used for dressings and gloves.

The main uses for chemical disinfectants in this connection are to keep sterile instruments free from further contamination; in emergency when other methods are not available and for non-boilable appliances, e.g. gum-elastic catheters and some electrical connections.

The disinfection of lavatories and drains is practically impossible and most disinfectant fluids poured down them only act as cleansing agents and deodorants.

Disinfectants and antiseptics

Strictly speaking, an antiseptic is a substance which prevents the growth of micro-organisms but does not necessarily kill them, so that their growth may be possible after the removal of the drug. Such action is sometimes described as **bacteriostatic.** A disinfectant or germicide kills bacteria and, by comparison with antiseptics, may be called **bactericidal.** All disinfectants are, therefore, antiseptics, but an antiseptic is not necessarily a germicide.

The term antiseptic is generally used for agents applied to living surfaces, while disinfectants are those used on inanimate objects.

It must be remembered, however, that a substance in strong concentration may be germicidal, but in weaker solutions may only act as an antiseptic, so that no exact distinction can be made between the two terms.

The following is a summary of some of the important factors upon which disinfectant and antiseptic action depends:

(1) The strength of the disinfectant.
(2) The time for which it acts.
(3) The temperature.
(4) The nature of the material in which it has to act. The presence of pus or other organic matter retards the action of some substances of this class.
(5) The type of the infecting organisms.

1. The strength of the disinfectant

It has just been mentioned that a substance in strong concentration may be bactericidal but in weaker solutions may only act as an antiseptic, i.e. as a bacteriostat.

This is a most important fact to realize, for many of the substances of this group are used in various strengths for different purposes, and dilution affects each disinfectant to a markedly different degree.

Thus, phenol in concentrated form acts very rapidly; in dilutions up to 1 in 100 it acts with reasonable rapidity; but in solutions weaker than this is almost ineffective and organisms will survive for many hours in a strength of 1 in 150. In other words the phenol in a 'carbolic bath', formerly given at the end of an infectious illness, was quite useless.

2. The time of action

Speaking generally, this varies with the concentration of the drug. The stronger the solution of the substance, the shorter the time required to kill bacteria.

The dyes, mercury salts and the salts of other metals tend to be slow in action, whereas disinfectants dependent upon the liberation of chlorine are relatively rapid.

3. Temperature

The action of disinfectants is, in most instances, increased to some extent by a rise in temperature. Therefore, preparations for external use should be employed at body temperature whenever possible.

4. The nature of the material

This specially applies to the presence of pus, blood, and other organic matter, such as necrotic tissue, which tend to decrease the activity of many antiseptics and germicides.

5. The type of the infecting organism

The most powerful disinfectants are germicidal to all organisms. On the other hand, some disinfectants, as well as the more powerful ones in weaker concentrations, show what may be called 'selective action'. That is, a disinfectant may be more effective against one organism than another.

For example, staphylococci are very susceptible to crystal (gentian) violet dye. Dyes of the flavine group are more active against streptococci than staphylococci. These facts may be of importance in the dressing and irrigation of wounds.

Important disinfectants and antiseptics

Much research has been carried out on these agents. The great difficulty has been to produce those which can be used not only outside the body but also on the human tissues, because so many substances which are lethal to bacteria also injure the tissues and are, therefore, of no value in disinfecting the skin or irrigating wounds, for they will do more harm than good.

The ideal requirements for a disinfectant are:

(1) to be strongly lethal to bacteria but non-injurious to human tissues (i.e. non-toxic and non-corrosive);

(2) to be easily soluble in water, saline and serum, and to act efficiently in the presence of blood, pus or dead tissue;

(3) to be inexpensive.

The disinfectants and antiseptics most commonly used can be classified roughly into several main groups:

(1) Acids and alkalis.
(2) Solutions of certain metallic salts.
(3) Various organic compounds (including alcohols and coal-tar products, etc.).
(4) The halogens, i.e. chlorine and iodine.
(5) Oxidizing agents, e.g. hydrogen peroxide.
(6) Dyes—(a) aniline type; (b) flavine type.
(7) Various other substances including ethylene oxide gas for sterilization'

1. Acids and alkalis

Strong mineral acids (such as nitric, sulphuric and hydrochloric acids) and alkalis (caustic potash and caustic soda) are corrosive and destroy all living matter. They also dissolve or damage many substances in common use. They are, therefore, unsuitable for application as disinfectants either to the surface of the body or on utensils in concentrated form.

They have been occasionally employed as caustics (i.e. to burn away tissue), for example, the application of strong nitric acid to warts.

In appropriate dilution they are sometimes employed in treatment. It will be recalled that the gastric juice contains hydrochloric acid (1·2 per cent) and that this is sometimes referred to as the 'antiseptic barrier' of the stomach. Dilute hydrochloric acid (10 per cent; dose up to 4 ml) is occasionally given in dyspeptic conditions and in some cases of pernicious anaemia, a disease in which hydrochloric acid is absent from the gastric juice.

There are a number of other weak acids not belonging to the mineral acid group which are non-corrosive and used in therapeutics for other purposes. The majority are given internally and are considered later. Others are employed externally for various purposes. The following are some which are given internally:

acetylsalicylic acid (aspirin)	lactic acid
ascorbic acid (vitamin C)	mandelic acid
citric acid	nicotinic acid.

Lactic acid is also used as an antiseptic in vaginal douches and pessaries.

Tannic acid was once used as an external application on account of its astringent properties and its power of tanning or coagulating proteins on an open surface, e.g. for burns. It has a serious toxic effect on the liver after absorption.

Boric acid
Boric acid, a white crystalline substance, is an antiseptic of feeble action which is non-irritant. A 4 per cent lotion may be used for irrigating the eye.

Ointments and dusting powders containing more than 5 per cent boric acid should not be applied to raw or weeping surfaces. Absorption of boric acid thus applied can have dangerous and even fatal toxic results.

It was formerly used as a preservative for food, but this is now illegal.

Salicylic acid

This occurs as colourless crystals and has some antiseptic properties, especially against fungi. For this purpose it is used in ointments in certain skin diseases, e.g. *Unguentum acidi salicylici compositum* (Whitfield's ointment). It is also used in foot-powders. In plasters or collodion, it is used for corns and warts.

Salicylic acid is not given internally, but its derivatives, sodium salicylate and acetylsalicylic acid (aspirin) are well known (see p. 159).

Acetic acid

This is an organic acid which is present in vinegar. Its only possible use as an antiseptic lies in the fact that a 2 per cent solution is an effective dressing for infections due to *Pseudomonas aeruginosa* (a good example of selective action previously mentioned).

2. Solutions of certain metallic salts

The metallic salts which can act as disinfectants are those which have the power of coagulating proteins, such as silver nitrate, copper sulphate and zinc sulphate.

Silver nitrate

This substance has special uses and may be employed in solid form or as a solution.

(a) In solid form it is used as a caustic (lunar caustic) to destroy excess of granulation tissue in an open wound or ulcer. The stick is slightly moistened and rubbed lightly on the area of granulation tissue, care being taken to avoid contaminating the surrounding skin. This process may be painful and produces a white appearance, which later turns black. When thus applied it destroys all the tissues and organisms with which it comes in contact.

NB.—Silver nitrate stains on the skin may be removed by mercuric chloride solution.

(b) As a solution for irrigating the bladder in chronic cystitis the strength may be gradually increased from 1 in 10 000 to 1 in 2000.

Copper sulphate

Copper sulphate was used in the now obsolete Benedict's test for glycosuria.

Zinc sulphate

This substance, and also zinc chloride, has been used in the form of antiseptic eye-drops. It has been given by mouth (220 mg doses) in the treatment of leg ulcers.

Mercury perchloride (mercuric chloride, corrosive sublimate)

This is a colourless, poisonous, antiseptic which must not be confused with mercurous chloride (calomel). Solutions of it and mercury biniodide may be artificially coloured to minimize the risk of being mistaken for water or other harmless liquid. Its solution is used in strengths up to 1 to 1000 for external purposes, but it should not be applied to steel instruments on account of its action on the metal.

There are a number of organic mercurial antiseptics which are less toxic and less irritating than the inorganic compounds. They include mercurochrome and merthiolate. Metaphen is a mercurial disinfectant.

NB.—some skins are sensitive to mercury and its use may result in dermatitis.

3. Various organic compounds
The alcohols

Chemically there are a number of different alcohols but only three require special mention, viz.:

ethyl alcohol;
methyl alcohol;
isopropyl alcohol.

Ethyl alcohol (Ethanol)

In its pure form and when free from any trace of water it is referred to as absolute alcohol.

Ethyl alcohol has maximum antiseptic properties as a 70 per cent solution, but in stronger or weaker concentrations is less effective. It is useful for rendering the unbroken skin aseptic, but it is painful when applied to raw surfaces and this, together with the fact that the presence of proteins reduce its activity, renders it unsuitable for application to wounds. Applied externally, however, alcohol hardens the skin and is useful in preventing bedsores. It evaporates quickly and is used in cooling lotions in the treatment of sprains and contusions. It is the type of alcohol present in fermented beverages (p. 263), and it is also the basis of a number of pharmaceutical preparations, e.g. tinctures and some liniments.

Absolute alcohol is a purer form which can only be purchased from a chemist on a prescription.

Surgical spirit is industrial methylated spirit with castor oil and other additives. Its methyl alcohol content makes it too toxic for internal use.

Methyl alcohol (wood alcohol, methanol)

When a chronic alcoholic falls upon hard times he may take to drinking methylated spirit, which is ethyl alcohol adulterated ('denatured') with methyl alcohol. Methanol is oxidized in the body to formaldehyde and then to formic acid, two very toxic substances. The symptoms of poisoning include headache, vertigo, vomiting, severe abdominal pain, back pain, muscle cramps, dyspnoea, restlessness, delirium, coma and circulatory collapse. Partial or total blindness, caused by the formaldehyde, may occur and is often permanent.

In the treatment of acute methanol poisoning the most urgent measure is to combat the severe acidosis caused by the formic acid. Large quantities of sodium bicarbonate may have to be given by intravenous infusion and continued for a while orally. Ethyl alcohol may also be useful in treatment because it reduces the conversion of the methanol into toxic metabolites; the dose is 1–1·5 ml/kg initially, followed by 0·5–1 ml/kg two-hourly for 4 days. Haemodialysis, if available, is an effective treatment for acute methanol poisoning and is indicated if the above measures are unsuccessful or if the blood methanol level exceeds 50 mg/100 ml.

Isopropyl alcohol (isopropanol)

70 per cent isopropyl alcohol is used as a skin cleanser prior to injections. It may be combined with 0·5 per cent chlorhexidine as in Sterets H Injection Swabs.

The coal-tar disinfectants

A large number of chemical substances are produced from coal tar. Many have germicidal properties and a number of others have various medicinal uses. Among the most important of the former are phenol (carbolic acid) and the cresols, which are the basis of the disinfectants of the lysol type.

Phenol

Pure phenol is a caustic which occurs in colourless crystals and has a characteristic pungent odour, but it is rarely used in this state.

Phenol is most commonly supplied in the form of a lotion (1 in 20), which may be further diluted for special purposes. It should not be employed as a dressing for open wounds as its absorption may either damage the tissues locally or cause general toxic symptoms.

A 1 in 20 solution is used for disinfecting excreta in typhoid fever and similar conditions.

A more modern preparation is 1 per cent clearsol, which is added in equal parts to the infected contents of bed pans or urinals and allowed to act for one hour before their disposal.

Liquefied phenol contains 80 per cent phenol and is sometimes used as a caustic. It must not be confused with phenol lotion (referred to above, which is usually of 1 in 20 strength).

Phenol is sometimes dissolved in glycerine instead of water. Solutions in glycerin are much less caustic (and of lower germicidal power) than those in water. Thus glycerin and phenol eardrops contain 7·5 per cent of phenol but under no circumstances should these be diluted with water which will render them caustic in action. It follows that the ear must be carefully dried after syringing with lotions before glycerin and phenol drops are instilled.

Phenol also has some local anaesthetic action, hence its value as a mouth wash or gargle in painful affections of the mouth and throat, for which it is also employed as a lozenge. As ear-drops it is, therefore, of value both on account of its antiseptic and anaesthetic properties.

Other preparations include:

glycerin of phenol
phenol ointment.

It should be noted that the correct modern term for this drug is **phenol** and that carbolic acid, no longer the 'official' name, should be dropped.

Lysol (solution of cresol with soap)

Lysol is a solution of cresol in soap. It is a powerful disinfectant and caustic. It may be employed undiluted for sterilizing instruments, which should be immersed for 5 minutes. Care should always be taken to avoid splashing the skin and especially the eyes, and it should be applied to utensils with a mop or by using rubber gloves. Utensils should then be rinsed with sterile water before use. Splashes of phenol or lysol on the skin should be immediately removed by swabbing with glycerin or olive oil. Water must be avoided.

Weaker solutions are also germicidal, but must be allowed to operate for longer periods.

It should not be employed on the skin in concentrations exceeding 2 per cent.

Sudol is a non-caustic proprietary form of lysol.

There are many proprietary preparations similar to lysol which are used for the same purposes, but in strengths appropriate for each, e.g. Izal and Jeyes' Fluid.

Chloroxylenol solution (Roxenol, Dettol)

This may be used (a) for cuts, 1 in 80 or 5 ml in 400 ml of water; (b) vaginal douche, 1 in 40; (c) mouth wash, 1 in 480 to 1 in 160, or 1–2 ml in 300 ml.

These agents are specially effective against streptococci. They have the advantage of being non-irritant and non-toxic even in concentrated form. A dilution of 1 in 10 is generally recommended for application to the skin. They may be used as a liquid, ointment or cream.

Chlorhexidine (Hibitane)

This is an important, non-irritating synthetic disinfectant which remains active in the presence of blood and body fluids and, therefore, has many uses.

It is prepared as a 5 per cent solution or concentrate (for dispensing only) and also as a powder, obstetric cream (1%), antiseptic cream (1%) and lozenge. It may be mixed with the detergent, cetrimide, to form a very useful wound cleansing agent (Savlon).

When combined with neomycin (Naseptin) if forms a useful cream for the treatment of nasal carriers of staphylococci.

Hexachlorophane (Phiso-MED)

This may be used for preoperative skin cleansing, routine hand washing and skin care generally. It is of value in the prevention and treatment of staphylococcal infections in the newborn. It can, however, be absorbed through the skin and may cause brain damage. Therefore, the treated infant should be bathed and the skin throughly rinsed before drying.

Dequalinium (Dequadin)

This has antiseptic properties and is used in lozenges and paint.

Hexetidine (Oraldene)

This (0·1% solution) is used as a mouth wash or gargle. It is effective against many bacteria and some fungi (e.g. *Candida albicans*).

4. The halogens

The term halogen (which is derived from two Greek words meaning 'salt producer') is used for the elements chlorine, iodine, bromine, and fluorine because their salts are found in sea-water. The disinfectant drugs of this group owe their germicidal power to the liberation of chlorine or iodine in small quantities.

Chlorine

Chlorine itself is a poisonous, intensely irritating, green gas which has no medicinal use in this form. The following compounds are, however, employed:

    chlorinated lime or bleaching powder
    hypochlorite solutions, which include eusol and Milton
    the chloramines.

Chlorinated lime or bleaching powder is a disinfectant and deodorant of special use in disinfecting faeces, deodorizing drains and lavatories, and as the basis of other preparations.

Eusol is a solution of chlorinated lime and boric acid which is used for the irrigation and dressing of wounds. It is non-irritating and non-toxic. Solutions tend to decompose on keeping and should not be more than 3 weeks old. Dressings are applied in the form of gauze soaked in eusol and should not be covered with waterproof material.

Milton is a pleasant proprietary preparation having sodium hypochlorite as a base which may be used for cleaning and irrigating wounds, as a dressing and for storing dentures and babies' feeding bottles.

Chloramine is a complicated organic compound containing chlorine and has similar uses to the former preparations.

Chlorine preparations are also used in the disinfection of drinking water and the water in public swimming baths. The unpleasant taste of the water may be neutralized by the addition of sodium thiosulphate (photographic 'hypo') after the chlorine has been permitted to act for a definite period.

Iodine

Iodine is an element which is in the form of bluish-black crystals. It is intensely irritating to the skin, which it stains a deep reddish brown. This may be removed by solutions of alkali or sodium thiosulphate.

In addition to its antiseptic properties, iodine and its salts have many other uses in medicine.

The disinfectant preparation most commonly employed is tincture of iodine (weak solution of iodine, 2·5 per cent). This is an alcoholic solution which must be distinguished from Lugol's solution. The latter is used for internal administration, especially in cases of thyrotoxicosis before operation, in doses increasing from 0·3 to 1 ml (see also p. 226).

Tincture of iodine is employed as a skin disinfectant. Preparations:

(a) for external use

strong solution of iodine

weak solution or tincture, of iodine

compound iodine paint, or Mandl's paint (sometimes used for sore throats)

iodine ointment

povidone–iodine (Betadine) solution and ointment;

(b) for internal use

aqueous solution of iodine and potassium iodide or Lugol's solution.

Radio-active iodine (^{131}I and ^{132}I) are used in the diagnosis and treatment of disorders of the thyroid gland.

Iodine compounds for x-ray diagnosis

There are a number of substances containing iodine which are opaque to x-rays and which can usually be introduced into the body without causing harm. They can be used for outlining the bronchial tree (bronchogram), the uterus (uterogram or hysterogram), the fallopian tubes (salpingogram), the spinal cord (myelogram), the gall bladder (cholecystogram), the urinary tract (urogram).

In the case of the cholecystogram the dye is usually taken by mouth and is excreted by the liver so that normally it fills the gall bladder. A urogram may be obtained by injecting the dye intravenously.

These compounds include:

(1) propyliodone (Dionosyl) which is used for bronchograms;

(2) sodium diatrizoate (Hypaque), which is used for intravenous and retrograde urograms and also for other radiographic procedures;

(3) Salpix and Endografin FL, for hystero-salpingography;

(4) 76 per cent Urografin or 70 per cent sodium iothalamate (Conray 420), for arteriography;

(5) Myodil, which may be injected intrathecally by means of lumbar puncture;

(6) Gall bladder dyes which include sodium ipodate (Biloptin, Oragrafin), Solu-Biloptin and iopanoic acid (Telepaque), which are given by mouth, and Biligrafin given intraveneously.

Iodoform

This is an organic compound, yellow in colour, with a strong odour which many persons find objectionable. It has the reputation of being an antiseptic, but its value is doubtful. It is sometimes used as a powder for insufflation into the ear. Mixed with bismuth subnitrate in the form of a paste (BIPP), it is sometimes used for packing wounds and sinuses. The maximum dose (external) of the paste is 4 g.

Whitehead's varnish may be employed to protect the skin from irritating discharges.

NB.—Some individuals are sensitive to iodine in any form. Toxic effects such as flushing, nausea, vomiting, skin eruptions and, rarely, collapse may be observed.

Fluorine

This element is present in natural water supplies and in places where the drinking water contains fluoride in a concentration of one part per million the incidence of dental caries (tooth decay) is lower than in districts having water supplies deficient in fluoride. In areas where the water supplies lack fluoride, the level can be artificially increased to 1 ppm (part per million), a process called fluoridation. In areas where this has been done, the incidence of caries has fallen to a level similar to that in areas where fluoride occurs naturally in the water at a similar concentration. The substances used to fluoridate water are sodium fluoride and sodium silicofluoride. Fluoride is incorporated into the enamel of teeth during their development (i.e. during the first 8 years of life and, in the case of the third molars, up to the age of 12 years), and protects it against attack by acids. It is also incorporated into the film (plaque) which normally covers teeth. This film contains bacteria which break down carbohydrate to acids which attack teeth. Fluoride inhibits the bacterial enzymes responsible for this breakdown. It may usefully be incorporated into toothpaste.

Sodium fluoride may be used to arrest otosclerosis (dose: 25 mg daily) and to strengthen bone in myelomatosis (dose: 40 mg thrice daily).

NB.—Fluoridated water should preferably not be used in the dialysis baths of artificial kidneys as it is claimed that it may result in osteomalacia. De-ionized water is preferred for haemodialysis.

5. Oxidizing agents

The most important drugs which owe their antiseptic properties to the liberation of oxygen in the presence of organic matter are hydrogen peroxide and potassium permanganate.

Hydrogen peroxide (H_2O_2)

This is used in the form of a solution which contains about 3 per cent of hydrogen peroxide but is described as '10 volumes'. This means that it can liberate 10 times its volume of oxygen, and a stronger solution of double this strength is described as being of '20 volumes'.

In the presence of organic matter or pus, bubbles of oxygen are liberated, and this has a valuable mechanical action in removing discharges from wounds in addition to its antiseptic property. It must be used with care in the irrigation of deep cavities, especially the thorax, and there must be a free outlet for drainage since the oxygen liberated may produce dangerous distension unless it can escape.

Hydrogen peroxide is used as a mouth wash and has a slightly bitter taste. Ater its use as ear-drops the meatus should be carefully dried by swabbing or its epithelium will become sodden. It also acts as an astringent and is a good haemostatic. It is used for bleaching fabrics and the hair, the latter being turned an easily recognizable, unnatural yellow colour not comparable in beauty with that of the natural blonde. It forms the basis of Sanitas.

Potassium permanganate

This occurs in the form of dark purple crystals. It is a disinfectant and deodorant and owes its power to the fact that in solution it gives off oxygen in the presence of organic matter. As it does so it turns brown, an indication that the solution has lost its efficiency. Permanganates form the basis of Condy's Fluid.

It is used in strengths of 1 in 5000 for application to wounds, ulcers, fungal infections, etc., and 1 in 10 000 as a vaginal douche, gargle and mouth wash. The solid was formerly applied to snake-bites but is no longer recommended. Permanganate stains in fabrics may be removed by applying sulphurous acid and then washing in water.

Preparations:

solutions of potassium permanganate, weak (1 in 8000), strong (1 in 2500).

6. Dyes

The most important germicidal dyes can be divided into two main groups which may be conveniently called (*a*) the aniline group and (*b*) the flavine group, thereby indicating their general chemical type.

(a) Dyes of the aniline group

Their main use is in disinfecting the skin and in the antiseptic treatment of wounds. Their action is relatively slow and, as has already been pointed out, is selective in character; that is, they only have a marked effect on certain organisms.

The most important dyes of this group are **crystal violet, magenta** and **brilliant green.** The green and violet dyes are sometimes used in combination in the form of Bonney's blue. They are most effective against staphylococci and are more useful in preventing infection than in the treatment of established sepsis, although they are of value in some cases of impetigo. Solutions may be either aqueous or spirituous. For application to the skin a 1 per cent solution is employed; for wounds, dilutions of 1 in 1000 to 1 in 2000 are used.

With acriflavine, they form the basis of triple dye jelly which may be used as a tanning compound in the treatment of small burns.

Crystal (gentian) violet capsules have been given internally for the treatment of thread worms.

Other dyes of this group employed for different purposes include:

congo red   indigo carmine   methylene blue

Indigo carmine, when given by intramuscular injection, is excreted by the kidneys and may be used as a test of renal efficiency. The principle is to observe the rate at which the dye is excreted from each kidney after ureteric catheterization.

Methylene blue is also used to test renal efficiency.

(b) Dyes of the flavine (acridine) group

These dyes are yellow in colour and show marked selective action against streptococci. The one most commonly used is **proflavine.** They are used both for application to the skin and for irrigating wounds. As distinct from many other germicides, their action is not decreased by the presence of blood and they do not interfere with the phagocytic power of the leucocytes. They are generally employed in strengths of 1 in 1000, but they must not be mixed with eusol, lysol or mercurial solutions. Stains are removed with dilute hydrochloric acid.

Indocyanine Green (Cardio-Green)

This belongs to neither of the foregoing groups of germicidal dyes, but is conveniently mentioned here. It is a water-soluble tricarbocyanine dye which is used as an indicator for determining cardiac output, intracardiac shunts, hepatic function and hepatic blood flow.

7. Other substances

Among the other disinfectants which have not so far been mentioned, the most important are formaldehyde and glutaraldehyde.

Formaldehyde

Formaldehyde itself is a pungent gas which irritates the eyes and mucous membranes of the respiratory tract. It is used in the form of a solution, formalin, which contains about 40 per cent of the pure substance. This is a powerful disinfectant but, in a solution of this strength, is unsuitable for application to the skin. It is useful for spraying the walls and furniture of infected rooms, and special fumigators for the liberation of the gas are employed to fumigate rooms. The room is sealed for 3 to 4 hours.

Formaldehyde has an important use in the sterilization of catheters which are exposed in a special box to its vapour. The vapour is obtained from formalin.

Glutaraldehyde

A 2 per cent aqueous activated solution (Cidex) is prepared by adding activator powder to a colourless solution, which changes to *green* to signify proof of activation. The expiry date, which is

2 weeks after the date of activation, should be clearly marked on the jug. After the 14-day expiry date, the solution should be discarded.

Bacteria and viruses are destroyed within 10 minutes of immersion in glutaraldehyde but it takes 3 hours to destroy all pathogenic spores.

The solution is used for sterilizing metal instruments, including those with lenses, and plastic and rubber anaesthetic and ventilation equipment. Instruments should be rinsed in sterile water before use.

Gas sterilization

Special automatic gas sterilizers using ethylene oxide are available. They are useful for disinfecting mattresses, pillows, clothing, and apparatus which might be damaged by other methods. Electronic cardiac pacemakers are sterilized in ethylene oxide gas.

In conclusion, the utmost care must be taken in the use of antiseptics and disinfectants. When employed they must be used in the appropriate strength and allowed to act for the correct time. So many are available that no one can be expected to know the details of all, but it should be regarded as a duty to be familiar with those in common use.

Although these substances are valuable, remember that unless correctly used they can afford a very dangerous false sense of security. Do not imagine that dipping the hands in a bowl of highly coloured liquid (reputed to be an antiseptic but probably inactive in the dilution employed) by the side of the typhoid or other infectious patient has any other value than to remind you to go and wash your hands at once, and properly, with soap and water. In any case, you should have been wearing rubber or disposable gloves!

Deodorants

Deodorants or deodorizers may be defined as substances which are used to destroy or remove disagreeable odours. Many of them are also disinfectants or antiseptics and have been mentioned in this connection. They may be used to get rid of odours from drains or from offensive discharges from wounds. For the former purpose, chlorinated lime and Jeyes' Fluid are examples of the most economical.

For wounds, hydrogen peroxide, Sanitas, eusol and Debrisan are useful.

Agents of the lysol and phenol types act as deodorants. Offensive smells can also to some extent be covered by the pungent odour of iodoform or by the burning of special deodorizing cones.

Special electrical apparatus which produces ozone is an efficient method of deodorizing a room. An Airwick is also useful.

A number of deodorant sprays with fancy names are available which, by their own potency, effectively mask unpleasant odours.

Chlorophyll tablets taken by mouth are optimistically claimed to deodorize the breath.

Cetrimide (Cetavlon) is a detergent which also has antiseptic properties (p. 00).

5 Drugs acting on the surface of the body

There are a number of specialized forms of treatment which are used in various skin and other conditions and also for the relief of superficial pain viz.:

Radiation: x-rays, radium, ultraviolet light
Heat:
  (a) cautery
  (b) radiant heat, infra-red rays.
Cold:
  (a) carbon dioxide snow (for warts and naevi)
  (b) evaporating lotions.

In addition, medicaments may be employed by local application in various forms including:

lotions and liniments;
ointments, creams and pastes;
paints, powders and poultices.

In order that the above may be applied to the skin a number of different bases or vehicles are employed to incorporate the medicaments used. These include:
(1) *Dusting-powders* consisting of powdered drugs mixed with starch, which absorbs moisture, or talc or Fuller's earth which do not.
(2) *Water:* (a) Soluble substances may be dissolved in water and applied in various strengths which are usually expressed as a percentage solution.
    (b) 'Shake lotions', such as calamine lotion, in which the substance does not dissolve but after application the water evaporates leaving the dried medicament in powder form on the skin surface.
(3) *Alcohol:* This is included in some lotions for the cooling effect which occurs with rapid evaporation. It is also used as a vehicle in some solutions, liniments and paints, e.g. tincture of iodine which has an antiseptic action.
(4) *Water-soluble vehicles and emulsifying agents:* These are non-

oily substances of complicated chemical structure (including glycols and stearates) which produce emulsions from which medicaments are easily absorbed. They include macrogols and substances such as lanette wax which assist in the mixture of watery and oily substances.

(5) *Oily and greasy vehicles:* These include soft and hard paraffin, also wool fat and the wool alcohols derived from it. They form the basis of ointments.

The majority of drugs used can be classified according to their main actions:

Antiseptic applications

Some of the antiseptic or bactericidal substances already mentioned in the previous chapters are suitable for external application in the form of lotions, paints or creams, etc. Among them are:

salicylic acid
formaldehyde (3%) lotion
copper and zinc sulphate lotion (astringent and mildly antiseptic)
brilliant green, magenta and crystal violet paints
cetrimide cream
chlortetracycline cream
proflavine cream
chlorhexidine (Hibitane) cream
hexachlorophane cream.

Ointments containing penicillin, streptomycin or sulphonamides carry a high risk of causing sensitization and are, therefore, contraindicated as local applications. Tetracycline, chloramphenicol and neomycin are less risky. Impetigo and local skin fissures are the types of condition treated in this way.

Antifungal preparations

There are numerous fungal infections of the skin, hair and nails, including ringworm and monilia infections. Local applications used in the treatment of conditions such as 'athlete's foot' include magenta paint, benzoic acid compound (Whitfield's) ointment, and zinc undecenoate dusting-powder and ointment. Proprietary preparations include Mycil (chlorphenesin), Asterol and Tina-derm (tolnaftate). Nystatin ointment is effective against superficial candidal infections. Clotrimazole (Canesten) and miconazole (Daktarin) creams are useful against a wide variety of fungal skin conditions.

Griseofulvin is an oral antibiotic used in ringworm and certain other fungal infections. The average adult dose is 500 mg daily for 3–10 weeks. Finger-nail infections may require longer treatment, up to 6 months.

Antiparasitic preparations

These include benzyl benzoate application used in the treatment of scabies. Crotamiton cream may also be used in this condition. Sulphur ointment, although effective, is liable to cause further dermatitis.

Applications of gamma benzene hexachloride (Lorexane, Quel-lada) and dicophane (DDT; dichloro-diphenyl-trichlorethane) are used for the treatment of lice infestation (pediculosis). Lice may be resistant to DDT and gamma benzene but may be destroyed by malathion lotion (Prioderm) or carbaryl lotion (Caryl-derm).

Antipruritics

Itching may be a symptom both of skin disorders and general disease such as diabetes, jaundice, drug intoxication and anxiety states. Lotions and creams such as phenol, calamine and crotami-ton (Eurax) have a local action. Antihistamine drugs by mouth may be helpful but when applied locally may cause sensitization.

Local steroid preparations such as hydrocortisone and predni-solone lotions and creams (up to 1 per cent) are valuable and may be combined with antibiotics such as tetracycline in infective skin lesions.

Steroids

Hydrocortisone and other steroids are used topically in the treatment of a number of skin diseases including eczema, derma-titis, acne, rosacea, lichen planus and psoriasis. Examples are:

hydrocortisone lotion (1%);
hydrocortisone cream (1%);

hydrocortisone ointment (1%);
betamethasone lotion (0·1%);
fluocinolone ointment (0·025%).

Caustics (Escharotics)

A caustic is a substance which has a burning or destructive action on living tissue. Its clinical use is limited. Many concentrated disinfectants are caustics and have been mentioned already. They include:

strong nitric, hydrochloric and sulphuric acids
glacial acetic acid and trichloracetic acid
silver nitrate, copper sulphate and zinc chloride
caustic potash and caustic soda (potassium and sodium hydroxides).

Strong acids have been used to destroy warts.

Silver nitrate is used to burn down excess of granulation tissue in a healing wound, in order that the epithelium may have an opportunity of growing over the surface of the granulation tissue from the sides of the wound. Silver nitrate may be applied to dog bites.

Copper sulphate is applied to the inner surface of the eyelids in trachoma.

Emollients

Emollients are bland oily substances applied to the skin or mucous membranes to protect them from irritation or to render them soft. They are therefore useful in the treatment of abrasions, chapped hands and healing surfaces. They also serve as vehicles for other drugs applied for various diseases in the form of ointments. (Not all ointments, however, are emollient in action.) The most important emollients are:

wool fat and Lanolin   soft paraffin (Vaseline)
olive oil   castor oil.
arachis oil

Barrier creams are preparations designed to protect the skin against irritant substances which may be encountered by industrial workers or nurses. They may also be used to protect the skin of patients from discharges. Silicone barrier creams are water-repellent and are used against water-soluble irritants. They are useful in the prevention of napkin rash and in the treatment of bedsores.

Demulcents

These are substances similar to emollients which are applied to mucous membranes and may be given internally. They are used for:

protecting inflamed mucous surfaces, e.g. white of egg or milk in the treatment of corrosive poisoning;
masking the unpleasant taste of certain drugs;
suspending insoluble drugs.

In addition to the above emollient drugs, milk, gelatin, starch, gum and tragacanth are all demulcents.

Sedative applications

When the skin is acutely inflamed wet dressings are often indicated. These include calamine lotion and sodium chloride solution (normal saline).

Starch poultices are useful for removing crusts such as may occur in severe impetigo of the scalp.

Soaps

Soaps are cleansing agents made by combining oils or fats with alkalis. There are three main types:

curd or animal soap made from animal fat and caustic soda;
hard soap made from vegetable oils and caustic soda;
soft soap made from vegetable oils and caustic soda or potash but containing glycerin; ether soap is a 40 per cent solution of soft soap in alcohol and ether.

Soapless washing powders for domestic use are special (sulphonated) fatty alcohols. These are also used in soapless shampoos.

Detergents and cleansing agents

These are cleansing agents for the skin. In addition to the use of ordinary soap and water, ether soap, spirit soap or a detergent when the skin is grimed with oil, it may be necessary to remove dirt or crusts from injured or inflamed skin by using olive oil, arachis oil or starch poultices.

Detergents are more effective cleansing agents than soap and water, and in addition many have mild antiseptic properties. Among the most important are:

Cetrimide (Cetavlon, CTAB)

This is generally used as a 1 per cent solution. A cream is also available. Napkins may be washed in 1 in a 1000 solution to prevent napkin rash.

Benzalkonium chloride (Roccal) has similar properties. Various strengths are employed according to the particular requirements.

A number of household detergents and washing powders are in use and are well advertised. These occasionally cause dermatitis in persons with a sensitive skin. Care should be taken not to employ them in concentrated form, and always to rinse the hands well after use or, preferably, to wear rubber gloves.

Astringents

These are drugs which check secretion and cause drying of a surface. They are most frequently used on mucous membranes and, therefore, in addition to their application to the mouth and throat, they are also given internally for their action on the bowel, especially in the treatment of diarrhoea.

Calamine lotion has a slightly astringent action and is used in the acute stages of eczema and to allay irritation in urticaria. Calamine liniment, various creams (e.g. ichthammol) and Lassar's paste are used in the later stages of eczema. Coal-tar preparations have mildly astringent and antiseptic properties.

Stimulating preparations

In order to stimulate the growth of granulation tissue in healing wounds, red lotion (*Lotio rubra*, containing zinc sulphate) or Debrisan may be applied. Cod-liver oil applied externally has similar properties. Preparations used on the unbroken skin include ichthammol ointment, zinc and coal-tar paste.

Softening preparations (Keratolytics)

It is sometimes necessary to soften the horny layers of the skin, and for this purpose pastes or ointments containing resorcin or salicylic acid may be used.

Dithranol is used for removing the scales of psoriasis. Stains produced by this substance may be removed with a solution of chlorinated lime.

Salicylic acid collodion is used in the treatment of corns.

Irritants

Depending upon the severity of their action, irritants may be classified as:

(1) rubefacients; (2) vesicants; (3) caustics (p. 57).

Rubefacients are drugs used to produce reddening or mild inflammation of the skin. By their action they cause the blood vessels to dilate so that the part to which they are applied becomes red and hot. For example, ammonia, camphor, menthol, oil of wintergreen (methyl salicylate), turpentine, all of which are employed in the form of liniments. Kaolin poultice also has a rubefacient action. It is mainly used for the relief of pain, e.g. pleurisy.

Counter-irritation

Remedies such as the liniments, poultices and paints already referred to, applied to the surface of the body with the object of relieving pain or congestion in an underlying organ by producing mild inflammation of the skin are called counter-irritants.

Pain resulting from a diseased organ is often felt in some part of the body wall rather than in the organ itself. As examples, the pain of a gastric ulcer may be felt in the epigastric region of the abdominal wall and is associated with excessive tenderness of the skin (hyperaesthesia) in that area. Pain in gall bladder disease may be felt in the right shoulder.

This phenomenon is called 'referred pain' and is due to the fact that the organ affected has a nerve supply from the same segment of the spinal cord as that of the area of skin in which the pain is felt.

Styptics or haemostatics
Drugs which check bleeding

Styptics are drugs applied *locally* to a bleeding surface with the object of checking haemorrhage. They are unlikely to be of marked effect except in oozing or capillary haemorrhage, bleeding from arteries requiring ligature or repair. Most astringents are also styptics, e.g.:

> solution of ferric chloride
> silver nitrate
> alum.

Hydrogen peroxide has a useful local haemostatic action. Adrenaline (1 in 1000) applied locally acts by causing the blood vessels in the bleeding area to contract. Caustics will stop haemorrhage but are not employed for this purpose.

Snake venom obtained from a viper (e.g. Stypven) is a very powerful haemostatic which may be applied on cotton wool in a dilution of 1 in 10 000. It may be used for plugging bleeding tooth sockets and may control bleeding in haemophilia.

The application of absorbable **gelatin sponge** to a bleeding surface promotes a clot which forms rapidly and adheres to the tissues. It may be moistened before use with saline and a wound closed over it. Complete absorption takes place in 4 to 6 weeks. Oxidized cellulose and calcium alginate are similarly employed and may, if necessary, be soaked in a solution of thrombin before use.

The treatment of haemorrhage is, however, a much wider subject annd involves the use of drugs given internally:
(1) Morphine is given to allay restlessness and thereby to cause a general lowering of blood pressure.
(2) Special haemostatic preparations, e.g.:
Epsikapron (aminocaproic acid); used to treat bleeding which is due to fibrinolysis (dissolution of the fibrin in clots).
(3) Special drugs such as ergot and ergometrine, and posterior pituitary extract (Pitocin, p. 237) are given to check bleeding from the pregnant uterus because they have a special action on this organ, causing its muscle to contract.
(4) In certain circumstances the tendency to excessive bleeding may be checked by the administration of vitamin K (menaphthone or phytomenadione) (p. 214). Vitamin K is necessary for the production of prothrombin and is given by injection as

a preoperative measure in cases of jaundice, in which absorption of the fat-soluble natural vitamin is impaired.

Drugs which prevent clotting (anticoagulants)

There are a number of substances which have a directly opposite *local* action to the styptics, namely they prevent blood from clotting. These include:

(1) Sodium and potassium citrates. They act by preventing the action of the calcium salts present in the blood by combining with them to form inactive compounds. Use is made of this in blood transfusion by collecting blood into 3·8 per cent citrate solution. Also, prothrombin times of blood are measured from samples collected into tubes containing sodium citrate solution.

(2) Sodium oxalate has a similar effect and is used together with sodium fluoride for preventing the clotting of blood taken for blood sugar estimation. The principal action of the fluoride is as a preservative.

(3) Lithium heparin, which is used in blood chemistry specimen tubes. Samples for measurement of electrolytes (including calcium) and enzymes, and for liver function tests are sent to the laboratory in these tubes.

(4) Sequestrine is used in sample tubes for blood counts.
   NB.—None of these substances are given internally to prevent blood coagulation. Citrates are metabolized by the body and hence do not affect coagulation. Oxalates and fluorides are poisonous in the amounts which would have to be given.

(5) Hirudin, a substance obtained from the leech, delays clotting. This explains why a leech bite continues to bleed for a considerable period.

(6) The anticoagulant drugs given *internally*, including heparin, phenindione (Dindevan) and nicoumalone (Sinthrome), are considered on p. 121.

Diaphoretics

The sweat glands are situated in the skin all over the body but are most abundant in the axillae, palms, soles and forehead, and have been estimated to number about 2 000 000. They are supplied by the sumpathetic nerves.

Drugs which increase the amount of perspiration are called diaphoretics but are not often employed as such. They may act:

(1) by stimulating the sweating centre in the central nervous system.
(2) by stimulating the sweat glands.

(3) by dilating the cutaneous blood vessels, which increase the blood supply to the glands.

It is not always possible to say exactly how and where each diaphoretic drug acts. The following are examples of diaphoretics:

Pilocarpine, a very powerful drug, which stimulates the nerves of the involuntary system supplying the sweat glands.
Alcohol, which acts by dilating the cutaneous blood vessels.

The main use of diaphoretics is to render a feverish patient with a hot dry skin more comfortable. The evaporation of the sweat also tends to cause a fall in the body temperature (i.e. diaphoretics have an antipyretic action).

Anhidrotics

These are drugs which diminish the amount of sweat. They include atropine and belladonna, and stramonium. They also cause dryness of the mouth.

Antipyretics

An antipyretic is a drug which reduces fever. There are a number of antipyretic drugs, but all have other actions for which they are employed, so that their antipyretic effect is incidental to their use for other purposes.

The normal temperature of the body is maintained by a balance between the heat produced and the heat lost, and this is controlled by the heat-regulating centre in the brain. Heat lost is dependent on (a) the amount of blood circulating in the vessels of the skin and (b) the amount of sweat secreted and the rate of evaporation.

A drug may therefore have an antipyretic effect:
(i) by acting on the heat-regulating centre;
(ii) by dilating the blood vessels in the skin;
(iii) by increasing the amount of sweat.

The drugs which have an antipyretic action include:
aspirin and sodium salicylate quinine all diaphoretics.

The methods employed when it is desired to lower body temperature are tepid sponging, a tepid bath, etc., details of which are given in books on Nursing.

6 Drugs acting on the alimentary system

Drugs acting on the mouth and pharynx

Drugs used for their action on the mouth and pharynx are most commonly employed in the form of mouth washes, gargles, paints or lozenges, which may be demulcent, antiseptic or sedative in character, e.g.:

Demulcent:	glycerin.
Antiseptic:	phenol (0·5%)
	hydrogen peroxide
	glycerin of thymol (as in Glycothymoline)
	crystal violet paint
	Mandl's paint
	hexetidine (0·1%) (Oraldene)
	chlorhexidine (0·2%) (Corsodyl)
	lozenges, e.g. Dequadin, Bradosol, Tyrozets.
Sedative:	benzocaine lozenge
	phenol or aspirin gargles, which have local anaesthetic effect
	Bonjela.
Steroid:	hydrocortisone pellets (Corlan) for ulcers in the mouth
	Bioral.

These preparations are generally used in various forms of stomatitis, pharyngitis and tonsillitis. They are palliative rather than curative.

Drugs acting on the salivary glands

Drugs may be given either to increase (sialogogues) or decrease (antisialagogues) the flow of saliva. Drugs may also decrease the flow of saliva and cause dryness of the mouth when given for other purposes. Thus atropine reduces the amount of saliva and this may be a troublesome side-effect of its administration.

Hyoscine and stramonium formerly used in large doses in the treatment of parkinsonism, also produece excessive dryness of the mouth which may be counteracted by giving pilocarpine, a drug which stimulates the flow of saliva.

Sialagogues (increasing flow): pilocarpine.

Antisialagogues (decreasing flow): atropine, hyoscine.

Drugs acting on the teeth and gums

Toothpastes are generally made of slightly abrasive powders, with soap, to which some antiseptic and a flavouring agent may be added. Fluoride may also be added to help to prevent caries.

Toothache due to dental caries may be relieved by inserting into the cavity a pledget of cotton wool soaked in oil of cloves which has a local anaesthetic action.

Various astringents, crystal violet or weak solution of iodine may be applied to the gums in cases of gingivitis.

Drugs acting on the stomach

In order to understand the various actions of drugs on the stomach it is important to recall the main points concerning its physiology.

The stomach is a hollow organ consisting of serous, muscular and mucous coats. The muscular coat (having circular, longitudinal and oblique fibres) gives it the power of peristaltic movement. The circular fibres also form the pyloric sphincter which relaxes at intervals to allow partially digested food to enter the duodenum.

The glands of the mucous membrane secrete pepsin, which converts proteins into proteoses and peptones; hydrochloric acid which acts as an antiseptic barrier and aids the action of pepsin; also rennin and the intrinsic factor essential for the absorption of vitamin B_{12}.

Hydrochloric acid may be absent (achlorhydria), diminished (hypochlorhydria) or increased (hyperchlorhydria).

The nerve supply of the stomach includes nerves passing to the vomiting centre in the medulla, which is also connected to the higher centres of the brain.

Drugs acting on the stomach can be considered according to whether they act (a) on its movements or (b) on the mucous membrane or its secretions, viz:

(1) Carminatives   ⎫ Acting on stomach
(2) Emetics   ⎬ movements
(3) Sedatives and anti-emetics ⎭

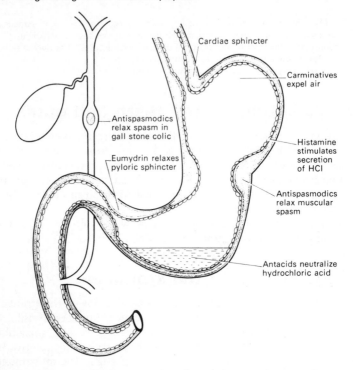

Fig. 6.1 Diagram illustrating the action of some drugs on the stomach, etc.

(4) Stomachics, including bitters—acting on the mucous membrane
(5) Antacids
(6) Other drugs used in peptic ulcer therapy.
(7) Substitutes
(8) Drugs used in radiography.

1. Carminatives

A carminative is a drug which aids the expulsion of wind from the stomach by increasing the tone of its muscle and stimulating its movements, e.g.

(i) the volatile oils such as oil of peppermint (0·2 ml).
(ii) aromatic spirit of ammonia (Sal volatile) (1–5 ml) in water.
(iii) various preparations of ginger (*Zingiber*).

2. Emetics

Emetics are drugs which produce vomiting and are therefore responsible for causing much more violent movements in the stomach muscle than carminatives.

Emetics acting directly on the stomach include:

ipecacuanha emetic draught paediatric, BP
ipecacuanha syrup USP (15 ml)
zinc sulphate (2 g)
mustard and water
Sodium chloride (common salt) solution is an emetic but its use as such should be avoided (e.g. in the emergency treatment of poisoning) because of the danger of inducing hypernatraemia (an excess of salt in the blood), which may be fatal.

An emetic acting directly on the vomiting centre is apomorphine 6 mg given hypodermically, but rarely used.
NB.—Excessive doses of many drugs will cause vomiting, and it is common after the administration of sulphonamides and nitrofurantoin, and in digitalis poisoning. In a number of persons the usual doses of morphine appear to stimulate the vomiting centre.

Emetic drugs are not often employed, as in most cases in which it is desired to empty the stomach of its contents it is preferable to wash it out with plain water after passing a stomach tube. In some circumstances, however, it may be necessary to use them. They may be employed to remove the contents of the stomach when it is over-distended with food. They are of value, as an emergency measure, in some cases of poisoning due to substances other than caustics, e.g. ipecacuanha as an alternative to gastric lavage in the emergency treatment of accidental poisoning in children. There is danger in using them after caustic poisoning because the violent contraction of the organ may cause rupture of its walls if they are severely damaged by the corrosive substance.

In order to appreciate their mode of action it is necessary to recall the physiological mechanism of vomiting.

There is a special vomiting centre in the medulla to which pass afferent (sensory) nerves from the stomach and other abdominal viscera. From the centre the efferent (motor) nerves are distributed to the muscle of the stomach, the diaphragm and the muscles of the abdominal wall, which take part in the muscular effort associated with vomiting. There is, therefore, a reflex arc through the vomiting centre from the sensory organ (the mucous membrane of the stomach) to the motor organs just mentioned. The centre is also connected to the higher centres of the brain, including those of sight and smell.

The causes of vomiting

The main causes of vomiting may be listed under the following headings:
(1) Peripheral, i.e. local or reflex irritation of the pharynx, stomach or other parts of the alimentary system by stimuli which pass to the vomiting centre.

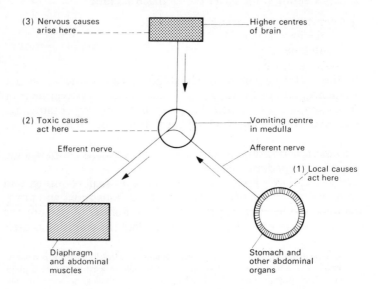

Fig. 6.2. Illustrating the mechanism of vomiting

(2) Central
    (i) drugs and toxins acting on the centre
    (ii) stimuli acting on the higher centres of the brain, e.g.
          (a) psychological and emotional factors such as revolting sights and smells, and anxiety states
          (b) organic brain disease (cerebral tumour, meningitis, concussion)
          (c) sea or motion sickness, due to impulses from the labyrinth
          (d) migraine.

3. Sedatives and anti-emetics

These are drugs which either tend to diminish the movements of the stomach or else to depress the vomiting centre. They include:

(*a*) Drugs of the antihistamine type, viz.:

promethazine (Avomine)
cyclizine (Marzine)
dimenhydrinate (Dramamine) } 25–50 mg.
meclozine (Ancolan)

(*b*) Drugs of the phenothiazine group:

promazine (Sparine) } 25–50 mg
chlorpromazine (Largactil) } as anti-emetics
perphenazine (Fentazin), 2–4 mg.

The first group are particularly useful in the prevention and treatment of travel sickness and both groups in vomiting due to other causes but they may increase the effect of alcohol. Cyclizine and similar drugs are reported to have caused fetal abnormalities in animals and, therefore, should be avoided in early pregnancy. Most of these drugs may be given by intramuscular injection.

(*c*) Metoclopramide (Maxolon, Primperan) acts locally and centrally. It may be given orally or by intramuscular injection in doses of 10 mg. Occasionally, a distressing adverse reaction occurs, with extrapyramidal symptoms, e.g. spasm of the facial muscles.

(*d*) Simple drugs which may be used include Chlorodyne (*Tinctura chloroformi et morphinae* 0·6 ml), atropine and belladonna.

Kaolin and morphine mixture may be used, especially if diarrhoea is present.

4. Stomachics, including bitters

These are given with a view to stimulating the appetite and the secretion of gastric juice, thereby improving digestion and aiding the general nutrition, especially during convalescence. They include gentian and nux vomica which are bitter and act mainly by suggestion.

5. Antacids

These drugs are given in order to neutralize hydrochloric acid in cases of gastric and duodenal ulcer and in the symptomatic treatment of heartburn. The most important are:

magnesia (magnesium oxide)   aluminium glycinate

magnesium carbonate   bismuth carbonate
magnesium trisilicate   calcium carbonate
aluminium hydroxide   sodium bicarbonate.

Sodium bicarbonate in the presence of hydrochloric acid liberates carbon dioxide and later stimulates the further secretion of hydrochloric acid, so is unsuitable for use alone as an antacid and may cause alkalosis in excessive dosage.

A number of the above substances may be mixed together to form special antacid powders and mixtures, e.g.:

magnesium trisilicate compound powder, BPC (dose 1–5 g)
magnesium trisilicate mixture, BPC (dose 10 ml).

Antacid tablets are convenient for carrying in pocket or handbag. They include aluminium hydroxide tablets, magnesium trisilicate compound tablets, Gelusil, Maalox and Neutrolactis. The dose of all of these is 1–2 tablets chewed when required.

Antacids may be mixed with milk solids, as in Nulacin, or with dimethicone, an anti-flatulent agent, as in Asilone.

6. Other drugs used in peptic ulcer therapy

(a) **Liquorice preparations.** These often heal gastric ulcers and may heal duodenal ulcers. Powdered block liquorice (as in Caved-S tablets) and the pure compound sodium carbenoxolone are both in use. The latter is given in tablet form (Biogastrone) for gastric ulcers and in special capsules (Duogastrone) for duodenal ulcers. These capsules rupture in the pylorus and release a concentrated solution of the drug into the duodenum. Carbenoxolone is thought to act by increasing the production of adherent mucus, which helps to protect the mucosa. Side-effects of carbenoxolone include oedema, hypertension and hypokalaemia in some patients. In elderly folk, and other patients thought to be at special risk from these side-effects, deglycirrhinized liquorice (Caved-S) is often preferred.

Doses: Biogastrone   Initially 2 tablets t.d.s. for 1 week, then
                        1 t.d.s., after meals.

         Duogastrone   1 q.d.s., 15–30 minutes before meals.

         Caved-S   2 tablets t.d.s., chewed and swallowed
                        after meals.

(b) **Bismuth.** De-Nol is a proprietary preparation containing a complex bismuth compound which is thought to allow healing of ulcers by forming a protective coat over them. It is therefore given on an empty stomach. The usual dose of 5 ml is diluted with 15 ml water and given 4 times a day, half an hour before meals and 2 hours after the last meal of the day.

(c) **Anticholinergic agents.** These have been used in the treatment of duodenal ulceration, to reduce acid secretion. They are now of little importance, however, because they are non-specific and act on the autonomic and central nervous systems to produce unwanted effects in organs other than the stomach.

(d) **Histamine H_2-receptor antagonists.** Histamine has long been recognized as a potent stimulant of gastric acid secretion. It acts on receptors in the gastric mucosa, known as H_2-receptors to distinguish them from the H_1-receptors elsewhere in the body which are concerned in allergic reactions. Ordinary antihistamines block the H_1-receptors but are inactive against H_2-receptors. Cimetidine (Tagamet) is one of a class of synthetic compounds which inhibit gastric acid secretion by blocking H_2-receptors. It is used in the treatment of peptic ulcers and reflux oesophagitis. The usual dose is 200 mg orally 3 times a day with meals and 400 mg at bedtime.

(e) **Other drugs used in the treatment of peptic ulceration** include gefarnate (Gefarnil) and metoclopramide (Maxolon).

7. Substitutes

Dilute hydrochloric acid (5 ml) may be given in water or orange juice with meals in cases of achlorhydria or hypochlorhydria and may be useful in checking the diarrhoea which sometimes accompanies these conditions.

8. Drugs used in radiography of the stomach

A suspension of barium sulphate, which is opaque to x-rays, is generally employed. It is swallowed as a 'barium meal', which can be followed by radiography in its course through the oesophagus, stomach, small and large intestines. In addition to showing the outline of the organs this also gives information about their rate of emptying. A 'barium enema' is given for examination of the rectum and colon.

Other drugs used for their action on the stomach

Atropine methonitrate (Eumydrin)

As its chemical name implies, this drug is a salt of atropine and has similar actions. It is of special value, however, in being less toxic and more effective in the medical treatment of congenital hypertrophic pyloric stenosis than atropine. By its action it helps to relax the hypertrophied pyloric sphincter and to allow the passage of the stomach contents into the duodenum. It is of value also in relieving the spasms of whooping cough. It may be given in the following way:

> 0·12 to 2 ml of 0·6 per cent alcoholic solution given on the tongue before each feed. This solution is very potent and must be used with great care. The container must be kept tightly closed to prevent evaporation and must not be confused with atropine methonitrate eye-drops. It is unsuitable for out-patients.

The gastric test meal

Hydrochloric acid may be absent from the gastric juice (achlorhydria), although the stomach is still capable of secreting it. In such instances, histamine will stimulate the glands of the gastric mucous membrane to secrete hydrochloric acid and thereby prove that the case is not one of true achylia gastrica. Unpleasant and dangerous side-effects are reduced by prior administration of an antihistamine. Betazole (Histalog), which causes less severe side-effects, is an alternative to histamine but the test agent now most often used is **pentagastrin** (Peptavlon). The dose of pentagastrin is 6 micrograms/kg by subcutaneous injection.

Drugs acting on the intestines

(1) Those promoting evacuation (the aperients, injections, enemata and suppositories).
(2) Those which lessen movements and spasm (sedatives).
(3) Antiparasitic:
   (a) antiseptics
   (b) anthelmintics.

The aperients

An aperient is a drug employed in medicine to assist the bowel to evacuate its contents and, in the majority of instances, it does so on account of its power of stimulating peristalsis and the movements of the bowel.

It will be recalled that the onward passage of the intestinal contents is due to two main factors: (i) peristalsis; (ii) the operation of the important gastrocolic reflex. When food is taken into the stomach this causes a reflex relaxation of the ileocaecal valve by which the contents of the lower ileum rapidly enter the caecum and, as a result, the contents of the colon are passed on into the rectum. The distension of the rectum thus produced gives rise to the natural desire to defaecate.

Aperients are sometimes classified according to the intensity of their action thus:

(1) Laxatives

These are relatively mild and result in the hastening of peristaltic action without altering the appearance or consistency of the stools. Simple lubricants such as liquid paraffin may also be included in this group.

(2) Mild purgatives

These are stronger in action, producing looser and, sometimes, repeated stools.

(3) Drastic purgatives

These are violent in action, often accompanied by pain and colic, and resulting in frequent and watery stools comparable with those of acute enteritis.

This classification is to some extent an artificial one because, in a number of instances, the effect produced is dependent upon the dose of the drug administered and, in excessive doses, some of the milder laxatives may act as drastic purgatives. However, from a practical point of view it is useful if the recognized doses of the various drugs are adhered to. The term aperient has here been used to cover all the groups.

Modes of action

Aperients act in various ways.
(i) The principal natural stimulus to peristalsis is the presence of faecal material stretching the muscle of the intestinal wall. Peristalsis is, therefore, more active if the amount of faecal residue is increased. In addition to taking cellulose material (fibre) in the diet, the bulk of the faeces may be increased by non-absorbable substances, such as agar and Isogel, which swell as they take up water present in the gut.

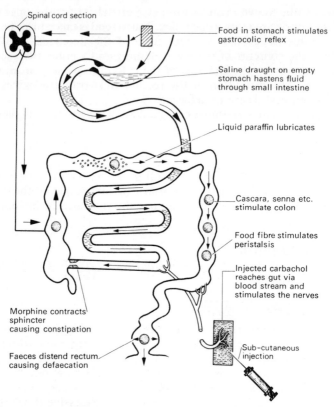

Fig. 6.3. Diagram illustrating the action of some aperients

(ii) Certain aperients, particularly those of the saline group, e.g. Epsom salts (magnesium sulphate), act mainly as hypertonic solutions which withdraw fluid via the mucous membrane of the gut. This fluid increases the bulk of the stool. At the same time the increased bulk of the stool causes more rapid peristalsis and so there is less time for the normal absorption of fluid from the lower bowel.

(iii) Others act by stimulating the nervous mechanism of peristalsis.

(iv) The drastic purgatives produce a definite inflammatory reaction in the mucous membrane of the intestine which results not only in stimulation of peristalsis but also in the outpouring of an inflammatory exudate. This also increases the relative bulk of the intestinal contents and, in addition, the hurried passage of the contents along the gut does not permit time for the normal absorption of fluid mentioned above. Frequent, copious and watery stools are, therefore, obtained.

In some instances the action of the drugs is more marked on the small intestine, in others it is on the large intestine. The main result, however, is to produce a rapid distension of the rectum with the contents of the gut from above, which is very similar to the effect of an enema distending the rectum when given from below.

Summary

The effects of aperients are:
(1) To increase the active movements of the intestine, i.e. to stimulate peristalsis and to hurry the passage of the intestinal contents.
(2) By mild irritation of the intestinal mucous membrane to increase slightly or greatly the amount of fluid exudate from the mucosa.
(3) To hasten the progress of the intestinal contents so that the normal absorption of water by the colon is partially prevented.
(4) To produce rapid distension of the rectum and the associated desire to defaecate.

Since the majority of aperients cause mild irritation of the mucous membrane of the gut it should be clear that their habitual use is undesirable. Their constant employment may cause the natural functions of the intestine to become sluggish so that a vicious circle is set up. It is a common experience that individuals who always employ aperients need to take constantly increasing doses of more powerful drugs.

In comparison with acute constipation associated with some temporary disorder or disease, chronic constipation (dyschezia) is, in most instances, due to faulty habits and failure to respond to the natural call to defaecate which occurs when the rectum becomes distended. The ideal treatment of chronic constipation is therefore not the regular administration of aperients but the gradual re-education of the bowel. This can generally be obtained by: (a) regular attempts at evacuation assisted by eating enough fibre (e.g. as bran) to increase the bulk of the faeces; (b) simple enemata from the use of which the patient is gradually weaned; (c) glycerin or bisacodyl (Dulcolax) suppositories are useful in some cases. Aperients may be of some value at the commencement of the course but should be dropped as soon as possible.

1. Laxatives

Fibre

As already mentioned, the natural stimulus to peristalsis is an adequate bulk of the faeces in the form of food residue consisting mainly of undigested cellulose. Wholemeal bread, whole-wheat cereals, bran, vegetables and fruits, especially figs and prunes, are all of value for this purpose.

Agar and other bulk laxatives

Agar is prepared from various seaweeds. It is not altered by digestion but has the power of absorbing water. In so doing it expands considerably in bulk and, by increasing the volume of the faeces, it promotes peristalsis. Agar is sometimes mixed with liquid paraffin to form an emulsion. Normacol, Isogel, Metamucil and various plant mucilages have a similar action.

Methyl cellulose in the form of granules (e.g. Celevac) also helps to retain water and thus adds to the bulk of the stools.

A bulk laxative (plantago seeds) is combined with senna in Agiolax. Usually, one or two heaped teaspoonfuls are swallowed unchewed with a drink, morning and evening, preferably before breakfast and after supper.

Lactulose

This is a sugar which passes unaltered from the mouth to the colon, where it is broken down into organic acids which promote peristalsis and have an osmotic effect. Lactulose is the principal constituent of Duphalac, of which the adult dose is 15 ml daily, after breakfast.

Liquid paraffin

This is a bland mineral oil which passes through the intestinal tract unchanged by the processes of digestion. It has no action on the mucous membrane of the gut, but acts as a simple lubricant, softening the faeces and aiding their passage through the bowel and rectum. There is no advantage in giving excessive doses and, when it appears to 'run through' the patient, the dose should be appropriately reduced. The usual dose is 30 ml at night, or possibly night and morning. Liquid paraffin should never be given to babies because of the risk of aspiration leading to lipoid pneumonia. This complication may also occur in elderly patients, in whom the cough reflex is weakened. Prolonged usage by any patient may lead to deficiency of the fat-soluble vitamins A, D and K by interfering with their absorption. When it is highly emulsified, liquid paraffin may be absorbed to a small extent and may be deposited in the mesenteric lymph nodes where it may cause a chronic inflammatory paraffinoma. It has also been suggested that prolonged use of liquid paraffin may induce cancer of the colon.

Magnesium hydroxide and Compound syrup of figs

These are laxatives especially useful for children (dose 2·5–10 ml).

2. Mild purgatives

In smaller doeses the following drugs will act as laxatives, but in full doses they are mild purgatives.

(a) Saline aperients

The saline aperients act fairly quickly and are best given in warm water on an empty stomach before breakfast.

Sodium sulphate (Glauber's salt; 15 g).

Magnesium sulphate (Epsom salts; 15 g).

Magnesium sulphate mixture, BPC (white mixture) contains magnesium sulphate (4 g), light magnesium carbonate (0·5 g) with peppermint emulsion and chloroform water. The dose is 10 ml.

(b) Drugs of the senna, cascara, rhubarb and aloes group

These are all mild purgatives of vegetable origin which do not produce inflammation of the intestine like the drugs of the drastic purgative group. As a rule they take 10 to 18 hours to produce an effect. Owing to some absorption from the bowel and subsequent excretion in the urine, rhubarb and senna tend to impart to the latter a yellow-brown colour.

Senna may be prepared from the leaflets or pods of the plant. It tends to produce more griping than other members of the group and its main action is on the colon.

Preparations include senna pods and syrup of senna, but the

effect of these preparations is unpredictable; it may be anything from inert to griping.

Standardized preparations of senna include senna tablets, BP (dose 1–4 tablets) and Senokot, which is available as granules, tablets and syrup. The correct dose is that which gives a comfortable formed motion and it has to be found by individual trial. For adults the dose of granules is usually one to two 5-ml teaspoonfuls. It is possible to 're-educate' the bowel so that the drug can be discontinued. It is a suitable purgative for use in pregnancy, but large doses should be avoided.

Danthron (as in Dorbanex and Normax) has an action similar to senna in stimulating colonic peristalsis.

Cascara sagrada is a bark from which the following important preparations are made:

cascara sagrada elixir (BPC, 2–5 ml)
compound cascara mixture (BPC, 10–20 ml)
cascara tablets (BP, dose: 1 or 2 tablets).

> **Rhubarb** (*Rheum*) is a rhizome from which compound rhubarb pill BP is made.
>
> It is also made up as rhubarb and soda mixture (BPC, 10 ml).
>
> **Aloes** is a dried juice obtained from the leaves of aloe plants. Preparations include:
>
> > Aloes and nux vomica tablet (BPC, dose: 1 tablet).

Bisacodyl (Dulcolax), one or two tablets of 5 mg, is a useful and popular aperient also employed as a suppository.

Castor oil (*Oleum ricini*). Applied to the surface of the body, castor oil is a bland substance having an emollient action. It is also used to allay irritation in the eye, and, mixed with zinc oxide, as an application to the skin.

In the intestines, however, it is altered in composition by the pancreatic enzymes and substances are produced which have a mildly irritating effect on the intestine, thereby giving the drug its aperient action. It may be given in capsules, as an emulsion, or mixture, and various methods have been devised for disguising its taste.

After its aperient action has passed off it tends to have a slightly constipating effect, hence its use in diarrhoea due to poisonous or unsuitable food, when it may be given with a view to emptying the intestine rapidly (2–6 hours) and then checking the condition by its constipating action. It is sometimes given after abdominal operations. Dose 5–20 ml.

3. Drastic purgatives or cathartics

These drugs are no longer employed. They include:

calomel.   jalap.   colocynth.

Drugs given by hypodermic injection

Certain drugs, having an action on the neuromuscular mechanism of the bowel whereby they increase the tone of the intestinal muscle and stimulate its movements, may be given by subcutaneous injection. They are useful in postoperative abdominal distension, and are also employed to stimulate the tone of the stomach muscle in acute dilatation of the stomach, and to aid expulsion of gas from the colon in intestinal distension and before x-ray examination. They include:

pituitary, posterior lobe injection (Pituitrin; 0·2–1·0 ml)
neostigmine injection (0·5–2 mg)
carbachol (0·25 mg).

Enemas

An enema consists of fluid for introduction into the rectum. Enemas may be given in order to empty the lower bowel, or for other purposes.

The main points to be remembered in the administration of rectal injections are:

(i) Collect all the required apparatus on a tray and cover with a towel before approaching the patient.
(ii) Whenever possible, place the patient in the lateral position. Enemas may be given with the patient on his back or in the knee-elbow position if necessary.
(iii) Do not insert the nozzle of a Higginson's syringe (if this instrument must be used) directly into the anus but attach a soft rubber catheter, which may be lubricated with a little Vaseline spread on gauze, and inserted into the rectum for two inches. The tube and funnel method is usually employed unless a modern prepacked disposable set is available.
(iv) Fluids should be injected at a temperature of 37 °C unless otherwise prescribed.
(v) After the removal of the catheter the patient should be lifted on to the bed-pan.

Contraindications. Enemas are generally contraindicated in myasthenia gravis, in which they may induce a crisis, and in Hirshsprung's disease, in which, unless they are isotonic, they may cause lethal derangements of fluid and electrolyte balance.

Types of enemata

(1) Those to be returned   warm water   arachis oil
                  (evacuant)   soap   phosphates.
(2) Those to be retained
    (*a*) anaesthetic, e.g. bromethol (Avertin)
    (*b*) steroid, e.g. prednisolone.
The following are some of the enemata which may be given:
(1) Warm water enema.
(2) Soap enema (30 g of soft soap to 500 ml of warm water).
(3) Phosphates enema BPC, contains the phosphate and acid phosphate of sodium. There are two formulations (A and B).
(4) Arachis oil enema. Up to 300 ml (5 to 10 ounces) of arachis oil are warmed in a water bath to 37 °C and run into the rectum by a tube and funnel. It should be retained from $\frac{1}{2}$ to 1 hour and may be followed in 4 hours by a soap enema if necessary. Olive oil may be used but is more expensive.
(5) Prednisolone (Predsol) enema and betamethasone enema (Retenema) are retention enemas which are used in the treatment of ulcerative colitis. They may be self-administered by the patient on retiring to bed each night, for 2 to 4 weeks.

Enema rash

Occasionally a patchy erythematous rash develops about 12 hours after an enema has been given. It usually appears on the face, buttocks and knees and may last for 24 hours. It is sometimes mistaken for scarlet fever or measles, but there is no pyrexia, it is not irritating and, as a rule, requires no treatment. Calamine lotion may be applied if desired.

Suppositories

Glycerine and bisacodyl (Dulcolax) are useful evacuant suppositories which are often used instead of enemata. They are valuable for elderly and bed-ridden patients provided the rectum is not full of impacted faeces.

Other drugs given in the form of suppositories are bismuth sub-gallate and hydrocortisone (e.g. Anusol and Anusol-HC supposit-ories) for their local action in minor ano-rectal conditions, penta-zocine and indomethacin for their analgesic effect, and aminophyl-line for its bronchodilator effect.

Intestinal sedatives

Intestinal sedatives have an opposite action to aperients, for they lessen peristaltic movement and diminish spasm. They are used in enteritis to check diarrhoea, to soothe the mucous membrane and to relieve colic. They may be classified thus:

(a) Soothing agents

Kaolin, chalk, bismuth salts and magnesium trisilicate are examples of drugs which help to protect the mucous membrane by their soothing action.

Kaolin and charcoal also absorb intestinal gases and prevent over-distension of the bowel, thus diminishing its movement and the colicky pains which are caused by the distension.

(b) Drugs acting on the nervous mechanism

Atropine and belladonna, and morphine and opium all act on the nervous mechanism. Atropine helps to relax spasm, while mor-phine has a general depressing effect on the muscular movements and tends to produce constipation.

Proprietary preparations which have an antispasmodic action on the alimentary tract include propantheline (Probanthine), Antrenyl, Merbentyl, Wyovin and mebeverine (Colofac).

Among the most useful remedies for diarrhoea are mixtures containing kaolin or bismuth salts and a small dose of morphine, e.g. *Mistura kaolin et morphinae* (p. 162), and Chlorodyne (p. 69). Codeine phosphate (30 mg) or diphenoxylate (Lomotil) are of value. Lomotil should not be given to children under 2 years of age. For infective cases sulphanamides or antibiotics are often employed.

(c) Drugs acting on the intestinal wall

Loperamide (Imodium) acts directly on the intestinal wall to inhibit excessive mobility and hence to relieve diarrhoea and the abdominal pains which may be associated with it. A first dose of 4 mg is followed by 2 mg after each loose stool up to a maximum of 16 mg in one day.

(d) Drugs acting on rectum and anus

These are usually in the form of suppositories or ointments which have an astringent or local anaesthetic action, e.g.:

   bismuth subgallate suppository
   benzocaine ointment
   hydrocortisone suppository.

Antiparasitic drugs

(a) Intestinal antiseptics.
(b) Anthelmintics.

1. Intestinal antiseptics

Under normal circumstances the presence of hydrochloric acid in the stomach helps to prevent the growth of bacteria, and in health this freedom from living organisms is maintained throughout the upper part of the small intestine. From the lower end of the ileum, however, the number of bacteria present increases and they are very numerous in the colon. Here they break down cellulose, which is unaffected by the digestive juices in the stomach and small intestine.

Sometimes bacteria pass through the gastric hydrochloric acid barrier and cause inflammation of the intestine (enteritis and colitis) or special conditions such as typhoid fever, bacillary dysentery and food poisoning. The bacteria which may be found in the intestines may, therefore, be classified as (a) pathogenic, or those responsible for disease of the intestines and (b) non-pathogenic, that is those organisms which are normally present in the intestines but cause no disease when they are confined to the bowel. They may, however, be harmful if they reach the peritoneum or other tissues. Included in this group are the organisms which assist in the digestion of cellulose in the colon. In certain circumstances these organisms may cause excessive putrefaction of the bowel contents or excessive fermentation, with the production of gas, some of which may be absorbed by kaolin or charcoal.

Common methods of treatment employed in a case of food poisoning or severe diarrhoea are:

(i) to allay the irritation of the mucous membrane by a mixture containing kaolin and morphine;

(ii) to relieve pain and spasm, if necessary, with morphine and atropine;

(iii) to absorb gas and intestinal toxins by charcoal or kaolin;

(iv) to replace the fluid lost from the body by diarrhoea by giving fluids orally, subcutaneously or intravenously, especially in infants;

(v) to avoid further irritation of the bowel by giving a light and easily digested diet commencing with milk, gruel, and arrowroot;

(vi) possibly to give one of the sulphonamides or antibiotics by mouth if a susceptible organism is found to be responsible for the condition.

Sulphonamides, including the insoluble ones which are not absorbed from the bowel such as sulphaguanidine and phthalylsulphathiazole (Thalazole), affect the growth of intestinal bacteria. A popular preparation is Guanimycin (a mixture of sulphaguanidine and dihydrostreptomycin). Tetracycline, chloramphenicol, etc., when given by mouth destroy many bacteria in the intestines (p. 000). If given for more than a few days, however, not only do they permit the overgrowth of many bacteria which are insensitive to them but they may also seriously affect the absorption of certain vitamins, particularly those of the vitamin B complex. Preparations of vitamin B must, therefore, be given at the same time if their administration is prolonged. Erythromycin may be valuable in cases of enteritis caused by staphylococci.

Obviously minor degrees of diarrhoea of short duration do not necessarily require any active treatment.

Treatment of special bowel infections

Dysentery

There are two types of dysentery:

(a) **Amoebic dysentery** caused by a single-celled organism known as the *Entamoeba histolytica*. In addition to general symptomatic treatment (fluid and electrolyte replacement) the following drugs may be employed:

(1) Metronidazole (Flagyl)—the drug of choice—in a dose of 800 mg t.d.s. by mouth for 5 days;

(2) Diloxanide (Furamide), 500 mg t.d.s. for 10 days, may be given in addition to metronidazole;

(3) Emetine hydrochloride, 60 mg subcutaneously daily for 4 days may be given in severe cases, especially if the patient vomits metronidazole;

(4) Tetracycline may be given in combination with the other drugs, in severe cases, in a dose of 500 mg 8-hourly.

Chloroquine is effective in the treatment of amoebic liver abscess, but is ineffective against amoebae in the bowel lumen or elsewhere.

(b) **Bacillary dysentery.** Often this is a mild self-limiting illness for which antimicrobial therapy is not recommended. Shiga dysentery tends to be more serious, however, and may warrant chemotherapy with one of the following drugs:

(1) Co-trimoxazole (Septrin);

(2) antibiotics, e.g. ampicillin, tetracycline;

(3) nalidixic acid (Negram).

Bacterial sensitivity tests are necessary as shigellae are often resistant, especially to sulphonamides and tetracyclines.

2. Anthelmintics

The intestinal canal may become the home of various parasitic worms. The ova or eggs of the parasites usually enter the human being (the host) in contaminated food or water. They reach the intestine, where they mature into the fully grown worm.

Drugs used in the treatment of worms are called **anthelmintics.** Those which actually kill the worm are sometimes referred to as **vermicides** while those which merely cause its expulsion from the body are called **vermifuges.**

The following are the most important varieties of worm found in the UK:

threadworms   tapeworms
roundworms   hookworms.

Threadworms (*Enterobius vermicularis*; enterobiasis)

These are common in children and inhabit the large intestine. Their successful eradication depends entirely upon the prevention of reinfection. Their presence is often associated with itching of the anus, for which benzocaine ointment may be applied. Other members of the household should also be checked for the presence of worms or ova.

Treatment

Any of the following drugs may be used:

(i) **viprynium** (Vanquin) is given as a single dose according to body weight (5 mg/kg). A repeated dose, after 2 weeks, is advisable. It stains the stools red;

(ii) **thiabendazole** (Mintezol). Dose: 25 mg/kg of body weight twice daily with meals for 1 to 2 days. Maximum daily dose: 3 g. It is effective not only against threadworm, but also against roundworms and other worms;

(iii) **mebendazole** (Vermox); a single dose of 100 mg, repeated after 2 or 3 weeks if necessary;

(iv) **piperazine,** e.g. Antepar. Dose (of base): 500–2000 mg, according to body weight, once daily for 7 days;

(v) **Crystal violet** given in enteric-coated capsules is effective. The adult dose is 60 mg t.d.s. with meals; for children up to 10 mg for each year of age. Two courses each lasting 8 days with an interval of a week are given.

Roundworms (*Ascaris lumbricoides*; ascariasis)

These resemble the earth worm in appearance and, in addition to entering the intestine, may occasionally wander into the stomach from which they may be vomited, or into the bile ducts when they produce jaundice. The larvae may reach the lungs and cause pneumonia.

Treatment

The following drugs are used:

(i) **Piperazine** (Antepar, Pripsen) is the drug usually prescribed. A single dose of 4 g may be given to an adult. For children the dose is calculated according to the age and weight. No purgative is necessary unless constipation is present;

(ii) **Bephenium** (Alcopar) is also an ascaricide. It is useful for mixed hookworm and roundworm infections;

(iii) **Mebendazole** (Vermox), a broad-spectrum anthelmintic, is highly-effective against ascaris. The dose is 100 mg twice daily for 3 days;

(iv) **Thiabendazole** (Mintezol) and mebendazole (Vermox) are active against roundworms, threadworms and whipworms.

If one member of a family has threadworms or roundworms other members almost certainly have them and should be treated.

Tapeworms (*Taenia solium, Taenia saginata*; taeniasis)

Drugs which may be used include:

(i) **Yomesan** (niclosamide) kills and partially dissolves tapeworms. Two tablets (2 g) are well chewed and followed by two more 1 hour later;

(ii) **dichlorophen** (Anthiphen) may be used against beef tapeworms but not against pork tapeworms. The dose for an adult is 6 g on each of two successive days. The worm is partially digested and there is no point in searching the stools for the head after dichlorophen. No starvation or purgation is necessary with either Yomesan or dichlorophen, but the tablets are best taken in the morning on an empty stomach;

(iii) **mepacrine hydrochloride.** This drug which is used in the treatment of malaria is also effective against tapeworms. 100 mg are given every 5 minutes for ten doses (total 1 g). It is often given via a tube directly into the duodenum as vomiting may occur when it is taken by mouth. Its action is less certain than that of male fern;

(iv) **Male fern.** In order that the anthelmintic drug may come into full contact with the worm, it is necessary for the stomach and intestines to be as empty as possible. The patient is, therefore, starved for 2 days, fluids only being given. Saline aperients are taken each morning. On the third morning male fern extract draught (BPC), 50 ml, is given and followed 2 hours later by 15–30 g of magnesium sulphate. If the bowels are not opened within an hour or so, a soap and water enema is administered.

The motions should be collected in warm water and a search made for the head of the worm. If it is not found the treatment should be repeated in 10 days.

Under no circumstances should castor oil be given after *Filix mas*, as a combination of these drugs produces very dangerous toxic symptoms.

Hookworms (*Ancylostoma*)

The ova of these worms may be found in the faeces of patients from tropical countries. The larvae bore their way through the skin and reach the duodenum via the blood vessels, lungs and trachea, causing anaemia and eosinophilia. **Bephenium** (Alcopar), 5 g, is given after an overnight fast and may be repeated each morning for two or three days.

Tetrachlorethylene, 0·1 ml/kg body weight up to 3 ml, may be used, but is more toxic. An overnight fast and a sline purge is required before administration of the drug. Another saline purge is given 1–2 hours after the drug.

Whipworm

Thiabendazole (Mintezol) or mebendazole (Vermox) is used.

Filariasis

Diethylcarbamazine (Banocide) is the drug of choice.

Schistosomiasis

Niridazole (Ambilhar) is employed except in S. japonicum infections. It is also used for guinea worms. Hycanthone, given as a single intramuscular injection, is another effective drug in schistosomiasis.

Trichiniasis

No drugs are very effective but emetine may be tried.

Hydatid disease (Echinococcosis)

Mebedendazole (Vermox) is reported to be lethal to the hydatid cysts. A dose of 400–600 mg is given three times a day for 21–30 days and the course is repeated if necessary.

Drugs acting on the liver and biliary apparatus

There are few drugs which can be used to alter the functions of the liver or to increase the formation of bile, but certain substances hasten the evacuation of bile from the gall bladder into the duodenum. They are called *cholagogues* and include:

sodium salicylate (2 g), sodium sulphate (16 g), and magnesium sulphate (5–15 g).

Sulphonamides and certain antibiotics (e.g. ampicillin) are the most effective biliary antiseptics.

The injection of adrenaline (1 in 1000) causes the liver to convert the glycogen stored in it into glucose, which passes into the blood. This fact is sometimes made use of in the treatment of hypoglycaemia due to overdosage of insulin.

A fatty meal or the administration of olive oil into the stomach or duodenum causes the gall bladder to empty its contents into the duodenum.

Glucose is said to have a 'protective' action on the liver and helps to diminish the damage done to the organ in various toxic states.

Bile acids

Chenodeoxycholic acid (CDCA) and ursodeoxycholic acid (UDCA) are naturally occurring bile acids which help to dissolve cholesterol gallstones. A synthetic form of CDCA is available as Chendol. The treatment is used only in cases in which the gallstones are radiolucent (clear on x-ray films) and the gall bladder is functioning. It is thought to act by inhibiting the synthesis of cholesterol in the liver, so that less cholesterol is secreted into the bile. Cholesterol-rich stones then slowly dissolve in the desaturated bile in the gall bladder. The process may take one to several years but the treatment is a useful alternative to surgery, especially in patients with severe heart or lung disease. CDCA is taken orally, usually three times a day with food, in a total daily dose of 13–15 mg per kg of body weight. Diarrhoea is a common side-effect. UDCA, obtained from Chinese bears, is effective in lower dosage and is much less likely to cause diarrhoea.

Cholecystography

Phenobutiodil (Biliodyl), Iopanoic acid (Telepaque), sodium ipodate (Biloptin), calcium ipodate (Solu-Biloptin) or iobenzamic acid (Osbil), when given by mouth, are absorbed in the alimentary tract and excreted by the liver into the bile. For a time they are stored and concentrated in the gall bladder. These substances are opaque to x-rays and an x-ray picture can therefore be obtained showing the outline of the gall bladder, provided it is functioning normally.

Technique

On the day before the examination is carried out, the amount of fat in the diet is reduced to a minumum. The patient has a light supper containing no fat at 7 p.m. At 10 p.m., 3 g of the dye dissolved in water are given, followed by further drinks of water. X-ray pictures are taken next morning. Often a second dose of the contrast medium is given 2–3 hours before the x-ray examination. During this period no food is allowed, but water may be drunk. The first meal is given one hour before the last x-ray. This consists of a fatty meal which should contain bread, butter, bacon and a cup of tea. Alternatively a fat emulsion containing nut oil (Prosparol; dose, 120 ml) may be used.

The gall bladder may not be visualized in some cases, such as when pyloric stenosis or conditions causing diarrhoea interfere with absorption of the dye. Seriously impaired liver function and inability of the diseased gall bladder to concentrate dye are other reasons for failure to visualize the gall bladder. Except in the case of seriously impaired liver function, the gall bladder may be outlined by dye injected intravenously. Iodipamide (Biligrafin) is used for this purpose and for visualizing the common bile duct; 20 ml of a 30 per cent solution or of a 50 per cent solution (Biligrafin forte) are injected intravenously over the course of 10 minutes.

Pancreas

Strong Pancreatin powder (Pancrex V) is used in cases of malabsorption due to disease of the pancreas, e.g. fibrocystic disease. It may be sprinkled on food or given in a liquid with each meal. The dose varies with the age of the child (up to 1 year, 0·5–1 g; 1 to 12 years, 1–2 g).

7 The action of drugs on the heart and circulation

In order to understand the action of drugs on the heart and circulatory system it is necessary to review certain aspects of the physiology.

(1) The heart muscle acts as a pump which supplies the motive force, driving the blood under pressure through the arterial system to all the organs and tissues of the body where it is distributed in the capillaries. The veins are the 'return' channels of the circulatory system.

The volume of blood passing through the heart each minute is called the cardiac output. In health cardiac output varies according to the immediate needs of the body, being increased on exercise by an increase in the rate and force with which the heart beats.

In cardiac failure, when the myocardium can no longer supply sufficient force, the cardiac output is reduced. This leads to:

(i) inadequate blood supply to the organs and tissues;

(ii) diminished activity of the kidneys causing salt and water retention and oedema;

(iii) venous congestion.

(2) In order to act efficiently the heart muscle must be adequately nourished. In particular, it requires oxygen and glucose to satisfy its metabolic needs. These reach it in the blood supplied to it through the coronary arteries. Diminution in the size of the lumen of the coronary arteries, either temporarily as a result of spasm or permanently owing to disease of their walls, will result in defective nutrition of the heart muscle, with either temporary or permanent effects on its efficiency.

(3) The pressure of blood within the arteries is dependent on (i) the force of the heart beat, i.e. the strength of the muscular contraction, (ii) the calibre of the arteries, (iii) the elasticity of the arteries, i.e. if the arteries are narrowed and inelastic the blood pressure is raised.

(4) The rhythm of the heart and the orderly sequence with which the various chambers contract is dependent on specialized conducting tissue in the heart.

The impulse for each cardiac contraction commences at the sinoatrial node (the pacemaker of the heart) near the entrance of the superior vena cava into the right atrium. It spreads over the muscle of both atria and reaches the atrioventricular node, from which it passes down the atrioventricular bundle of His. In the interventricular septum, the bundle of His divides into right and left branches and distributes the impulse to the right and left ventricles respectively.

The bundle of His can only pass a certain number of impulses per minute, that is to say, a definite period must elapse after one impulse has passed before the bundle is able to transmit the next. This period of rest during which no impulse can pass is called the refractory period.

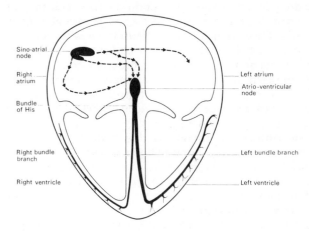

Fig. 7.1. Illustrating the spread of the impulse for contraction from the sinoatrial node over the atria to reach the atrioventricular node, whence it passes down the bundle of His and is distributed to the ventricles

(5) The constant rate of the heart is maintained because the sinoatrial node is under the influence of two sets of nervous impulses which normally are equally balanced.

Parasympathetic nerve fibres reaching the heart in the vagus (Xth cranial) nerve carry impulses which tend to slow its rate (inhibitors).

Sympathetic fibres from the cardiac plexus tend to increase its rate (accelerators).

Therefore, drugs which tend to paralyse or depress the parasympathetic or vagus will permit over-action of the sympathetic and the rate of the heart will be increased. Those which stimulate the vagus (parasympathetic) will slow the rate.

Conversely, stimulation of the sympathetic fibres will also increase the heart rate, while their depression will slow the rate by permitting over-action of the vagus.

As an example, adrenaline, which stimulates the sympathetic, will increase the rate of the heart if given by injection or if its secretion by the adrenal glands is naturally increased as it is in states of fear or violent emotion.

Drugs acting on the heart

Among the important drugs acting on the heart itself are those of the digitalis group, and the condition on which they have the most beneficial and dramatic effect is atrial (auricular) fibrillation.

In atrial fibrillation, the atrial muscle loses its power of contracting as a whole, and instead of one impulse commencing at the sino-atrial node spreading in an orderly fashion over the atrial muscle to reach the atrio-ventricular node at the rate of approximately 72 per minute, a series of irregular contractions occur which are scattered over the atria. Each of these small contractions produces an impulse which passes to the atrio-ventricular node. In atrial fibrillation, therefore, this node is bombarded with impulses at the rate of about 400 per minute.

Owing to the refractory period, however, the bundle of His transmits only some of these irregular impulses. The ventricle therefore contracts at irregular intervals at a rapid rate (often up to 130 or more beats/minute).

Since the contractions of the ventricle occur at irregular and rapid intervals, it follows that it can never be filled completely nor will it contain the same amount of blood for each beat. Therefore the output per beat is small and variable in quantity. This means that the pulse will be irregular both in rhythm and volume. Some of the heart beats will be so small that the pulse-wave produced will be imperceptible at the wrist. Therefore the rate of the pulse counted at the wrist will not be a true indication of the rate of the ventricles. Hence the importance of taking and recording the rate at the apex in cases of atrial fibrillation.

The digitalis group

Drugs of the digitalis group act:

(i) on the bundle of His in atrial fibrillation. Their action is a depressing one, that is, they reduce its power of conducting impulses. In other words, they increase the refractory period. By this means, the bundle of His allows fewer of the irregular impulses bombarding the atrioventricular node to pass and, by adjusting the dose of the drug, this number can be reduced to 70 or 80 per minute or even lower.

In this way the ventricular rate is slowed. Slowing of the ventricle means better filling of the ventricle and an increased out put per beat. Consequently, the efficiency of the heart as a pump is increased and the general circulation is improved.

(ii) Digitalis acts directly on the myocardium and increases the force of contraction. It thereby increases cardiac output and reduces the raised venous pressure and the venous congestion in congestive heart failure.

The improvement in the circulation has other beneficial effects:

(1) The circulation in the coronary arteries is increased and the nutrition of the heart is improved.

(2) The circulation in the kidneys is improved and the output of urine is increased, a factor important in the reduction of cardiac oedema. This explains the diuretic action of digitalis in heart disease.

(3) Oedema is also diminished by reason of the improved circulation in the more distant and dependent parts of the body.

Summary

The action of the digitalis group of drugs may be summarized:

(i) Digitalis is of special value in atrial fibrillation.

(ii) It acts by depressing the bundle of His and increasing its refractory period.

(iii) Thereby it slows ventricular rate, increases the output per beat and improves the circulation.

(iv) Digitalis also has a general tonic effect on the heart muscle, increasing the force of ventricular contraction and the cardiac output. It is, therefore, of value in other cases of cardiac weakness. Its most dramatic effect, however, is in atrial fibrillation.

(v) Improvement in the circulation has a beneficial effect on various symptoms, e.g. the urinary output is increased; oedema is diminished.

(vi) It has an action on the vagus nerve and sino-atrial node which also contributes to the slowing of the cardiac rate.

(vii) In therapeutic doses digitalis has little action on the normal heart.

Digitalis

Digitalis is obtained from the foxglove and was first used in the treatment of heart disease by William Withering in 1785. Many preparations exist, from the simple powdered leaves, now rarely used, to pure substances (glycosides) such as digoxin, digitoxin, lanatoside C and medigoxin (Lanitop).

The following are commonly used:

Digoxin tablets (Lanoxin) (0·25–1·0 mg); Lanoxin PG (0·0625 mg)

Digoxin injection, BP, for intravenous or intramuscular use (2–4 ml)

Digitoxin (Digitaline Nativelle) tablets (0·1 mg).

NB.—0·1 mg of digitoxin and 0·1 of medigoxin are both approximately equivalent in therapeutic effect to 0·25 mg of digoxin.

Methods of administration of digitalis

Treatment of atrial fibrillation with digitalis may be divided into stages:

(i) Initial doses for reduction of heart rate to about 70.

(ii) Maintenance doses.

(iii) Urgent cases.

Initial doses

Provided no digitalis has been taken within 2 or 3 days, a full dose of digoxin is given.

Maintenance doses

These are adjusted to maintain the pulse and apex rate between 60 and 80 per minute.

Urgent cases

In very urgent cases, rapid results are obtained by giving digoxin; e.g. 1 mg by mouth will slow the heart rate in 6 to 8 hours. If necessary, 0·75 to 1·0 mg may be given intravenously in 10 to 20 ml of normal saline. The heart rate begins to fall in 10 minutes and the maximum effect of the dose is apparent in less than 2 hours. Digoxin should not be given by subcutaneous injection.

Notes on the administration of digitalis

(1) During the treatment of atrial fibrillation with digitalis both the apex rate and the pulse rate should be recorded.
(2) The urinary output should be carefully measured.
(3) Elderly patients usually require a reduced dosage, because toxic effects occur more readily in old age.

Toxic symptoms

These may be due to over-dosage, cumulative effect or idiosyncrasy. They include:

(i) undue slowness of the pulse and apex beat, e.g. below 60;
(ii) paired beats (*pulsus bigeminus*) and other rhythm changes;
(iii) nausea and vomiting, anorexia and diarrhoea;
(iv) diminished urinary output.

Other drugs of the digitalis group

These are very much less frequently employed than digoxin but are useful when patients show intolerance to the latter drug. They include strophanthus, ouabain and lanatoside.

Quinidine sulphate (60–300 mg)

This is a drug allied to quinine in composition. It acts directly on the heart muscle and suppresses excitable foci. It therefore tends to prevent ectopic beats and paroxysmal tachycardia. For this purpose (prophylaxis), quinidine sulphate is usually given in a dose of 200 mg 3 or 4 times daily by mouth. It was formerly used, in higher doage, for the conversion of atrial fibrillation to sinus rhythm, but direct current electric shock therapy (dc cardioversion) is now preferred.

Kinidin Durules are sustained-action tablets of quinidine bisulphate (250 mg). The usual dose is 1 to 3 Durules twice daily (morning and evening).

Rarely, quinidine provokes a **hypersensitivity reaction,**

manifested by urticaria, and pyrexia. Very rarely, thrombocyto-penia occurs.

Over-dosage

Over-dosage of quinidine may cause blurring of vision, impair-ment of hearing, dizziness, vomiting and headache. This state is known as cinchonism. Over-dosage can also cause heart block, premature beats, ventricular tachycardia and ventricular fibrilla-tion.

Procainamide (Pronestyl) (500 mg to 1 gram)

This is a synthetic substance having somewhat similar actions and uses to quinidine in paroxysmal tachycardia. It may be given orally or by very slow intravenous injection (up to 10 ml, and not exceed-ing 50 mg per minute), during which a check on the blood pressure and electrocardiogram is maintained.

Lignocaine (Xylocaine)

Lignocaine has a similar action but is less likely to cause hypo-tension. It is given intravenously to reduce or abolish ventricular ectopic beats resulting from myocardial infarction. An initial single dose of 50–100 mg is usually followed by an infusion of 1–4 mg per minute until there has been no significant ectopic activity for 24 hours. Lignocaine is metabolized in the liver. Smaller doses are therefore usually adequate for patients with liver disease.

Disopyramide (Rythmodan)

Disopyramide is effective in the treatment of many disturbances of cardiac rhythm, especially ventricular arrhythmias. The drug may be given orally (300 to 800 mg daily in divided dosage) or by slow intravenous injection. Disopyramide has a mild anti-cholinergic action which may cause a dry mouth and blurred vision.

Verapamil (Cordilox)

This drug is given by slow intravenous injection, in a dose of 5 mg, to stop a paroxysm of supraventricular tachycardia. An oral dose of 40 to 80 mg three times a day may prevent recurrences.

Mexiletine (*Mexitil*)

Mexiletine is effective in the treatment of ventricular premature beats and ventricular tachycardia. It is particularly useful intravenously when lignocaine has failed to stop the arrhythmia and orally for the prevention of recurrences. The oral maintenance dose is 200 or 250 mg 3 or 4 times a day.

Beta-adrenergic-receptor blockade

The sympathetic nervous system and free circulating catecholamines (adrenaline and noradrenaline) act on receptors which are present in certain tissues. The receptors are of two distinct types—alpha (α) and beta (β). *α-Receptors* are generally *excitatory* in function, so that their stimulation causes, for example, contraction of the smooth muscle in the walls of blood vessles and hence vasoconstriction. *β-Receptors* are generally *inhibitory* in function so that their activation causes relaxation of the smooth muscle in the walls of blood vessels and bronchi, resulting in vasodilatation and bronchodilatation. This is the mechanism by which adrenaline and similar compounds (sympathomimetic amines) dilate the bronchi and relieve bronchial asthma.

The β-receptors in cardiac muscle are exceptional in being excitatory. Their stimulation by adrenaline causes the heart to beat more rapidly and more forcibly. This can be prevented by blockade of the β-receptors with certain drugs which are therefore called β-adrenergic-receptor blocking agents or 'beta-blockers'. The approved names of these agents all end in '... olol', as in propranolol and oxprenolol or '... alol' as in acebutalol and sotalol. β-blockers are used principally in the treatment of:

angina
hypertension
and cardiac arrhythmias.

They are also used as an adjunct in the treatment of thyroid over- and under-activity, in the control of essential tremor, and in the management of Fallot's tetralogy, hypertrophic obstructive cardiomyopathy (HOCM, a disease of cardiac muscle) and phaeochromocytoma (a tumour which secretes adrenaline and noradrenaline). For the latter condition, it is used in conjunction with an α-receptor blocking drug.

β-Blockers are generally **contraindicated** in *heart failure* (in which the heart may be relying on sympathetic stimulation) unless this can be controlled with digitalis, in the presence of second- and third-degree *heart block*, in states of *metabolic acidosis* (e.g. diabetic ketosis) and in patients with *asthma* or *chronic bronchitis*. However, some β-blockers (e.g. metoprolol and atenolol) act more on the β-receptors in the heart than on those in the bronchi and are there-fore said to be cardioselective; these can often be given to asth-matics without provoking bronchospasm. Some β-blockers (e.g. oxprenolol) have a slight stimulant effect on the myocardium and are reputed to be less likely than others to aggravate heart failure. These and other differing properties of β-blocking agents partly account for their number.

In diabetics, β-blockers may mask the symptoms and signs of hypoglycaemia (e.g. tremulousness, sweating and tachycardia) which are due to increased sympathetic activity.

Side-effects

These are usually minor and transient and include lassitude, in-somnia, nausea, diarrhoea and cold extremities. Rashes occasion-ally occur and practolol lost favour because of these and other side-effects, including 'dry-eye' which sometimes progressed to corneal scarring.

One of the therapeutic actions of β-blockers is to reduce the heart rate, but an excessive fall (to below 55 beats per minute) indicates the need for a reduction in dosage. Excessive bradycardia can be counteracted with atropine (0·25–2 mg intravenously), fol-lowed by a β-receptor stimulant, such as isoprenaline in an initial dose of 25 micrograms by slow intravenous injection.

Examples of β-blockers, with their starting doses for the treat-ment of hypertension, are:

propranolol (Inderal)	40 mg b.d. or t.d.s.
oxprenolol (Trasicor)	80 mg b.d.
pindolol (Visken)	5 mg t.d.s.
sotalol (Beta-Cardone, Sotacor)	80 mg t.d.s.
acebutalol (Sectral)	100 mg b.d.
timolol (Blocadren)	5 mg t.d.s.
metoprolol (Betaloc, Lopressor)	100 mg b.d.
atenolol (Tenormin)	100 mg daily.

Circulatory stimulants

Circulatory stimulants are drugs which are given to improve the circulation. They are generally employed in acute conditions such as shock.

They may be roughly classified into two main groups:

(i) Those which raise the blood pressure by their action on the arteries (vasoconstrictors or vasopressors).

(ii) Those which stimulate the heart directly.

(a) **Adrenaline** and noradrenaline are examples of drugs which stimulate the α-receptors in the walls of small arteries. They cause constriction of the arteries by stimulating the plain muscle in their walls to contract. The result of this general arterial constriction is a rise in blood pressure.

Noradrenaline (Levophed) is usually given in a slow intravenous drip, 4 ml of a 1 in 1000 solution being added to 1 litre of saline or 5 per cent dextrose solution (p. 119). Its main use is when the blood pressure is low in surgical shock.

Metaraminol (Aramine), 0·5 to 5 mg intravenously, 2 to 10 mg intramuscularly, is a vasoconstrictor used as an adjunct in the treatment of hypotension due to drugs, surgery, or haemorrhage. It is contraindicated in most cases of heart disease, diabetes and thyrotoxicosis.

(b) Certain drugs stimulate the sympathetic β-receptors of the heart and cause an increase in the rate and force of contraction of this organ. Adrenaline, isoprenaline and orciprenaline are such substances. A long-acting preparation of isoprenaline, Saventrine is useful in the treatment of complete heart block although an electronic pacemaker is usually preferable.

Digitalis is a drug which stimulates the heart to contract more forcibly but does not increase the heart rate. It is therefore said to have an *inotropic* action. In cases in which it also slows the heart, it is said to have a negative *chronotropic* action.

Drugs acting on the arteries

The drugs in this group which dilate the arteries are called vasodilators. Advantage is taken of this effect for different conditions, i.e.

(i) Drugs are sometimes used especially for their power of dilating the coronary arteries.

(ii) They may be used for their action in dilating the peripheral arteries in the limbs and the cerebral arteries.

(iii) They may be employed with the definite intention of lowering blood pressure.

Drugs used to dilate the coronary arteries
The nitrites and nitrates

These drugs are used especially in the treatment of angina pectoris, both in acute attacks and with a view to reducing their frequency. Their main action is to dilate the peripheral veins, thus reducing venous return, and the arterioles, thus reducing peripheral resistance. In this way, the work of the left ventricle, and its oxygen demand, is reduced. Coronary arteries narrowed by atheroma cannot be effectively dilated, but healthy collateral vessels can be and this is another way in which these drugs act.

Glyceryl trinitrate tablets (trinitrin, 0·5 mg)

This is the most important drug used in the treatment of angina pectoris, the pain of which is rapidly relieved. It is of greatest value when taken before an exertion which the patient knows, by experience, would usually cause pain. The tablets are placed under the tongue or chewed very slowly but not swallowed whole. The drug is absorbed by the mucous membrane of the mouth, but has little effect if it enters the stomach.

Its action is more prolonged than that of amyl nitrite (i.e. up to 15 minutes). Kept in a well-closed glass or metal (not plastic) container with a metallic-foil-lined lid, in a dark, dry, cool place, tablets can be expected to remain potent for 2 years from the date of their manufacture. In less favourable conditions they may lose their potency very rapidly.

Amyl nitrite capsules

This is a volatile liquid given by inhalation. It is supplied in glass capsules containing 0·2 ml which are broken in a handkerchief and then inhaled. Its action in angina pectoris is rapid but brief. It also dilates the other arteries of the body, and this can be observed in the flushing of the face and felt in the throbbing of the head after inhalation. It is sometimes used to relieve biliary and renal colic and hiccough.

Other vasodilators

Pentaerythritol tetranitrate (Peritrate, Mycardol) and sorbide nitrate (Isordil) are long-acting nitrate preparations taken three or four times a day in the hope of preventing anginal pains. They are contraindicated in glaucoma.

Other drugs used to prevent anginal attacks are the β-blockers (e.g. propranolol 160–240 mg daily), nifedipine (Adalat, 10–20 mg three times daily), prenylamine (Synadrin, 60 mg three times daily) and perhexilene (Pexid, 100 mg 1 to 4 times daily).

The β-blockers act by preventing excessive sympathetic stimulation of the heart. Both the rate and the force of contraction of the heart are reduced. The work of the heart and its oxygen requirement are therefore diminished.

Prenylamine depletes the stores of catecholamines (adrenaline and noradrenaline) in the myocardium. The myocardial oxygen demand during physical or mental stress is consequently reduced.

Nifedipine reduces myocardial oxygen consumption, lowers peripheral (arteriolar) resistance and thus the workload of the heart, and dilates coronary arteries.

Perhexilene reduces the tachycardia which is induced by exertion and produces a decrease in the work of the left ventricle and in myocardial oxygen consumption.

Drugs used to reduce blood pressure (antihypertensive drugs)

These fall into three groups:

  diuretics
  sympathetic-inhibitors
  vasodilators.

A general principle is to combine drugs with different sites of action to obtain the greatest therapeutic benefit with the minimum of side-effects. It is therefore common for a hypertensive patient to be taking moderate doses of several antihypertensive drugs rather than a large dose of any one.

Diuretics

By themselves these exert a substantial antihypertensive action and, in mild cases of hypertension, are often the only drugs required. They also potentiate the effectiveness of all other anti-hypertensive agents, so that they form a basis for treatment of all grades of hypertension. The long-acting diurectics, which need be taken only once daily, are generally most suitable and most effective. Examples are:

bedrofluazide (Aprinox) 5–10 mg daily
chlorthalidone (Hygroton) 50 mg daily
clorexolone (Nefrolan) 10–25 mg daily
xipamide (Diurexan) 20 or 40 mg daily.

Hypertensive patients with potassium deficiency can be prescribed either a potassium supplement, such as Slow-K, or a potassium-retaining diuretic agent, such as amiloride. Combined preparations are available, eg.:

Navidrex-K (cyclopenthiazide 0·25 mg and potassium chloride 600 mg)
Neo-naclex-K (bendrofluazide 2·5 mg and potassium chloride 630 mg)
Moduretic (hydrochlorothiazide 50 mg and amiloride 5 mg).

Sympathetic-inhibitors ('adrenolytic agents')

These drugs inhibit the sympathetic nervous system at various levels. Those acting on the autonomic centres in the brain are said to be *centrally acting* and include the **veratrum alkaloids** (e.g. Veriloid) and **clonidine.**

Clonidine (Catapres) has both central and peripheral sites of action. It is started orally in a dose of 0·05 mg 3 times a day and the dose is increased every second or third day. An injectable form is also available for slow intravenous injection in a dose of 0·15 mg.

Some antihypertensive drugs act by blocking the ganglia of the autonomic nervous system and are known as *ganglion-blocking agents*. The blockade of the sympathetic ganglia prevents vessel-contracting (vasoconstrictor) nervous impulses from being transmitted. The resulting dilatation of the arterioles reduces the peripheral resistance and consequently lowers the blood pressure. Unfortunately, the ganglionic blockade is unselective and the parasympathetic ganglia are blocked as well as the sympathetic ganglia. The blockade of the parasympathetic ganglia causes undesirable effects such as dryness of the mouth, blurring of vision due to impairment of accommodation, difficulty in micturition, constipation and occasionally paralytic ileus. Ganglion-blockers are rarely used now except by the parenteral route, for the treatment of hypertensive emergencies. For this purpose, **trimetaphan** (Arfonad) may be given by intravenous infusion or **pentolinium** (Ansolysen) may be given subcutaneously. However, even these are infrequently used for the emergency treatment of hypertension, since there are effective injectable antihypertensive agents which are not ganglion-blockers. These include **diazoxide** (300 mg by rapid intravenous injection), **sodium nitroprusside, labetalol** and **hydrallazine.**

Drugs which selectively inhibit the peripheral sympathetic nerve fibres and which do not affect the parasympathetic nerves are known as *post-ganglionic adrenergic inhibitors*. Examples of these, with their usual dose ranges, are as follows:

> **reserpine** (Serpasil) 0·3–0·5 mg daily
> **methyldopa** (Aldomet) 500 mg to 2 g daily
> **guanethidine** (Ismelin) 20–160 mg daily
> **bethanidine** (Esbatal) 30–100 mg daily
> **debrisoquine** (Declinax) 10–300 mg daily.

All of the above listed drugs are taken in divided dosage, apart from guanethidine, which is long-acting and is therefore taken only once a day.

The remaining group of drugs which inhibit the action of the sympathetic nervous system is of those which block the receptors in the walls of the arterioles or in the myocardium. They are known as *adreno-receptor blockers* and are divided into two subgroups, according to whether they block the α-receptors or the β-receptors. α-Blockers include phentolamine and phenoxybenzamine, which are used respectively in the diagnosis and control of hypertension due to a phaeochromocytoma and prazosin (Hypovase) which may be used in any form of hypertension.

Much more extensively used in the treatment of hypertension are the *β-blockers* which probably act mainly by reducing the force of myocardial contraction. Beta-blockers reduce not only the cardiac output at rest but also the increase in cardiac output induced by exercise and catecholamines (adrenaline and noradrenaline). Beta-blockers may also act by suppressing plasma renin activity and by a central action on the brain. Examples are:

> **propranolol** (Inderal) 20–1000 mg daily in 2 or 3 doses
> **oxprenolol** (Trasicor) 80–480 mg twice daily

pindolol (Visken) 5–15 mg 3 times a day
sotalol (Sotacor) 240–600 mg daily in 2 or 3 doses
metoprolol (Betaloc, Lopressor) 100–200 mg twice daily
acebutalol (Sectral) 400–1200 mg daily
atenolol (Tenormin) 100 mg daily.

The β-blockers have the advantage over the ganglion-blockers and the post-ganglionic adrenergic inhibitors (e.g. guanethidine) of not causing postural hypotension. The latter is an unpleasant and disabling condition which causes giddiness, faintness or actual syncope on assuming the erect posture. It is the principal factor limiting the dosage of many antihypertensive agents.

Labetalol (Trandate) is unique in having both alpha- and beta-adrenoreceptor blocking properties. The peripheral arterioles are dilated by the blockade of the α-receptors and reflex cardiac stimulation is prevented by the beta-blockade. It is claimed to be safer than pure β-blockers in patients with bradycardia or asthma. The usual oral dose is 200 mg 3 times a day.

Vasodilators

These drugs dilate arterioles and thereby reduce peripheral vascular resistance.

Prazosin (Hypovase) is an effective antihypertensive agent which dilates arterioles probably largely by blocking α-adrenergic receptors. The dose is usually 2–5 mg 3 times a day. Dosage increments are made at 4- to 6-weekly intervals to a maximum of 20 mg daily. Occasionally, syncope occurs in a hypersensitive patient in the early stages of treatment with this drug, usually within 30 to 90 minutes of the first dose. For this reason, treatment is initiated with 0·5 mg doses and patients are advised to take their first dose with food in the evening, when they are staying at home. It is usually possible to continue the drug without further episodes of syncope. Common side-effects include dizziness, drowsiness and lack of energy.

Hydrallazine (Apresoline) has a direct action on the smooth muscle in the walls of arterioles. Partial α-receptor blockade may contribute to the effect. The oral dose is 25 to 100 mg twice daily, usually in conjunction with a β-blocker or other antihypertensive agent. The drug may be given in hypertensive emergencies, by slow intravenous injection of 20–40 mg, repeated as required.

Diazoxide (Eudemine) also has a direct vasodilating effect on arterioles. It is used primarily by the intravenous route (by the rapid injection of 300 mg), for the control of hypertensive crises.

Sodium nitroprusside (Nipride) is another direct-acting vasodilator, used by intravenous infusion to control hypertensive crises and to reduce the blood pressure in cases of aortic dissection.

It is important to remember that diuretics increase the effect of all antihypertensive drugs, the dose of which may have to be reduced by as much as a half when diuretics are, for any reason, added to a patient's treatment.

Drugs used for their action on the peripheral arteries

(i) Alpha-adrenergic-receptor blockade

Certain drugs block the alpha-adrenergic receptors in the walls of the arterioles and so reduce or abolish the vasoconstrictor effect of the sympathetic nervous system. Vasodilatation results. Alpha-adrenergic-blocking agents increase the flow of blood in the skin rather than in muscles, however, and are therefore of use in cases of Raynaud's phenomenon, chilblains and superifical ulcers rather than in cases of intermittent claudication.

Phentolamine (Rogitine) is a short-acting alpha-adrenergic blocker and is used mainly in the diagnosis of phaeochromocytoma, a tumour of the adrenal medulla which secretes excessive quantities of adrenaline and noradrenaline and thereby causes hypertension.

Phenoxybenzamine (Dibenyline) is a powerful and long-acting alpha-adrenergic blocker but is not often used because side-effects are common.

Thymoxamine (Opilon) may be given by direct injection into veins or arteries or may be given orally as a 40 g tablet, one 4 times a day.

Hydergine, an ergot derivative, antagonizes alpha-adrenergic cerebral vasoconstriction and is therefore a cerebral vasodilator.

(ii) Drugs acting directly on the vessel wall to produce vasodilatation

These include ethyl alcohol, nicotinic acid, inositol nicotinate (Hexopal), nicotinyl tartrate (Ronicol), papaverine and bamethan (Vasculit).

Tolazoline (Priscol) has both an alpha-adrenergic-blocking effect and a direct vasodilator effect on peripheral vessels but, even so, blood flow is increased more in skin than in muscles. The oral dose is 1 or 2 25 mg tablets 4 times a day.

None of these drugs is very effective in intermittent claudication. Progressive walking exercise may produce improvement by increasing the collateral circulation. Some patients, in whom the obliterative changes are mainly in the larger arteries, benefit from arterial surgery–disobliteration or grafting procedures.

Cyclandelate (Cyclospasmol), isoxsuprine (Duvadilan) and Cosaldon are all vasodilators which are optimistically marketed for the treatment of cerebrovascular disease. If diseased arteries could be dilated then there would indeed be an enhanced oxygen supply to the areas of brain supplied by those vessels. An alternative to increasing the oxygen supply is to increase the *utilization* of oxygen by the deprived tissues; this is the rationale for the use of naftidrofuryl (Praxilene).

Antihistamine drugs

Histamine is a substance which is liberated in the tissues especially in allergic conditions such as hay fever and urticaria and which has an action on the local circulation directly opposite to that of adrenaline. It has a powerful action in dilating capillaries, and may increase their permeability so that plasma escapes into the tissues producing local oedema such as is seen in urticaria.

There are a number of drugs, known as antihistamines, which block the action of histamine. They include:

Thephorin	(phenindamine)	25–50 mg
Phenergan	(promethazine)	25–75 mg
Benadryl	(diphenhydramine)	50 mg
Anthisan	(mepyramine)	100 mg
Piriton	(chlorpheniramine)	4 mg.

They are given 1 to 3 times a day according to their duration of action and should be taken after meals. They sometimes produce marked drowsiness and should not be taken before driving a car or undertaking work requiring special skill unless their precise effect on the individual is known. The patient must be warned that antihistamines enhance the effect of alcohol and sedatives.

In addition to their value in allergic conditions (hay fever, drug rashes and angioneurotic oedema), these drugs are useful in paralysis agitans, travel sickness and for the itching of obstructive jaundice. They are also used in the form of ointments to relieve irritation in some skin conditions and insect bites but, applied locally, they may themselves cause dermatitis in sensitive patients.

In anaphylactic shock an intravenous preparation (e.g. Piriton, 10 mg) may be used in addition to an intravenous injection of hydrocortisone hemisuccinate and a subcutaneous injection of adrenaline.

Drugs used to reduce serum lipid levels

These drugs, which are known as **hypolipidaemic agents,** might reasonably be classified as Drugs acting on the Blood (Chapter 8), or as Drugs used in Disorders of Metabolism (Chapter 14). However, they are used principally in the hope of preventing or reducing atheromatous disease of the coronary and peripheral arteries and are therefore included in this chapter. High serum cholesterol or triglyceride levels are 'risk factors' for the development of coronary heart disease.

Young people with excessive blood levels of these lipids (hyperlipoproteinaemia) are given dietary and, in severe cases, drug therapy. If hyperlipoproteinaemia is diagnosed in childhood or youth, the patient may have the advantage of early treatment.

Among the hypolipidaemic agents are **clofibrate** (Atromid-S), 500 mg to 1 g twice daily, which principally reduces triglyceride levels, and **cholestyramine** (Cuemid, Questran), 4 g 3 or 4 times daily, and colestipol (Colestid), 15–30 g daily in divided doses, which reduce cholesterol levels. All three of these drugs tend to cause constipation, which can often be counteracted by including more fibre (e.g. bran) in the diet. Clofibrate should be given in reduced doses, if at all, to patients in renal failure, in whom it may cause severe muscle weakness and tenderness. Cholestyramine is used not only to reduce the serum level of cholesterol but also to relieve pruritis in cases of incomplete biliary obstruction. It is an anion-exchange resin and acts by binding bile acids in the intestine so that they cannot be reabsorbed.

8 Drugs acting on the blood

Blood consists of red corpuscles, white cells and blood platelets floating in plasma.

The red cells (erythrocytes)

The **red corpuscles** or erythrocytes which number $5.0 \times 10^{12}/1$ (5 000 000 per cubic millimetre), are biconcave discs containing haemoglobin. Haemoglobin consists of a protein globin, combined with an iron-containing pigment. The red corpuscles are developed in the bone marrow from large nucleated cells called proerythroblasts (pro-normoblasts), which as they mature become smaller in size and are called normoblasts. Normoblasts become filled with haemoglobin, lose their nuclei and are then discharged as the fully developed erythrocytes into the general circulation.

In order that the proerythroblast may develop into the normoblast, a special blood-forming or erythrocyte maturing factor is necessary. This is produced by the interaction of the intrinsic factor (of Castle) in the gastric juice with an extrinsic factor in the diet (liver, meat and eggs) which is now known to be vitamin B_{12} and which is stored in the liver. The two factors work together, as originally suggested by Castle, and, in this way, the intrinsic factor aids the absorption of the extrinsic factor (vitamin B_{12}) from the terminal ileum. Folic acid is also necessary for red-cell synthesis. It is present in green vegetables, liver, kidney and yeast, and is absorbed in the jejunum.

In order that sufficient haemoglobin may be manufactured in the body to fill the normoblast and permit its development into the fully formed red corpuscle, there must be an adequate supply of iron. This is normally taken in the diet especially in liver, meat, eggs, oatmeal, peas, beans and wholemeal bread. It is absorbed mainly in the duodenum and upper jejunum.

In disease, the red corpuscles may either be deficient (anaemia) or excessive in number (polycythaemia). Anaemia may be defined as a deficiency in the number of red corpuscles or in the amount of haemoglobin, or both. Anaemia may be due to:

defective blood formation
excessive blood loss
excessive blood destruction.

Drugs used for defective blood formation

Anaemia due to defective red-cell maturation (megaloblastic anaemia)

Deficiency of vitamin B_{12} or folic acid results in a macrocytic anaemia with a megaloblastic marrow. Dietary deficiency of both vitamins is responsible for cases of tropical macrocytic anaemia. In the UK dietary deficiency is rare, but folic acid deficiency may occur in elderly people and vitamin B_{12} deficiency may occur in strict vegetarians (vegans) and in elderly people. Other causes of deficiency are as listed below:

Vitamin B_{12} deficiency

(1) Pernicious (Addisonian) anaemia, in which there is absence of intrinsic factor and hence no absorption of the vitamin B_{12}.
(2) Total (or, sometimes, partial) gastrectomy.
(3) Malabsorption states, e.g. Crohn's disease.
(4) Infestation with the fish tapeworm as the result of eating raw fish, as in Japan.

Folic acid deficiency

(1) Malabsorption states, e.g. tropical sprue.
(2) Macrocytic anaemia of pregnancy.
(3) Haemolytic anaemias and leukaemia.
(4) Folic acid antagonists, e.g. methotrexate, which is used against leukaemia, and phenytoin, primidone and barbiturates which are used as anticonvulsants.
(5) Alcoholic cirrhosis of the liver. In these cases, folic acid deficiency is due to an inadequate diet.

Vitamin B_{12}

This may be given: (i) by intramuscular injection, which is the usual, more efficient and economical method or (ii) by mouth, which is much less reliable. Different preparations are available for each form of therapy. Treatment is divided into two stages:
(1) The therapeutic stage, when large doses are employed until the blood count has reached normal. Injections are given on

alternate days for 1–2 weeks, then weekly until the anaemia has been corrected.

(2) The maintenance stage, which is continued indefinitely by monthly injection.

Vitamin B_{12} (**cyanocobalamin,** Cytamen) is usually given by intramuscular injection in doses of 250 to 1000 micrograms. The dose of hydroxocobalamin (Neo-Cytamen) is usually the same as for cyanocobalamin but the interval between maintenance doses can be as long as two or three months. For oral administration Cytacon tablets may be used. None of these preparations has any value as a 'tonic'.

Folic acid

This is one of the factors in the vitamin B complex which, although it will restore the blood picture in pernicious anaemia to normal, will not prevent the development of neurological complications. It should not, therefore, be used in this condition.

It is, however, valuable in the treatment of macrocytic anaemia in malabsorption states, malnutrition and pregnancy. Dose: 5–20 mg daily, but for prophylactic use in pregnancy, 350 micrograms daily is sufficient. For use in pregnancy, a daily dose of folic acid, 350 micrograms, and iron, 100 mg, is combined in one tablet e.g. Iron and Folic acid BNF, Folex-350, and Pregaday. Folic acid is usually given by mouth.

Defective haemoglobin formation

Defective formation of haemoglobin is due to lack of **iron.** This may result from a deficiency of iron in the diet or defective absorption of iron from the alimentary tract. It may also occur after loss of blood by haemorrhage, when haemoglobin is lost from the body in the red corpuscles and an additional quantity of iron is required for the manufacture of new supplies. Because of fetal requirements, iron should be given during pregnancy.

(1) Iron is usually given by mouth 3 times daily, e.g.:

ferrous sulphate tablets (200 mg).
ferrous gluconate tablets (300 mg).
ferrous fumarate (Fersamal, 200 mg).

NB.—These daily doses should not be exceeded. Special proprietary preparations have little advantage.

(2) Imferon is an iron-dextran complex which may be given by

intramuscular injection. The usual dose is 5 ml. When given by intramuscular injection, great care must be taken to see that none of the solution remains in the needle track. Otherwise some permanent staining of the skin may result. Jectofer, an iron–sorbitol–citric acid complex, is another intramuscular iron preparation.

(3) Occasionally, iron–dextran (Imferon) is given as a total dose infusion (TDI) in normal saline. The prescribed quantity of iron–dextran is added to sodium chloride injection in such proportions that the final concentration of iron–dextran does not exceed 5 per cent volume for volume. A test dose is given in order to detect those individuals who might have an anaphylactoid reaction to the infusion.

Iron poisoning

Mothers should be warned that there is a danger of young children mistaking iron tablets for sweets which will result in severe toxic or even fatal symptoms. The treatment of acute iron poisoning is to administer Desferal intravenously (25 mg/kg) in saline. The drug can also be given by mouth.

Excessive blood loss

In severe haemorrhage there is loss of red corpuscles, haemoglobin and fluid (plasma), and the ideal treatment is their replacement by blood transfusion. The loss of fluid, which is even more important than the loss of haemoglobin, can be made up by intravenous infusions of plasma, dextran and other fluids until cross-matched blood is available.

Residual anaemia due to deficiency of haemoglobin requires treatment with iron. Folic acid and vitamin B_{12} are of no value in anaemia of this type because there is no deficiency of anti-anaemic factor.

Excessive blood destruction

There are many causes of haemolytic anaemia, in which the red cells are broken up (lysed). In haemolytic disease of the newborn, treatment consists of exchange transfusion of blood. In other haemolytic anaemias, steroids (e.g. prednisone) may be prescribed or splenectomy may be advised.

Aplastic anaemia

This is due to an absence (aplasia) or diminution (hypoplasia) of bone marrow activity. It may be congenital or may be caused by poisons, drugs (e.g. chloramphenicol) or irradiation. It usually necessitates regular blood transfusions but may remit spontaneously or respond to treatment with an anabolic steroid, e.g. oxymetholone (Anapolon). It is thought that this acts by stimulating the production of erythropoietin in the kidney. Erythropoietin increases the red cell production rate. Oxymetholone is used in preference to testosterone because of its lesser tendency to cause undesirable side-effects such as virilization, acceleration of bone ageing in children, and liver damage.

Excessive blood formation

In a disease known as polycythaemia vera in which the spleen may be enlarged, and also in certain other circumstances, the number of red corpuscles may be considerably increased above the normal (up to 8 or $10 \times 10^{12}/l$). Symptoms are relieved by venesection, which is repeated as often as necessary. Radioactive phosphorus (^{32}P) is the most effective treatment for this condition.

The white cells (leucocytes)

There are two important varieties of white cell, the polymorphonuclear leucocyte, having a granular cytoplasm (granulocyte), and the lymphocyte. The former develop in the bone marrow, the latter in the lymphoid tissue (e.g. the lymph glands and spleen). The normal number of white cells in the blood is $4 \cdot 0 - 11 \cdot 0 \times 10^9/1$ (4000 to 11 000 per cubic millimetre), of which about 70 per cent are polymorphonuclear leucocytes and 30 per cent lymphocytes. If the total number of white cells is less than $4 \cdot 0 \times 10^9/l$, the condition is known as leucopenia, if more than $11 \cdot 0 \times 10^9/l$ it is called leucocytosis.

Leukaemia is a disease in which very large numbers of abnormal white cells (e.g. up to $100 \times 10^9/l$ or more) are present in the blood.

Acute leukaemias

Acute leukaemias are classified as lymphoblastic, myelogenous and undifferentiated (indeterminate). The lymphoblastic variety responds best to treatment.

Acute lymphoblastic leukaemia

Drugs used to induce remission

Two drugs are usually used in combination.

In lymphoblastic leukaemia, steroids (e.g. **prednisone** 40 mg daily by mouth) are given together with **vincristine** (Oncovin). The latter drug, a product of the periwinkle plant, is injected intravenously in a once-weekly dose of 1·5 mg per square metre of body surface area.

Additional drugs, used in some cases of lymphoblastic leukaemia, are daunorubicin (Cerubidin), colaspase (Crasnitin) and adriamycin.

When remission has been induced, the cranium is irradiated with x-rays and methotrexate is injected intrathecally to prevent leukaemic meningitis. Vincristine does not cross the blood-brain barrier in therapeutic amounts.

Continuation (maintenance) therapy

Relapse soon occurs unless treatment is continued with other drugs after remission has been induced with the drugs mentioned above. Weekly doses of methotrexate (Amethopterin) or daily doses of 6-mercaptopurine (Puri-Nethol) frequently prevent relapse. High-dose methotrexate therapy may result in ulceration of the mouth, pharynx and intestine, which can be prevented with folinic acid (Calcium Leucovorin). Other drugs used for continuation therapy, in cases of acute lymphoblastic leukaemia, are cyclophosphamide (Endoxana), thioguanine (Lanvis), hydroxyurea and cytarabine (Cytosar). The latter drug is also of value in the treatment of herpes encephalitis, in which it is used in combination with dexamethasone.

Acute myelogenous leukaemia

Drugs used to induce remission are cytarabine (Cytosar) and daunorubicin (Cerubidin) together, or cytarabine and thioguanine (Lanvis) together.

Continuation therapy, after induction of a remission, may be quite complex. In addition to chemotherapy, attempts may be made to stimulate the patient's immunity mechanisms. This treatment, called **immunotherapy,** may be specific, using irradiated leukaemia cells, or non-specific, using BCG vaccine.

Chronic myeloid leukaemia

Any of the following drugs may be used, but busulphan is usually tried first:

busulphan (Myleran), 65 micrograms/kg of body weight daily by mouth;
radioactive phosphorus, ^{32}P;
dibromomannitol, 750 mg daily, in divided doses, for 4–6 days;
hydroxyurea (Hydrea), 80 mg/kg of body weight twice weekly by mouth;
mitobronitol (Myelobromol), 250 mg daily initially.

Chronic lymphatic leukaemia

Chlorambucil (Leukeran), 0·2 mg/kg of body weight daily by mouth or cyclophosphamide (Endoxana).
Prednisone as a temporary measure.

The nurse is not expected to commit these doses to memory; they are given merely for reference. There are, in any case, alternative dosage schemes. Apart from the drugs mentioned, supportive treatment is important in leukaemia. This may include fresh whole blood and platelet transfusions and treatment of infections.

Drugs producing leucopenia

In addition to their reduction in diseases such as typhoid fever, the white cells, especially the polymorphonuclear leucocytes, may be seriously diminished (granulocytopoenia) or completely absent (agranulocytosis) as a result of the toxic action of certain drugs.

The most important drugs liable to produce severe leucopenia (granulocytopoenia or agranulocytosis) are:

thiouracil and its derivatives	chloramphenicol
	troxidone
the sulphonamides	methoin
amidopyrine	phenylbutazone (Butazolidin)
gold salts	radioactive substances.

Drugs producing thrombocytopenia

Some drugs may interfere with the production of platelets, which results in purpura, e.g.:

phenylbutazone   quinine
chlorpropamide   quinidine
tolbutamide   digitoxin
barbiturates   sulphonamides.

The volume of the blood

The total volume of the blood is made up by the plasma and the blood cells. It may be decreased by loss of both in severe haemorrhage. The fluid portion alone may be diminished in states of dehydration due to excessive fluid loss from the tissues in severe vomiting, diarrhoea, diabetic coma, severe burns and insufficient fluid intake, i.e. the plasma becomes more concentrated.

The treatment of these conditions necessitates the replacement of fluid by one of the following means:
(i) Blood transfusion, indicated when both plasma and red corpuscles have been lost by haemorrhage.
(ii) Plasma transfusion, especially in cases of shock but also of value after haemorrhage.
(iii) Dextran by intravenous infusion.
(iv) Normal saline by rectal, subcutaneous, intravenous or intraperitoneal injection in cases of fluid loss.
(v) Normal saline with glucose by rectal or intravenous infusion.
(vi) Water or half-strength normal saline by mouth.

Blood transfusion

The main indications are:
(1) Severe haemorrhage
   (a) accidents
   (b) before and after operation
   (c) conditions such as haematemesis, abortion and post-partum haemorrhage.
(2) Medical conditions
   (a) severe hypochromic anaemia
   (b) some cases of septicaemia
   (c) haemophilia
   (d) occasionally in pernicious anaemia.

It has been found that, for purposes of blood transfusion, individuals may be divided into four basic (ABO) groups, and it is only when they belong to the same group that their bloods will mix properly. If blood from the wrong group is transfused the red cells in it are destroyed with very serious and often fatal results to the recipient. It is, therefore, most important to discover the group to which the patient belongs and to select a suitable donor. It is also necessary to test the blood for Rhesus factor (Rh).

In view of the danger to life if blood of the wrong group is given, any nurse handling bottles of blood for transfusion must be particularly careful to see that they reach the right patient, as confusion can occur, especially if more than one transfusion is going on at the same time. Before each bottle is given, its label and group should be checked by 2 persons and compared with the known group of the patient.

Table 8.1. Blood groups

International	AB	A	B	O
Percentage of persons	5	40	10	45

In most instances, the blood of group O donors may be given to any patient without causing ill effects, and they are, therefore, referred to as universal donors, but even with these donors a preliminary test must be made to ensure compatibility.

As a rule, 1000 ml or more of blood are given as a single transfusion in units of 500 ml.

The continuous drip method is generally used, and by this means as much as 3 litres (about 5 pints) or more is commonly given over a period of 24 hours at the rate of about 40 drops a minute.

The basis of modern blood-transfusion technique is to collect blood from a donor into a vacuum bottle containing a special preservative such as acid citrate dextrose (ACD) or citrated phosphate dextrose (CPD). Blood thus obtained can be stored in a refrigerator for about 2 weeks. Nevertheless, blood deteriorates within a few days of storage and from the fourth day contains many deposits of fibrin strands and micro-aggregates of platelets and leucocytes. These particles, if infused, form micro-emboli in the lungs and secondarily in other organs. An in-line microfilter should therefore be used, interposed between the blood packet and the infusion set, for all transfusions of whole blood which has been stored for more than 4 days.

Packed cell transfusion

'Concentrated human red blood corpuscles' is whole human blood from which 40 per cent of the plasma has been removed. This form of transfusion may be used in certain cases of anaemia when it is especially desirable to raise the haemoglobin rapidly without introducing a large amount of fluid into the circulation.

Plasma transfusion

Plasma will keep longer than citrated blood containing red cells and therefore plasma may be withdrawn from citrated blood after the red corpuscles have fallen by sedimentation to the bottom of the collecting bottle, and stored for a long period.

Plasma is of great value in restoring the blood volume in cases of shock. It may be stored in dry form. Dry plasma is rendered suitable for intravenous infusion by dissolving 20 g in 500 ml of sterile distilled water and using it at once. While dried plasma is a volume expander, it does not correct coagulation factor defects, for which fresh frozen plasma is required. Rhesus negative females should receive only Rh-negative plasma.

Dextran injection

This must not be confused with dextrose. Dextran 70 (average molecular weight 70 000) is sometimes given intravenously in cases of severe haemorrhage when blood is not available for transfusion and also in cases of shock as a temporary measure. It is made up in dextrose or saline solution to have the same osmotic pressure as blood. Its main effect is to increase the blood volume and it has the advantage over normal saline that it is not so rapidly excreted and, therefore, exercises its action for a longer period after injection. Dextran 110 (average molecular weight 110 000) is also available. These high-molecular-weight dextrans cause the red blood cells to form rouleaux which cause difficulty in blood grouping. Blood samples for grouping and cross-matching should therefore be taken before starting the dextran infusion.

Low-molecular-weight dextran—Dextran 40 average molecular weight 40 000)—is used not to restore blood volume but to improve blood flow. It is rapidly excreted and has only a short-lived effect on plasma volume.

The dextrans are supplied in 5 per cent dextrose or 0·9 per cent sodium chloride solution. The prescriber must state not only which dextran but also which solvent is required.

Plasma protein fraction (PPF)

This is the plasma expander of choice when the serum albumin level is below 25g/l, in septicaemia, and in profound haemorrhagic shock where there is an increased likelihood of pulmonary oedema.

Haemacel

This is another plasma volume substitute (plasma expander) used in hypovolaemic shock. It is a preparation of modified gelatin and is free of some of the problems (e.g. in blood grouping and cross-matching) encountered with dextrans.

Electrolyte and water replacement solutions (saline solutions, etc.)

The blood and tissue fluids normally contain a more or less constant concentration of various salts, and one of the functions of the kidneys is to keep this at a steady level. If the concentration of salts in the blood is increased there will be a passage of fluid from the tissues to the blood until the salt concentration of both is again equal (i.e. a passage from the weaker to the stronger to produce equality).

The effect produced by this concentration of salts (and other substances) is called osmotic pressure, and, in the example just given, the osmotic pressure in the blood would be greater than that in the tissues and, as a result, water would be withdrawn from the latter until the osmotic pressures of the blood and tissue fluids were equal.

Solutions of salts and other substances are frequently injected into the blood stream for various therapeutic purposes, or they may be applied externally to wounds, etc. Depending on their strength (concentration) such solutions may have the same osmotic pressure as the blood, when they are said to be isotonic (*iso* = equal). Their strength may be less than that of the blood and, if injected, would have a weakening or diluting effect (hypotonic), or they may be stronger solutions (hypertonic). Hypotonic solutions are not often used in Therapeutics.

Sodium chloride injection (normal or isotonic saline)

The term saline used in this connection refers to a solution of sodium chloride or common salt, and normal saline is a sterile solution of sodium chloride in water having a strength of 0·9 per cent.

The concentration of sodium chloride being the same as that of the various salts in the blood, when normal saline is injected intravenously it does not affect the balance which exists between the blood and tissue fluids—unless this is already abnormal and the saline is given to restore the balance to normal.

Hypertonic saline

This is a solution of sodium chloride in water exceeding the strength of normal saline (0·9 per cent). Various concentrations are employed according to the purposes for which they are needed.

When given by intravenous injection, the effect will be to raise the salt concentration in the blood so that it is higher than that in the tissues. The result of this is the withdrawal of fluid from the tissues.

For example, 30 ml of 30 per cent saline (or 50 ml of 15 per cent) may be injected intravenously in cases of raised intracranial pressure. The effect is withdrawal of fluid from the brain into the blood. In consequence the brain shrinks in size, thus lowering the tension within the cranium. A similar effect is produced by intravenous glycerol or more slowly by the rectal injection of hypertonic magnesium sulphate solution (175 ml of 25 per cent).

Hypertonic saline is also applied as a wound dressing and by its hypertonic action promotes the flow of tissue fluids into the wound.

Sodium chloride and dextrose injection (glucose–saline solution)

This consists of 4 per cent glucose and 0·18 per cent sodium chloride.

Being isotonic it may be injected intravenously or intramuscularly or subcutaneously with hyaluronidase (Hyalase).

Dextrose injection

Dextrose injection (5 per cent) may be given intravenously. In addition to water it supplies calories having food value.

Hypertonic glucose solutions up to 40 per cent are sometimes used for special purposes.

Potassium chloride injection

Potassium supplements may be required in patients on long-term diuretics, which increase potassium excretion, and in cases of starvation and severe diarrhoea and vomiting. Because it is cardio-toxic and an irritant it must be diluted 50 times with sodium chloride injection before being given intravenously.

Sodium lactate injection and sodium bicarbonate injection

These are sometimes required to combat acidosis.

Hartmann's solution

This may be given orally, subcutaneously or intravenously in the treatment of gastro-enteritis in children and other conditions when acidosis is present. It contains lactic acid and the chlorides of sodium, potassium and calcium.

Hyaluronidase (Hyalase)

This is an enzyme found in various animal tissues and may be described as a 'spreading factor'. That is to say, it increases the permeability of the capillaries and tissues so that substances injected into the latter can be more easily dispersed and more rapidly absorbed into the blood stream.

It is of particular value when intravenous therapy is impossible. Hyaluronidase has many uses, in particular the administration of subcutaneous saline (e.g. in infants) and for pyelograms when a vein cannot be used. 1 ml containing 1000 units in distilled water, is injected into the site of the proposed infusion. The solution must be freshly prepared.

The anticoagulant drugs

Substances such as potassium citrate which can prevent clotting when added to blood after it has been withdrawn from the body have already been mentioned (p. 62).

The ability of blood to clot is one of Nature's processes which protects the individual against excessive bleeding as a result of injury.

The actual mechanism is a complicated one and involves the interaction of a number of substances present in the blood, the liver and the tissues. It may be briefly simplified in the following way:

Prothrombin + thromboplastin + calcium → thrombin.
Thrombin + fibrinogen → fibrin clot.

Blood platelets play an important role and red cells are enmeshed in the final fibrin clot.

In greater detail:

(1) Blood platelets + factors VIII, IX, XI and XII + calcium → thromboplastin.
(2) Thromboplastin + factors V, VII and X + calcium → activated thromboplastin.
(3) Prothrombin + activated thromboplastin + calcium → thrombin.
(4) Thrombin + fibrinogen + calcium → fibrin clot.

Coagulation of blood within the blood vessels, or thrombosis, is not an uncommon pathological condition. There are drugs which can be given internally which prevent or diminish the risk of clotting within the body. These are referred to as anticoagulants and are of two main types:

(1) Heparin.
(2) The oral anticoagulants (Dindevan, Sinthrome, Marevan).

The two groups of drugs act at different stages of the clotting process.

1. Heparin

This is an anticoagulant substance prepared from beef lung. It acts rapidly and is soon eliminated from the system. It is usually given by intravenous injection in doses of 8000 to 10 000 units every 6 hours. In order to facilitate this a special needle with a non-leaking diaphragm may be left in the vein if desired, or 1500 units per hour may be given in a saline infusion, after a starting dose of 5000 units. If the administration of heparin is prolonged, the dosage is controlled by estimating the clotting time of the blood.

Heparin may be given by intramuscular injection, using a very fine needle, but there is risk of local haematoma formation. It is absorbed slowly and its action is less reliable when given by this route.

Heparin may also be given subcutaneously to prevent deep venous thrombosis in patients undergoing surgery. 5000 units in a 0.2 ml injection are given 2–6 hours preoperatively and every 8 hours postoperatively. Suitable preparations are Minihep and Calciparine.

Over-dosage

The antidote to over-dosage is the intravenous injection of protamine sulphate, 50 mg of which will neutralize the effect of 5000 units of heparin. A blood transfusion may also be given

2. Oral anticoagulants

These substances differ from each other somewhat in chemical composition but all act by preventing the formation of prothrombin and other factors (VII, IX and X) in the liver. Thus they take some time to act since the clotting factors present in the blood must first be used up.

Phenindione (Dindevan)

This belongs to the indanedione group of drugs and is given in doses of 100 mg b.d. followed by 50 mg usually twice daily.

Nicoumalone (Sinthrome)

This is supplied in 1 mg and 4 mg tablets. The average dose is 1st day 8–16 mg, 2nd day 4–12 mg, 3rd and subsequent days 1–6 mg.

Warfarin sodium (Marevan)

Initial dose 25–50 mg; subsequent doses 3–15 mg daily.

Since these drugs take 24 to 36 hours to become effective, it is a common practice to commence anticoagulant therapy with heparin for 24 to 36 hours, during which the first tablets of Dindevan or Sinthrome are beginning to act. Their dosage is controlled by estimations of the blood prothrombin time, which should be kept at 2 to $2\frac{1}{2}$ times the control time, or the 'Thrombotest' value which should be kept at 7·5 to 15 per cent of the control.

Over-dosage

This may be followed by bleeding into the skin and mucous membranes (purpura), the presence of red cells in the urine (haematuria), vaginal haemorrhage or excessive haemorrhage from recent wounds or operation sites. The treatment is to stop the drug at once and to give blood transfusions and intravenous vitamin K_1 (phytomenadione), 5 to 20 mg. (Ordinary water-soluble vitamin K is ineffective in this condition.)

Haemorrhagic effects may result not only from over-dosage of an anticoagulant but also from giving certain drugs to patients who are receiving anticoagulant therapy. These drugs include aspirin, phenylbutazone, chlorpropamide, clofibrate and broad-spectrum antibiotics.

Anticoagulants are used in the treatment of coronary artery thrombosis, pulmonary embolism, and thrombosis of veins in the limbs, etc. They do not dissolve thrombus once it has formed, but prevent the extension of thrombosis.

Thrombolytic agents

Anticoagulants prevent the formation or extension of thrombus but do not 'dissolve' existing thrombi. The human body has its own chemical mechanism, known as the fibrinolytic system, for lysing (breaking up) fibrin and hence dissolving thrombus. Certain drugs, known as thrombolytic agents, activate the system and accelerate the process. These drugs are streptokinase (Kabikinase) and urokinase (Ukidan), both of which are enzymes. They activate the patient's plasminogen, converting it to plasmin. The plasmin breaks down the fibrin which binds the thrombus together. Consequently, the thrombus 'dissolves', a process known as thrombolysis. Unfortunately, streptokinase being a product of bacteria causes the formation of antigens in man, so that a second course of treatment may result in an allergic reaction.

Sclerosing agents

These act by causing fibrosis and hence obliteration of the lumens of veins.

Ethanolamine oleate injection is given intravenously in a dose of 2 to 5 ml in the treatment of varicose veins.

Sodium tetradecyl sulphate (Sotradecol, STD) is used in the now more usual injection treatment of varicose veins. After injection of the sclerosant into a perforating vein, a wedge of plastic foam is placed over the site and firm bandages are applied. This is called injection–compression sclerotherapy.

Phenol injection, oily, is given in volumes of 0·5 to 1·5 ml, by injection into the submucosal layer of the rectum, in the treatment of haemorrhoids (piles).

9 Drugs acting on the respiratory system

For purposes of therapeutics it is convenient to consider separately the lower respiratory tract, consisting of the trachea, bronchi and alveoli of the lungs; and the upper respiratory tract which includes the nose, pharynx and larynx.

The object of respiration is the interchange of gases between the blood and the atmosphere, oxygen being absorbed and carbon dioxide (and water) being excreted by the lungs.

The rate and depth of respiration is controlled by the respiratory centre in the medulla oblongata in such a way that the concentration of oxygen and carbon dioxide in the blood is normally kept constant. This is done in the following way: the respiratory centre is especially sensitive to the amount of carbon dioxide in the blood. If this rises above the normal (e.g. as a result of exercise) the respiratory centre is stimulated so that the rate and depth of respiration are increased. The increase in the respiratory movements results in a greater intake of oxygen and an increased excretion of carbon dioxide, so that the concentration of the latter in the blood tends to fall to normal once more.

Other substances may also influence the respiratory centre. They may produce similar stimulation, with increased movements, or alternatively they may depress the centre so that breathing becomes slower and shallower.

The respiratory tract is lined with ciliated epithelium, the cells of which also secrete mucus. The bronchioles have plain muscle fibres in their walls.

There are two troublesome features which occur in a number of disorders affecting the respiratory system, viz.:

(1) Cough.

(2) Bronchospasm.

A cough may be a voluntary act or a reflex act with a cough centre in the medulla. The stimulus provoking a cough may arise from irritation or inflammation in the pharynx, larynx, trachea, bronchi, lungs or pleura. It may be (*a*) dry and unproductive; (*b*) loose and with sputum:

(*a*) Sometimes it is desirable to suppress a distressing dry cough

125

by means of a sedative linctus containing drugs which depress the cough reflex by acting on the centre.

(b) Expectorant or mycolytic drugs may be needed to loosen sticky sputum.

Drugs stimulating the respiratory centre

The stimulants of the respiratory centre are used to counteract its depression in various types of poisoning, after anaesthesia and in other conditions in which respiratory failure may be evident. They include:

nikethamide (Coramine)	doxapram (Dopram)
aminophylline (p. 134)	caffeine
bemegride (Megimide)	ethamivan (Vandid).

Nalorphine (Lethidrone) and **naloxone** (Narcan) are opiate antagonists and not general respiratory stimulants. They cannot reverse respiratory depression caused by non-narcotic drugs.

Carbon dioxide

Carbon dioxide (CO_2) is a colourless gas which plays a number of important parts in the economy of Nature. It is an oxide of the element carbon and is produced when carbon is burnt in the presence of sufficient oxygen. It must not be confused with carbon monoxide (CO), a very poisonous oxide of carbon which is, for example, emitted in the exhaust fumes of cars, as a result of the incomplete combustion of petrol.

Carbon dioxide is present in the atmospheric air, i.e. inspired air (0·04 per cent), and in expired air (4 per cent). It is soluble in water. In the manufacture of 'soda water' the gas is dissolved in water under pressure. Owing to the escape of carbon dioxide the solution effervesces when the pressure is withdrawn. Beer, champagne and effervescing mineral waters ('aerated waters') also give off carbon dioxide.

It can be compressed by pumping it into steel cylinders and, by special methods, can be converted into a solid, soft, snowlike substance, 'carbon dioxide snow', which only remains solid at a very low temperature and quickly vaporizes at room temperature.

The main medical use of carbon dioxide is as a respiratory stimulant. Mixtures containing 5 to 10 per cent of carbon dioxide with oxygen are administered by inhalation. The additional concentration of carbon dioxide thus produced in the lungs leads to an increase in the amount in the blood. The respiratory centre is, therefore, stimulated so that respiration is increased in frequency and depth. A mixture of carbon dioxide 5 per cent with oxygen 95 per cent may be administered at the end of an operation under general anaesthesia.

It may be useful in helping the expansion of the lungs after any portion has been collapsed, e.g. postoperative 'atelectasis', and after abdominal operations when the action of the diaphragm may have been impaired.

A solution of carbon dioxide in water, e.g. 'soda water', has a mildly stimulating effect on the mucous membrane of the stomach, improving the appetite and causing a feeling of well-being. The increased blood supply to the mucous membrane caused by this stimulating effect hastens the absorption of water and other substances which accounts for the rapid absorption of alcohol from sparkling wines such as champagne and may explain their exceptionally exhilarating effect.

In solid form, **carbon dioxide snow,** which can be produced in the shape of a cone or pencil, is applied to the skin in the treatment of naevi, moles, warts, etc., on which it has a freezing action. If contact is too prolonged blister formation may ensue.

Oxygen

Although not a respiratory stimulant, oxygen may be conveniently considered here on account of its use in cases of respiratory failure.

The atmosphere (inspired air) contains 20 per cent oxygen and the expired air 16 per cent. The 4 per cent oxygen absorbed via the alveoli of the lungs into the blood is conveyed in the red corpuscles to the tissues as oxyhaemoglobin.

The amount of oxygen carried to the tissues may be **decreased** by:

(a) Diseases of the lungs and disorders of the pulmonary circulation, whereby the blood fails to acquire sufficient oxygen during its passage through the lungs.

(b) General circulatory failure with stagnation of blood in the peripheral parts.

(c) Deficiency in the oxygen-carrying power of the blood due to decrease in the amount of haemoglobin or red corpuscles, i.e. anaemia.

(d) Defective oxygen-carrying power of haemoglobin by its

conversion into carboxyhaemoglobin in carbon monoxide poisoning.

The amount of oxygen in the blood can only be **increased** by increasing the amount of oxygen in the alveolar air. This may be done by the administration of oxygen by inhalation.

Oxygen may be given in the following ways:

(1) The oxygen tent, which is expensive to operate and impedes medical and nursing care. It is also a much greater fire risk than is other apparatus. It is used for children and rarely for adults, e.g. those who because of facial injuries or burns cannot wear a mask or cannula.

(2) Nasal cannulae and oxygen masks. These devices provide a low oxygen concentration or a high one. A high oxygen concentration must not be given if there is a danger of inducing carbon dioxide narcosis, as in chronic bronchitics with a high arterial carbon dioxide tension ($Pa\text{CO}_2$). The respiratory centre in such patients is accustomed to a high blood level of carbon dioxide, by which it is no longer stimulated, and is being driven largely by hypoxia. Deprived of this hypoxic stimulus, ventilation becomes shallower and more carbon dioxide is retained until the patient lapses into unconsciousness. Patients with chronic airways obstruction must therefore be given only low concentrations of oxygen, e.g. 24 per cent. Patients without ventilatory failure may be given high concentrations of oxygen (e.g. 60 per cent), which they may badly need.

Devices for oxygen therapy may be divided into two types, those which give controlled oxygen therapy and those which provide uncontrolled oxygen therapy. The inspired oxygen concentration is not, however, entirely uncontrolled with the latter devices.

(a) **Controlled oxygen therapy devices.** These use the HAFOE (high air-flow with oxygen enrichment) principle. They include **Ventimasks** (24, 28 and 35 per cent oxygen models), **Ventimasks Mk 2** (5 models providing oxygen concentrations from 24 to 60 per cent), **Mixomasks,** and the **Bard Inspiron-Accurox range** of oxygen masks and dilutors.

(b) **Uncontrolled oxygen therapy devices.** These are acceptable for patients who are not relying upon hypoxia for their respiratory drive. They are commonly employed postoperatively and after myocardial infarction. Examples are **MC** (Mary Catterall), **Hudson, OTU** (Harris), and **Edinburgh** masks, and **nasal cannulae.** Although in the category of un-controlled oxygen therapy devices, the Edinburgh mask was designed for low flows primarily for use in respiratory failure. It is extremely comfortable, which is important if a patient has to wear an oxygen mask for several days. Nasal cannulae are a modern development from Tudor Edwards' spectacles. They are useful in patients who are intolerant of a mask and have the advantage of continuing to supply oxygen to patients while they are eating, drinking and expectorating. In patients in respiratory failure, treatment is given initially with a con-trolled therapy mask delivering 24 per cent oxygen. If the patient's condition improves, a mask providing 28 per cent oxygen is substituted. If the improvement is maintained, nasal cannulae may be substituted for the mask, using a low flow of oxygen to give restricted rather than controlled oxygen therapy. The flow of oxygen through the cannulae is adjusted according to the results of arterial blood gas analyses.

The administration of oxygen by any method requires some sort of flow meter with a fine adjustment valve in order that economical and efficient use may be obtained. The amount of oxygen usually required is 2 to 6 litres per minute.

In many hospitals, oxygen is piped to each bedside from a central supply. Others have to make do with cylinders.

(*a*) A 100 cubic foot oxygen cylinder with a rate of flow of 4 litres per minute will last about 12 hours.

(*b*) No oil or lubricant must be put on the high-pressure valves as this may cause fire.

(*c*) Under no circumstances should matches or cigarettes be brought near to a patient having oxygen.

Oxygen given by the tube and funnel method does not raise the oxygen content of the alveolar air sufficiently to have any effect. It therefore has no use other than impressing anxious relatives that something is being done, and is a waste of oxygen.

The greatest care must be taken to discriminate between (*a*) pure oxygen and (*b*) oxygen and carbon dioxide mixtures. The latter should only be used when specially ordered.

Particular care is also necessary not to administer oxygen for too long or in too great a concentration to premature and newborn infants. An excess may cause blindness due to a condition known as retrolental fibroplasia.

Hyperbaric oxygen

This is oxygen administered under pressure, usually thrice atmospheric pressure or less. It may be used either in a large chamber of compressed air shared by the patient's attendants or in an individual tank only large enough for the patient. The former chamber is known as a walk-in pressure vessel and the latter is known as a single-patient pressure vessel or hyperbaric bed. In the large chamber, oxygen is administered in the usual manner by a closely fitting mask or by endotracheal tube; the high atmospheric pressures ensures a high concentration of dissolved oxygen in the tissues. Surgical operations may, if necessary, be performed in the chamber. In the hyperbaric bed, the patient sits or lies alone for short periods (up to 2–3 hours). In this, the oxygen itself is usually the compressing gas and the need for a mask is obviated.

Hyperbaric oxygen is used principally for the treatment of gas gangrene and carbon monoxide poisoning but may also be used in some cases of the 'bends', air embolism, chronic skin ulcers and surface infections.

Hyperbaric oxygen finds a special use in radiotherapy as a tumour sensitizer. Hypoxia frequently affords partial protection to at least some of the malignant cells in a tumour. Hyperbaric oxygen raises the oxygen tension within the hypoxic regions of the tumour and makes them more radiosensitive. The patient is wheeled beneath the radiotherapy machine after being sealed in a one-person hyperbaric vessel filled with oxygen to a pressure of 3 atmospheres absolute. Occasionally a patient refuses treatment because of claustrophobia. Oxygen convulsions are another occasional complication. Attendants observe stringent precautions against the risk of fire in the vessel. The technique improves the survival of patients with tumours of the head and neck or advanced carcinoma of the cervix.

Drugs which depress the respiratory centre

There are a number of drugs which slow the rate and diminish the depth of respiration. They are not, however, employed therapeutically to produce this result and this action must be regarded as a side-effect of their uses for other purposes, for example:

　　all general anaesthetics
　　morphine

alcohol
barbiturates
chloral and other hypnotics in toxic doses.

Cough-suppressants

Drugs which reduce the excitability of the cough centre and are thereby effective in diminishing a dry and unproductive cough include:

morphine and opium   methadone (Physeptone)
diamorphine (heroin)   pholcodine (Ethnine, etc.)
codeine

These drugs are often employed in various linctuses which are made up with syrup. The dose is usually 5 ml:

squill opiate linctus
codeine linctus
Physeptone linctus
pholcodine linctus.

Other linctuses contain noscapine; an example is Extil. There are in fact an enormous number of proprietary cough medicines, the respective merits of which are difficult to compare.

Sucking a sweet or medicated lozenge (e.g. liquorice) will often help a troublesome cough.

Drugs affecting bronchial secretion
Expectorants

An expectorant may be defined as a drug which aids the expulsion of mucus from the respiratory tract either by increasing its secretion or by 'loosening' it so that it becomes less tenacious and sticky.

Recent research indicates that many of the drugs which were formerly regarded as increasing the amount of mucus secreted, probably do not act in this way and that they owe their usefulness to their 'loosening' effect, which makes expectoration of sputum easier. There is little doubt, however, that in practice the so-called cough mixture is appreciated by the patient and that it helps to relieve his symptoms.

In smaller doses, a number of emetic drugs (p. 67), such as ipecacuanha, act as expectorants. Potassium iodide in addition to other effects, also appears to increase and loosen secretion from the respiratory mucous membrane. It will be remembered that one of the symptoms of 'iodism' is that of a common cold in which the flow of mucus from the nose and bronchi is increased (p. 30).

The following are among the important expectorants and one or more are often combined in cough mixtures:

ammonium bicarbonate   potassium iodide
ipecacuanha   squill.

An example is ammonia and ipecacuanha mixture, known also as Mistura Expectorans.

Squill

In addition to its effect on the heart which, in appropriate doses, is similar to that of digitalis, squill acts as an expectorant by reason of its irritating effect on the bronchial mucous membrane. It is, therefore, more suited to cases of chronic than of acute bronchitis. It is an irritating drug and in large doses acts as a gastro-intestinal irritant and irritant to the kidneys.

Bronchial secretion may be loosened and expectoration helped by the following 'mucolytics':

(a) Sodium chloride compound mixture (*Mist. sodii chlor. co.*) taken in hot water.

(b) Steam inhalations to which may be added benzoin (Friar's balsam) inhalation.

(c) Water-mist inhalations, produced by bubbling oxygen through water in a special apparatus. The liquefaction of mucus is increased if ascorbic acid and an oxidizing agent are added to the water.

(d) Aerosols containing detergents, e.g. Alevaire.

(e) Nebulized 20 per cent solution of acetylcysteine (Airbron),

(f) Carboxymethylcysteine (Mucodyne) is available as syrup or capsules to be taken orally. Adult dose: 15 ml of syrup or 2 capsules 3 times a day initially.

(g) Bromhexine (Bisolvon) reduces sputum viscosity ('thickness') by disrupting the feltwork of acid mucopolysaccharide (AMPS) fibres which make mucoid sputum viscid. It is therefore used in chronic bronchitis. Dose 8 to 16 mg 3 times a day.

Anti-expectorants

By this term is meant drugs which reduce bronchial secretion; the most important being belladonna and its alkaloid, atropine.

Atropine is used before general anesthetics, especially ether, in order to prevent excessive bronchial secretion. It is also occasionally given in cases of pulmonary oedema (see also p. 192).

Bronchodilators

These are mainly used in the treatment of bronchial asthma and in some cases of bronchitis, when the plain muscle of the walls of the bronchioles is contracted and in spasm or oedema narrows the airways and causes respiratory distress.

There are two main groups of drugs, viz.:
(1) Sympathomimetic drugs which act on the beta-adrenergic receptors in the bronchi.
(2) Anticholinergic drugs.
(3) Drugs derived from theophylline which act directly on the bronchial muscle.

(1) *Sympathomimetic drugs*
(see also p.187)

(a) Unselective

These, which stimulate all β-receptors including those of the heart, include adrenaline, isoprenaline and ephedrine. They are of relatively short duration of action but this is slightly increased if they are combined with atropine methonitrate.

Adrenaline

Subcutaneous injection of 1 in 1000 solution may be given in doses up to 1 ml.

Isoprenaline

This has a similar action to adrenaline and may be given as a 20 mg tablet which is allowed to dissolve under the tongue.

Both these and similar drugs can be used in an aerosol spray for inhalation but patients should be warned of the dangers of over-dosage from too frequent use.

Ephedrine may be given by mouth (15–60 mg) but may cause insomnia and urinary retention in older subjects. It can, however, be very useful in children

(b) Selective

These drugs act particularly on the bronchial receptors and, in the doses used, have little or no effect on cardiac receptors. They therefore have less tendency than unselective agents to cause palpitation.

They include salbutamol, terbutaline and rimiterol.

Salbutamol (Ventolin)

Oral dose: 4 mg 3 or 4 times a day; inhalation (aerosol) dose: 100 or 200 micrograms; subcutaneous and intramuscular dose 250 micrograms; intravenous infusion 3–20 micrograms per minute.

Terbutaline (Bricanyl)

Oral dose: 5 mg 3 times daily; inhalation (aerosol) dose: 250 or 500 micrograms; subcutaneous dose: 250 micrograms.

Rimiterol (Pulmadil)

By inhalation (aerosol): 200–600 micrograms.

(2) *Anticholinergic drugs*

Bronchodilatation may be achieved by blocking parasympathetic activity in the bronchi. A suitable preparation is ipratropium.

Ipratropium (Altrovent)

Aerosol dose: 20–40 micrograms 3 or 4 times daily.

(3) *Drugs acting directly on bronchial muscle*

Theophylline

Derivatives of this drug can be very useful. They include; aminophylline, choline theophyllinate (Choledyl) and theophylline sodium glycinate (Englate).

Aminophylline (Cardophyllin or theophylline with ethylenediamine). This drug has a number of actions. Bronchospasm is relieved, hence it is often employed in the treatment of bronchial asthma, especially if there has been no relief from adrenaline or isoprenaline. It is also of value in nocturnal dyspnoea in heart disease ('cardiac asthma') when one or two suppositories may be given at night. Intravenous aminophylline will often abolish Cheyne-Stokes breathing. It also has a mild diuretic action. It may be given by mouth (up to 500 mg), but may cause gastric irritation, or by suppository, or slow intravenous injection (250 mg in 10 ml). Intramuscular injection is often painful.

Choline theophyllinate (Choledyl). This drug has an action similar to aminophylline but is less irritating to the stomach. Dose: 100–400 mg.

Theophylline sodium glycinate (Englate) available in tablets and as a linctus is useful for mild bronchospasm.

Both Choledyl and Englate are useful drugs in acute or chronic bronchitis when the chest is wheezy.

Sodium cromoglycate (Intal) is used in bronchial asthma but is not a bronchodilator. It inhibits allergic reactions in the bronchi and is, therefore, employed prophylactically. It is supplied in capsules (Spincaps) which contain powder for inhalation via a special insufflator (the Spinhaler). The contents of one Spincap are inhaled every 3 to 6 hours. Spincaps of *Intal Compound* contain isoprenaline in addition to the cromoglycate. Sodium cromoglycate (Nalcrom) is also used in the treatment of ulcerative colitis, albeit with less success.

Steroid inhalers

Certain corticosteroids are used as aerosols in the management of asthma because they are highly active at body surfaces in doses which have no significant systemic effects. The disadvantages of systemic steroids (see p. 233) are thereby avoided. They are not primarily bronchodilators and may act by reducing inflammatory oedema of the bronchial mucosa and by diminishing the excessive secretion of mucus.

Beclomethasone dipropionate (Becotide) is administered in a dose of 50–200 micrograms by inhalation 3 or 4 times a day.

Betamethasone valerate (Bextasol) is administered 2 to 4 times a day in doses of 100–200 micrograms'

Oral corticosteroids (e.g. prednisone) are used in severe cases of asthma, not responding adequately to other measures.

Intravenous steroid preparations may be required in status asthmaticus.

Inhalant therapy in asthma

Nowadays, this is usually provided by aerosols, which use an inert gas (freon) as the propellant. The canisters are small and easy to carry in pocket or handbag. Some 'hand-pumps', worked by squeezing a rubber bulb, are still in use, however.

Inhalant therapy is of two distinct kinds, viz:
(1) that which is used when required, for **acute attacks,** e.g. iso-prenaline salbutamol;
(2) that which is used regularly for **prevention** of attacks, e.g. 'Intal' and 'Becotide'.

If the distinction is not made clear to patients, they may fail to benefit from treatment. There is a tendency to use inhalers only during an actual asthmatic attack. Consequently, inhalers in the second category may be ignorantly forsaken in disgust because they do not relieve acute bronchospasm.

Pulmonary antiseptics

Drugs such as creosote and guaiacol which were formerly used as pulmonary antiseptics have long been replaced by sulphonamides, cotrimoxazole, penicillin, and other antibiotics such as tetracycline which are selected according to the sensitivity of the organisms found in the sputum in bronchitis, pneumonia, lung abscess and bronchiectasis.

Drugs used in radiography of the chest

Propyliodone (Dionosil) and similar preparations (p. 47) are introduced into the trachea from which, by adjusting the position of the patient, they run into the bronchi of either lung. The following methods may be employed: (i) a nasal catheter is passed so that its end over-hangs the larynx and the liquid drops down; (ii) the liquid is dropped from a special syringe over the back of the tongue; (iii) it is injected into the trachea through the cricothyroid membrane after local anesthesia. General anaesthesia may be needed for children.

Propyliodone is opque to x-rays and is of value in the diagnosis of bronchiectasis, lung abscess and new growth of the lung. About 16 ml are required for each lung in an adult. It has the advantage over its predecessor, iodized oil (Lipiodol), of not remaining for long periods in the bronchi and alveoli.

Drugs acting on the nose and nasal sinuses

While it is not possible to give in detail all the drugs which are employed in affections of the nose, the following are the most important methods of application.

Nasal drops

Among the best known are ephedrine nasal drops which have a vasoconstricting action and thereby help to shrink a swollen and congested mucous membrane. They are of value in hay fever and sinusitis and also in acute otitis media where they decongest the mucous membrane around the opening of the Eustachian tube and allow drainage from the middle ear.

Oily solutions should not be instilled into the nose as they interfere with the action of cilia, and liquid paraffin may cause lipoid pneumonia.

Drops should be instilled with the patient lying down with the head extended and breathing through the mouth.

Many proprietary nasal decongestants are available, e.g. Neophryn, Antistin-Privine and Otrivine.

Nasal sprays (*Nebulae*)

Watery solutions are employed and sprayed into the nasal cavities by an appropriate atomizer or used as nasal drops.

Ephedrine, xylometazoline (Otrivine) and oxymetazoline are used for catarrhal affections of the nose and for nasal sinusitis. These substances are preferable to others (e.g. adrenaline and naphazoline), which cause severe 'rebound' congestion of the nasal mucosa.

Corticosteroid sprays (e.g. Beconase Nasal Spray) are used in the treatment of hay fever and other types of allergic rhinitis.

Inhalations

Inhalations of menthol (120 mg; 4 or 5 small crystals), also menthol and benzoin and menthol and eucalyptus or compound tincture of benzoin (*Tinctura benzoini composita*—Friar's balsam), 4 ml added to 500 ml (1 pint) of boiling water, are commonly employed. They are of value in sinusitis, acute nasal catarrh, laryngitis, tracheitis and bronchitis.

Some drugs may be given by inhalation because they are absorbed from the respiratory tract, e.g. ergotamine inhalation in an aerosol spray used in migraine.

Insufflations and snuffs

These are occasionally employed, a special powder insufflator being used in some cases, e.g.:

> disodium cromoglycate (Rynacrom) for hay fever prevention
> posterior pituitary snuff (Di-Sipidin) for diabetes insipidus
> menthol snuff for nasal catarrh.

Local anaesthetics

Lignocaine and adrenaline injection BP may be used.

Cocaine (5 to 10 per cent), which is never injected, may be used to produce local anaesthesia by plugging the nasal cavity with strips of 1·5-cm ($\frac{1}{2}$-inch) gauze soaked in the solution.

Cocaine ointment may also be applied on a wool-coated probe.

Caustics

Chromic acid, trichloracetic acid, silver nitrate or the electric cautery may be applied to ulcers in the nasal mucous membrane; or to a bleeding-point to stop epistaxis.

Drugs applied to the larynx

Various drugs are applied to the larynx by inhalations, insufflations and sprays.

Inhalations

Menthol and Friar's balsam are used as in the treatment of nasal conditions.

Sprays

Lignocaine, 2 ml of a 4 per cent solution, may be sprayed on to the larynx, after the pharynx has been rendered insensitive by sucking a benzocaine compound lozenge containing 100 mg benzocaine, in order to produce anaesthesia for bronchoscopy.

10 Drugs acting on the urinary system

The urinary system is formed by the kidneys, ureters, bladder and urethra. The kidneys are excretory glands and consist of cortex and medulla which are made up of Malpighian bodies and tubules. The ureter, the bladder and the urethra form the ducts and reservoir via which the urine reaches the exterior.

The processes employed by the kidneys in the formation of urine are:

(1) Filtration of water and salts through the Malpighian bodies.
(2) Secretion of various substances by the tubules.
(3) Absorption of water and substances excreted by the first two processes but required by the body to maintain the composition of the blood at a constant level.

The primary function of the kidneys is to keep the composition of the blood constant by:

(i) the excretion of water;
(ii) the excretion of the end products of protein metabolism;
(iii) the excretion of salts;
(iv) the excretion of drugs, toxins and chemical substances which may be harmful.

The kidneys are therefore of great importance in dealing with the subject of drugs. Many drugs given internally by mouth or injection, are excreted by the kidneys either in their original form or after they have been changed by chemical action in the body (e.g. by the liver).

Some of these drugs have no effect on the urinary tract; others have a beneficial action in certain conditions and are given for this action. Finally, some have a harmful effect, especially when used in toxic doses, and may produce serious urinary symptoms such as haematuria.

Diseases of the urinary tract

These include congenital abnormalities, traumatic and mechanical conditions, acute or chronic inflammation of the kidneys (nephritis and pyelonephritis), of the bladder (cystitis) and of the urethra (urethritis), tuberculosis and new growths. Abnormal products of metabolism may also be excreted in the urine. Medical treatment may be required for many of these conditions. Further, it may be necessary to modify the excretory functions of the kidneys in order to relieve symptoms caused by disease of other organs, e.g. the removal of fluid in cases of oedema.

Drugs increasing the output of urine (diuretics)

A diuretic is a substance which increases the output of urine. These agents act on the kidneys and increase the output of water and also certain electrolytes such as sodium and chloride.

The amount of urine normally excreted depends on three factors:
(i) The fluid intake.
(ii) The fluid lost by the evaporation of sweat.
(iii) The amount lost via the bowel.

The most obvious physiological diuretic is water. In some cases, when the kidneys are normal this is the most suitable method of producing an increased urinary flow. On the other hand, diuretics are given in order to eliminate surplus fluid already present in the body, i.e. oedema. This occurs when water and salt are retained in the body particularly in the following conditions: (a) congestive heart failure, (b) pulmonary oedema and congestion, (c) ascites in cirrhosis of the liver, (d) nephrotic syndrome.

The processes employed by the kidneys in the formation of urine have already been mentioned. A diuretic may act in one of the following ways:
(i) Increasing the filtration of water and salts through the Malpighian bodies by generally improving the blood supply to the kidneys. Blood transfusion and saline infusions will do this in cases of surgical shock and dehydration. Caffeine (and theophylline derivatives) and digitalis will improve the renal circulation in cardiac failure.
(ii) By osmosis, preventing the reabsorption of water in the renal tubules. An abnormally high glucose load acts in this way to cause polyuria in diabetes mellitus. Urea can be given therapeutically to produce a diuresis in certain cases. However, mannitol (intravenously) is the chief **osmotic diuretic** used in medicine. It is also used in the prevention of acute renal tubular

necrosis when perfusion of the kidneys is inadequate due to severe hypotension.

(iii) By preventing the reabsorption of sodium and accompanying water by the renal tubules thereby producing an increased excretion of sodium (natriuresis) and of water (diuresis). All of the commonly used diuretics act in this way.

In addition to prescribing diuretics to reduce oedema it may sometimes be necessary to restrict salt intake. Less often it is necessary to restrict fluid intake also. In addition to the increased sodium excretion, which is one of the objects of administering diuretics, there is increased potassium loss. This may result in general muscular weakness, especially in the nephrotic syndrome and cirrhosis of the liver. To counteract this loss, potassium supplements are often required. To assess this need, periodic estimations of the blood electrolytes may be required.

Mercurial diuretics have been superseded by convenient oral diuretics of high efficacy and low toxicity. Acetazolamide (Diamox) quickly loses its diuretic effect if given in the repeated doses needed to clear oedema; it is principally used in the treatment of glaucoma, in daily doses of 250 to 1000 mg.

The **major oral diuretics** may be classified as follows:

(1) *Moderate diuretics*

(*a*) the thiazides, e.g. chlorothiazide (Saluric);
(*b*) chlorthalidone (Hygroton);
(*c*) clorexolone (Nefrolan);
(*d*) metolazone (Zaroxolyn).

(2) *Potent diuretics*

These are also known as loop diuretics because, unlike the others, they act on the loop of Henle in the kidney tubule.
(*a*) frusemide (Lasix);
(*b*) ethacrynic acid (Edecrin);
(*c*) bumetanide (Burinex).

(3) *Potassium-sparing diuretics* (potassium-conserving diuretics)

Unlike those in the first two groups, these drugs tend to conserve potassium in the body. By themselves they are very mild diuretics.

However, they augment the action of other diuretics and prevent potassium loss so that they are useful when used together with say a thiazide or frusemide.

(*a*) spironolactone (Aldactone);

(*b*) amiloride (Midamor);

(*c*) triamterene (Dytac).

Two types of diuretic are sometimes combined in one tablet, e.g. Dytide (triamterene and a thiazide) and Moduretic (amiloride and a thiazide).

Potassium supplements are not usually required when a potassium-conserving diuretic is being used; they may under these circumstances cause dangerously high potassium levels.

Potassium-sparing diuretics must be used with great caution in chronic renal failure and not at all in acute renal failure because potassium retention may be lethal.

Principles of diuretic therapy

(1) Except for those in the third group, diuretics are usually given in a once-daily dosage. Those in the first group produce a slow diuresis over the course of 12 to 24 hours whilst the potent diuretics produce a brisk diuresis which is completed within 6 hours, indeed often within 4 hours.

(2) Intravenous forms of the 3 potent diuretics are available for the treatment of acute pulmonary oedema and, in very high dosage, for the treatment of renal failure.

(3) All diuretics, with the exception of those in the third group, cause loss of potassium in the urine and may lead to potassium deficiency. Therefore, when they are being used for their diuretic effect, potassium supplements are usually prescribed with them. The potassium is best given as the chloride salt, e.g. Slow-K, two to six 600-mg tablets daily. A diet rich in potassium (e.g. containing oranges and bananas) will help to prevent potassium deficiency but is seldom adequate by itself when diuresis is considerable.

(4) Potassium-conserving diuretics may cause dangerous hyperkalaemia and are not therefore generally used (*a*) together with potassium supplements or (*b*) in cases of renal failure, in which potassium retention is a feature.

Problems of diuretic therapy

Diuretics are among the least toxic drugs in general use, and they
infrequently cause troublesome side-effects. The nurse should,
however, know about them. The complications of diuretic therapy
may be conveniently divided into three groups—diuretic, metabolic and toxic. Complications of the diuretic action include
potassium deficiency, magnesium deficiency, hyponatraemia (low
serum sodium level), a state of alkalosis with a low serum chloride
level, excessive salt and water loss resulting in a low blood volume,
postural hypotension and oliguric renal failure, and acute retention of urine in the elderly male with prostatic symptoms.

Metabolic complications include hyperglycaemia and an increase in serum uric acid levels. Patients on diuretic therapy
should have their urine periodically tested for sugar. Patients who
are already diabetic may need more insulin or oral hypoglycaemic
agents when they are treated with diuretics.

Toxic complications are very uncommon and include rashes,
thrombocytopenia (thiazides), acute haemorrhagic pancreatitis
and deafness. The latter is induced by high doses of frusemide
given quickly by intravenous injection and by high doses of ethacrynic acid given orally to patients with renal failure. To avoid
loss of hearing, the rate of infusion of frusemide should not exceed
250 mg per hour. The incorporation of a burette into the giving-
set facilitates accurate dosage.

Doses of diuretics

chlorothiazide (Saluric)	500 mg to 1 g once or twice daily
bendrofluazide (Aprinox)	2·5–10 mg daily
polythiazide (Nephril)	1–4 mg daily
chlorthalidone (Hygroton)	50–100 mg daily or 100–200 mg on alternate days
clorexolone (Nefrolan)	10–100 mg daily
metolazone (Zaroxolyn)	5–80 mg daily
frusemide (Lasix)	20 mg to 2 g daily
ethacrynic acid (Edecrin)	50–400 mg daily, usually 50–150 mg daily
bumetanide (Burinex)	0·5–40 mg daily, usually 1–4 mg daily
spironolactone (Aldactone)	25–100 mg 4 times daily

amiloride (Midamor)   5–10 mg once or twice daily
triamterene (Dytac)   150–250 mg daily or on alternate days,
               , in divided doses.

Non-diuretic uses of diuretics

Diuretics are often used for some purpose other than ridding the body of excess water. The commonest alternative use for diuretics is in the control of **hypertension.** Most often, the moderate diuretics are used for this purpose, because of their prolonged action and the need for only one dose a day. They have an anti-hypertensive action of their own and will also potentiate the effect of other antihypertensive agents. A reduction in the dosage of the latter agents is therefore often necessary when a hypertensive patient starts diuretic therapy.

An unexpected use for diuretics is in some cases of **diabetes insipidus** where, paradoxically, they are used for their anti-diuretic effect.

Thiazides are used to reduce urinary calcium levels in cases of **idiopathic hypercalciuria,** in which a high urinary calcium content is causing urinary calculi.

Frusemide, ethacrynic acid and triamterene cause an increase in urinary calcium excretion and are therefore used to reduce serum calcium levels in cases of **hypercalcaemia.**

Methods of reducing general oedema

One of the causes of generalized oedema is the retention of sodium within the body which, in turn, causes the retention of an excess of fluid in the tissues.

In treating such cases the following methods are employed:
(1) Diuretics to increase fluid output by the kidneys.
(2) Restricted sodium intake (low-salt or, rarely, a salt-free diet).
(3) Restricted fluid intake.
(4) The use of cation-exchange resins.
(5) Peritoneal dialysis with a solution containing 6·36 per cent dextrose.

> **Certain cation exchange resins** prevent the absorption of sodium from the alimentary canal and can, therefore, be used to assist the effects of the other forms of therapy, e.g. Katonium, average dose 15 g twice daily with meals. It is important to check the blood electrolytes during their use.

Other methods of removing surplus fluid from the body include:

paracentesis thoracis

paracentesis abdominis

incisions on the dorsal surfaces of the oedematous feet (Southey's tubes were formerly used).

Drugs rendering the urine alkaline

The urine is normally slightly acid in reaction, i.e. it turns blue litmus red.

In addition to this method of indicating the reaction of urine (or any other liquid), the reaction may also be stated in terms of what is called the hydrogen-ion concentration or pH. A solution which is neutral is described as having a pH of 7. Acid solutions have a pH of less than 7 (e.g. pH 5) while alkaline solutions have a pH greater than 7 (e.g. pH 9). Special indicators are required to determine pH accurately.

It is sometimes desirable to render the urine alkaline, for example to hinder the growth of organisms, especially *Escherichia coli* which does not flourish in alkaline urine. Alkalis are therefore given in some cases of cystitis, particularly in the acute stages.

Alkalis, usually given in mixture form, include:

potassium citrate
sodium citrate
sodium bicarbonate.

Drugs rendering the uric acid

Drugs are occasionally given to make the urine acid in order to permit the efficient action of other drugs which are only effective in an acid medium. For example, mandelic acid and its preparations are only effective as urinary antiseptics against *Escherichia coli* in acid urine (pH 5·5).

Acid sodium phosphate or ascorbic acid may be used.

Urinary antibacterial agents

Urinary antibacterial agents are drugs which, when given by mouth, are excreted by the kidneys and have the power of inhibiting the growth of organisms in the urine. The most important urinary antibacterials are:

sulphonamides   co-trimoxazole   antibiotics.

The sulphonamides

In addition to their action on streptococcal, pneumococcal, meningococcal and other infections in various parts of the body, drugs of this group are of special value in infections of the urinary tract due to *Escherichia coli*. They are, therefore, used in the treatment of pyelonephritis and cystitis. They are also effective against the gonococcus (p. 285). Most soluble sulphonamides act as urinary antiseptics. **Sulphamethizole** (Urolucosil), 100–200 mg every 4 hours, is specially employed for this purpose.

Sulphonamides act by interfering with synthesis of folate in bacteria. Bacteria have to synthesize their own folate because they cannot absorb it from their environment. Folate is necessary for the growth of bacteria and sulphonamides therefore stop them from growing. Sulphonamides are thus said to have a *bacteriostatic* action. Another drug has been made specifically to block the next step in bacterial folate metabolism, in case the organism overcomes the action of the sulphonamide. This antibacterial drug is called trimethoprim. It too is bacteriostatic when used alone. When used together with a sulphonamide, however, the effect of the combination is *bactericidal*. Septrin and Bactrim are combinations (mixtures) of sulphamethoxazole and trimethoprim, and have the approved name of co-trimoxazole. The usual dose is 2 tablets twice daily for adults and children over 12 years. A paediatric suspension is also available. Coptin is a mixture of sulphadiazine and trimethoprim; the adult dose is one tablet or 10 ml of suspension 12-hourly.

Antibiotics

Various antibiotics may be used depending on the organism present in the urine and its sensitivity. Streptomycin may be useful in special cases, but it must be remembered that *Escherichia coli* is insensitive to penicillin. Ampicillin is a useful antibiotic for urinary tract infections (see p. 272).

Carfecillin (Uticillin) is an antibiotic of the penicillin series which is rapidly absorbed, when taken orally, and hydrolysed to carbenicillin, which achieves a high concentration in the urine. The level achieved in the blood is insufficient for the treatment of systemic infections and carfecillin is therefore used only for urinary tract infections. The dose is 500 mg to 1 g 3 times a day.

Penicillin hypersensitivity is a contraindication to the use of either ampicillin or carfecillin.

Other urinary antibacterials

Nitrofurantoin (Furadantin), 5–8 mg/kg body weight. This substance is active against both Gram-positive and Gram-negative organisms, including staphylococci and *Proteus* species. The average adult dose is 100 mg 4 times daily, with meals or milk (since it is a gastric irritant). Rarely, neuritis or hepatic damage may follow its use.

Nalidixic acid (Negram) 1 g 6-hourly, is bactericidal to many Gram-negative organisms found in urinary tract infections. It may give a false positive test for sugar in the urine.

Mandelic acid

Mandelic acid or one of its preparations acts as a urinary antiseptic when excreted into the urine. It is essential, however, to have a certain degree of acidity present which is measured, not by litmus, but by a special indicator recording the hydrogen-ion concentration or pH. This should not exceed 5·5. Mandelamine is a proprietary preparation given in a dose of 1 g 4 times a day.

Hexamine is hydrolysed in the urine and releases formaldehyde, which is bactericidal. Hexamine hippurate (Hiprex), 1 g 2 to 4 times daily, may be useful especially in chronic urinary tract infections resistant to antibiotics and other antibacterial agents. If the urine is alkaline, acidification may be necessary, e.g. with ascorbic acid 500 mg 4 times a day.

Drugs acting on the bladder

The urinary antiseptics and alkalis already mentioned are given by mouth in cases of cystitis. Hyoscyamus may be included in alkaline mixtures because it has a sedative action on the bladder and helps to relieve the symptoms of frequent or painful micturition.

Local applications are also used for washing out the bladder, particularly in cases of chronic cystitis and after operations involving the bladder.

One litre of sterile fluid at a temperature of 43 °C (110 °F) from a bottle about 1 metre (3 feet) above the patient is generally employed, e.g.:

  sodium bicarbonate (1 to 2 per cent)
  dilute acetic acid (0·5 per cent)
  potassium permanganate (1 in 4000)
  silver nitrate (1 in 10 000, increasing to 1 in 2000)
  noxytiolin (Noxyflex S; 2·5 per cent)
  chlorhexidine (1 in 5000).

Cholinergic drugs such as carbachol have an action on the muscle of the bladder causing it to contract and may be useful in the treatment of postoperative retention of urine.

Emepronium bromide (Cetiprin) is an anticholinergic drug

which increases bladder capacity and delays the desire to void urine. It is of value in treating an 'irritable' bladder, especially after prostatectomy or radiotherapy and may relieve frequency and incontinence in the elderly. It should be swallowed with an adequate volume of water to avoid oesophageal pain and possibly oesophageal ulceration. Dose: 200 mg 3 times a day. For nocturnal frequency, 200 mg on retiring is adequate.

Drugs acting on the urethra

The main condition requiring treatment is urethritis, which may be 'non-specific' or due to the gonococcus or to other causes.

Intramuscular injection of a single dose of procaine penicillin (1·2 or 2·4 mega-units), or of ampicillin (2 g) is usually effective in gonorrhoea. Probenicid (1 or 2 g) may be given orally to block the renal excretion of the antibiotic and thus to increase the duration of its bactericidal action. Other antibiotics may be useful, e.g. tetracyclines.

The organism or organisms responsible for non-specific urethritis often remain unknown although Chlamydia trachomas is probably responsible in about 50 per cent of cases. The condition is usually treated with a tetracycline or erythromycin. Local applications are sometimes employed, e.g. urethral irrigations with potassium permanganate, 1 in 8000.

In order to produce local anaesthesia of the urethra, 2 per cent lignocaine jelly (Xylocaine gel) or lignocaine and chlorhexidine gel is used.

Drugs used in the diagnosis of urinary conditions

The efficiency of the kidneys may be investigated by testing their power of excreting various substances.

1. Urea

Urea is normally excreted by the kidneys and the urine contains approximately 2 per cent.

Urea concentration test

No fluid is taken for several hours, the bladder is then emptied and the patient given 15 g of urea by mouth dissolved in 100 ml of water. The urine is collected 1 and 2 hours later. The amount of urea in each specimen is then estimated. If the concentrating power of the kidneys is normal, the first specimen should contain at least 1·5 per cent and the second 2 per cent of urea.

Urea clearance test

There are several methods of performing this test, which depends on comparing the blood urea with the output of urea in the urine.

2. Creatinine

This is a breakdown product of the creatine found in muscle. It is freely filtered by the kidney and its clearance from the plasma can be determined by a simple formula. The creatinine clearance provides an approximate estimate of the glomerular filtration rate (GFR). This indicates how much renal tissue is functioning.

Creatinine clearance is determined from the plasma creatinine concentration and from the urinary excretion of creatinine. Urine is collected over a timed period, preferably of 24 hours. As with all tests involving a 24-hour urine collection, the nurse should ensure that at the start of the test (e.g. at 9 a.m.) the bladder is emptied and the urine is discarded. *All* urine passed during the next 24 hours is collected in a bottle. The patient must be *asked* to empty his bladder into the bottle at the end of the test (e.g. at 9 a.m. the following day) to complete the collection.

3. Dyes

Various dyes given by intrasmuscular or intravenous injection are excreted by the kidneys and colour the urine (p. 50).

By passing ureteric catheters after cystoscopy, the urine from each kidney can be collected separately and the time taken for the dye to appear in the urine from each kidney can be estimated. A delay will indicate damage to one or both kidneys.

The dyes used include:

indigocarmine,	intramuscular, 50–100 mg
	intravenous, 8–16 mg
methylene blue,	intramuscular, 1 ml of 5 per cent solution.

4. Radio-opaque substances

An outline of the urinary tract obtained by x-rays after the introduction of a radio-opaque substance is called a urogram or pyelogram. This may be obtained in the following ways.

(a) Excretion or intravenous urography (pyelography)

The intravenous injection of:

meglumine iothalamate (Conray 280) 60 per cent or
sodium iothalamate (Conray 325 or 420) 54 or 70 per cent or
sodium diatrizoate (Hypaque) 45 or 65 per cent (25 per cent for children) or
sodium metrizoate (Triosil) 60 or 75 per cent or
Urografin 370 (a mixture of diatrizoates).

These iodine-containing substances are excreted by the kidneys and, being opaque to x-rays, radiograms taken 5, 10, 30 and 50 minutes after injection show the outline of the pelvis of the kidneys, the ureters and the bladder.

When these substances are being injected, care must be taken that none of the fluid escapes from the vein or a painful arm will result.

(b) Instrumental or retrograde pyelography

A cystoscope is passed and the orifices of the ureters in the bladder determined. After a catheter has been introduced into one or both ureters, 5 to 10 ml of sterile, 12·5 per cent solution of sodium iodide or 45 per cent Hypaque are injected, the injection ceasing when the patient complains of pain in the loin. The solution is opaque to x-rays and in this way the outline of the pelvis of the kidney is obtained.

Drugs altering the colour of the urine

Normal urine is described as straw-coloured, amber or like pale sherry. The following abnormalities of colour may occur:

Bright yellow; due to nitrofurantoin.

Pink or red: due to rhubarb, senna, phenolphthalein, Dorbanex or phenindione.

Black or brown: due to bile, to poisoning with phenol or lysol or to disseminated melanoma. Rarely the urine of patients taking methyldopa or levodopa may darken on exposure to air.

Blue or green: due to methylene blue.

Drugs used in the treatment of renal failure (uraemia)

(1) Intravenous glucose and insulin for the rapid but temporary reduction of a high serum potassium level.

(2) Cation-exchange resins (see p. 000) to eliminate· excess potassium from the body, e.g. Resonium-A 15 g 3 times a day by mouth or 30 g by retention enema.

(3) Loop diuretics in high dosage, e.g. frusemide 250 mg to 2 g.

(4) A mixture of all the essential amino acids may be given in tablet form (Kidnamin) to patients with renal failure. Given with a high-calorie, low-protein diet, they aid the body to utilize urea for protein synthesis.

(5) Chlorpromazine and metoclopramide are valuable anti-emetics for relieving nausea and vomiting in renal failure.

(6) Dialysis solutions.

NB.—All drugs which are normally excreted by the kidneys must be given in reduced or carefully controlled doses in cases of renal failure. Toxic concentrations will otherwise build up in the blood. Examples are streptomycin, gentamycin and digitalis.

Peritoneal dialysis

Peritoneal dialysis solutions are sterile electrolyte solutions made hypertonic by the inclusion of dextrose 1·36 per cent or 6·36 per cent. The 1·36 per cent dextrose solution is ordinarily used but when the patient is 'waterlogged' with oedema fluid, the stronger solution is used. The electrolytes in the solution are sodium chloride, sodium lactate, calcium chloride, magnesium chloride and sodium metabisulphate. These are present in concentrations approximately the same as in normal extracellular body fluid. Potassium chloride may be added if necessary; it is not included in the dialysis solution as supplied because hyperkalaemia is usually present in renal failure.

A trocar or stylet-catheter (e.g. Trocath) is introduced into the peritoneal cavity by puncture in the midline of the abdomen, a little below the umbilicus, after emptying the bladder. The peritoneal dialysis fluid should be warmed before being run through the peritoneal catheter and into the patient. One litre of dialysate is exchanged every half hour. An accurate record must be kept of input and output and of the patient's weight.

11 Drugs acting on the nervous system

The nervous system may be divided into three main portions:
(1) The brain and spinal cord or central nervous system.
(2) The nerves or peripheral nervous system.
(3) The involuntary (autonomic) system.

The functioning elements of the system are different types of nerve cells and their fibres.

Nerve cells and fibres are sensitive to the action of various drugs which reach them via the blood and the cerebrospinal fluid. Their activities may be stimulated, depressed or altered in function by the action of drugs.

Drugs which depress the central nervous system

One of the features of a number of drugs, which in full doses have the effect of depressing the nervous system, is that in small doses they often have an apparently stimulating action. This is shown, for example, in the exhilarating effect of small or moderate doses of alcohol and in the excitement stage manifested during the induction of general anaesthesia.

It may be that in small doses such substances do have an initial stimulating effect. However, it must be remembered that the highest centres of the brain, namely those which are concerned with consciousness and behaviour, are the first to be affected and, normally, these centres exercise a restraining influence on the activities of an individual. It is, therefore, much more likely that these drugs exercise their depressing effect from the commencement and that the apparent stimulation is merely the result of removing the controlling action of the higher centres.

As the dosage of such drugs is increased, other centres or levels of nervous activity are depressed. Sensation is dulled, consciousness is lost, the cough and vomiting reflexes are abolished. Finally, in toxic doses, the vital centres such as the respiratory and vasomotor centres are affected, and if these are completely paralysed death ensues.

From the point of view of therapeutics these drugs may be divided into the following groups:

(1) Hypnotics or drugs used to produce sleep.
(2) Analgesics
    (a) simple analgesics, e.g. aspirin
    (b) analgesics with hypnotic properties, e.g. morphine.
(3) Psychotropic drugs. There are two main groups of these drugs:
    (a) tranquillizers which are used to relieve anxiety
    (b) antidepressants, used to treat depression.
(4) Drugs which stimulate the nervous system.
(5) Anticonvulsants used in the treatment of epilepsy.
(6) Drugs used in the treatment of Parkinson's disease.
(7) Drugs used in the treatment of migraine.
(8) A miscellaneous group some of which are used in the treatment of special symptoms.

1. Hypnotics

A hypnotic drug is one which is used to induce sleep. An analgesic relieves pain. Drugs having both actions are therefore used to treat insomnia or sleeplessness when the patient is unable to sleep on account of pain.

Insomnia

The inability to secure sufficient sleep, or failure to obtain sound restful sleep, is a problem which frequently presents itself for treatment, and it is not solved by simply prescribing one of the many available hypnotic drugs.

The first step is to ascertain, if possible, the underlying cause. A simple method of grouping cases is:

(1) Primary—where no physical cause can be found, e.g. anxiety states.
(2) Secondary—where pain, physical discomfort such as indigestion, irritation of the skin (pruritus), frequency of micturition, cough, or some organic disease, is the cause.

In the second group, treatment is given for the underlying cause and its symptoms before, or at the same time as, active measures are adopted to procure sleep.

General management

A careful history of the patient's habits must be obtained so that any undesirable factors or contributory causes may be eliminated. Thus the sufferer may lack adequate exercise and fresh air during the day.

(1) He should sleep in a quiet room, adequately ventilated but kept at a comfortable and even temperature. The blinds should be drawn, doors and windows wedged to prevent rattling and clocks removed (but occasionally the monotonous ticking of a clock is an aid to drowsiness).

(2) The bedclothes should be light but warm. As a rule, a spring mattress is best, but it is not always wise to change the type of bed to which the patient is accustomed. Night clothes should be comfortable.

(3) A warm bath on retiring promotes sleep in some individuals but refreshes and rouses others.

An electric blanket or bed-socks are often of value, especially if coldness of the extremities is noticed.

(4) Overloading the stomach shortly before bedtime is undesirable and a light evening meal is often preferable to a heavy dinner. In such circumstances, soup, Bovril, hot milk or a preparation such as Ovaltine may be taken just before retiring, or during the night if the patient wakes, provided it is kept hot in a Thermos flask and the patient does not have to rouse himself to prepare it.

(5) Tea and coffee at night should be avoided. Some individuals extol the virtues of whisky or brandy as a night-cap. Unfortunately, however, alcohol causes early morning restlessness and so makes sleep less sound.

(6) Patients who complain of wakefulness on account of excessive mental activity on retiring, should pass their evenings quietly and games such as competitive cards should be avoided. Quiet reading of unsensational literature may be recommended, while the effect of a walk, but not vigorous exercise, before bedtime may be tried.

(7) Many people sleep best on their right side; some prefer one pillow, others like a number.

(8) The patient often fears the consequences of insomnia more than the lack of sleep, a dread which in itself may produce an anxiety state. Reassurance is, therefore, of great importance. He should be told that life will not be lost on this account nor will he lose his reason.

It is clearly wrong to attempt to force the patient to sleep with potent drugs without first attempting to remove the underlying cause. Drugs may be necessary in some cases, however, if only for a short period.

The following are hypnotic drugs:

(1) the barbiturates
(2) chloral hydrate, dichloralphenazone (Welldorm), and tri-clofos (Tricloryl)
(3) the benzodiazepines, e.g. nitrazepam (Mogadon)
(4) glutethimide (Doriden)
(5) methyprylone (Nodular)
(6) methaqualone (Revonal)
(7) Mandrax (methaqualone and diphenhydramine)
(8) ethchlorvynol (Serenesil).

Generally, the benzodiazepines and chloral or Welldorm are preferred for their safety.

(1) The barbiturates

There are a large number of drugs derived from barbituric acid which have a depressing effect on the central nervous system and are used as hypnotics.

In addition to their use as hypnotics and general sedatives in anxiety states, certain of them, e.g. phenobarbitone, are employed in the treatment of epilepsy to depress the irritability of the cerebrum. They are no longer widely favoured for any of these purposes.

Dependence on barbiturates may develop and some patients habitually take relatively large doses. In such instances sudden withdrawal may result in fits.

Cases in which an over-dose was taken accidentally or with suicidal intent were fairly frequent when these drugs were commonly used.

Neither barbiturates nor other hypnotics should be taken with alcohol as the combination may cause serious depression of the central nervous system, to the extent of coma.

The barbiturates fall into three main groups, viz.:

(1) Short action (3 to 6 hours), rapid excretion, e.g.:

		Dose: mg
quinalbarbitone	Seconal	200
hexobarbitone	as in Evidorm	500
cyclobarbitone	Phanodorm	400

(2) Intermediate action (4 to 8 hours), e.g.:

amylobarbitone	Amytal	300
pentobarbitone	Nembutal	200
butobarbitone	Soneryl	200

(3) Long acting (8 to 16 hours), e.g.:

phenobarbitone	Luminal	120
methyl phenobarbitone	Prominal	200

Among the many other drugs containing barbiturates are Carbrital, Sonalgin and Tuinal (a mixture of quinalbarbitone and amylobarbitone).

The sodium preparations of the various barbiturates are more soluble than the other forms and act more quickly. Soluble phenobarbitone (sodium) may be given by intramuscular injection (200 mg).

Barbiturates should be used with special caution in:
(1) Allergic patients (asthma, angioneurotic oedema).
(2) Defective renal or hepatic function.
(3) Diabetes.
(4) Thyrotoxicosis.
(5) Old age.

Phenobarbitone and other barbiturates have an interesting action on the liver where they 'induce' enzymes. As a result, anticoagulant drugs may be detoxified more rapidly and hence lose their effect. Bilirubin conjugation and excretion are enhanced, so that phenobarbitone may be of value in the treatment of Rhesus haemolytic disease of the newborn.

Features of barbiturate poisoning

These include:

Increasing coma.
Depression of the respiratory centre with slow, shallow breathing.
Abolition of the tendon and eye reflexes.
Fall in blood pressure.
Later, bronchopneumonia.

Treatment of barbiturate poisoning

(1) *Ensure a clear airway and adequate ventilation.* Endotracheal intubation and perhaps the use of a mechanical ventilator may be necessary.
(2) *Gastric lavage* should be performed if less than 4 hours have elapsed since the over-dose was taken.
(3) In the more severe cases of phenobarbitone or barbitone

poisoning, active measures can be taken to aid the elimination of the drug from the body.

Forced diuresis is feasible if the patient is without cardiac or renal disease. Large volumes of normal saline and 5 per cent dextrose solution, specified quantities of sodium bicarbonate and potassium chloride, and a slow drip of 20 per cent mannitol solution (500 ml over 12 hours) are administered intravenously. A careful watch is kept on the patient's clinical condition, fluid balance and serum electrolytes.

Haemodialysis is indicated in phenobarbitone poisoning if the initial blood barbiturate level is greater than 15 mg/100 ml.

(2) Chloral hydrate (300 mg to 2 g)

This is a drug which occurs in crystalline form and is usually dissolved in water and given in the form of a mixture or draught, but its bitter flavour is not easy to conceal. The Official Preparations are chloral mixture and chloral elixir, paediatric.

Chloral is a very effective hypnotic, especially for children and the elderly, which does not predispose to habit formation. It is quite safe to give to cardiac patients in ordinary doses, although at one time this was thought to be inadvisable.

Dichloralphenazone (Welldorm) and triclofos (Tricloryl) are close relatives of chloral and are both available in tablet or elixir form. Triclofos is tasteless and dichloralphenazone is less unpleasant than chloral to take.

(3) The benzodiazepines

Nitrazepam (Mogadon) and flurazepam (Dalmane) are benzodiazepines with a hypnotic effect lasting about 8 hours. Temazepam (Normison, Euhypnos) has a short half-life and is therefore unlikely to cause drowsiness the next day. The advantages of the benzodiazepines over barbiturates are:
(a) they are very safe, even after massive over-dosage
(b) They have less tendency than barbiturates to cause confusion in the elderly
(c) they have less severe hangover effects
(d) they do not affect anticoagulant therapy.

The doses are: nitrazepam 2·5–20 mg (average 5 mg); flurazepam 15–30 mg; temazepam 10–30 mg.

(4) Glutethimide

Glutethimide (Doriden) has a hypnotic effect for about 6 hours.

The dose is 250–500 mg. The tablets should be protected from light. In cases of glutethimide over-dosage, the doctor has to keep a watch for papilloedema.

(5) Methyprylone
Methypyrlone (Noludar) also has a hypnotic effect lasting about 6 hours. Dose: 200–400 mg.

(6) Methaqualone
Methyprylone (Revonal) is given in a dose of 200–400 mg. Over-dosage of this drug characteristically causes increased muscle tone, myoclonia and convulsions.

(7) Mandrax
Mandrax contains methaqualone (250 mg) and an antihistamine, diphenydramine (25 mg). Dose: 1 tablet.

(8) Ethchlorvynol
Ethchlorvynol (Serenesil) is given in a dose of 500 mg. An over-dose of this drug can usually be diagnosed from the characteristic odour of the gastric aspirate.

Other hypnotics

Paraldehyde (oral dose 2–8 ml)
This is a colourless liquid, with a characteristic pungent odour and unpleasant taste, which should be stored in the dark. It is, however, a very safe hypnotic. Its duration of action is relatively short and it is excreted in the breath so that it can be smelt some hours after its administration.

Paraldehyde is given by intramuscular injection for the treatment of status epilepticus (dose 5–10 ml), but a **plastic syringe must not be used.**

It is now rarely prescribed in mixture form for oral administration and is only slightly soluble in water. The bottle must be carefully shaken as the bulk of the paraldehyde tends to float on the top of the mixture.

It can also be given per rectum, when double the oral dose may be ordered.

Accidents have sometimes happened, and proved fatal, because the dose intended for rectal administration has been given intramuscularly.

The bromides

Bromides are crystalline salts which are soluble in water, e.g.:

potassium bromide
sodium bromide
ammonium bromide

They have a general sedative effect on the nervous system. In order to produce sleep they may be given with chloral.

Bromides are now rarely used.

'Bromism' (p. 159) may develop in persons especially sensitive to bromide (idiosyncrasy) and in cases of over-dosage. The symptoms include skin eruptions which resemble acne or eczema. Bromides are not well tolerated by the elderly and, therefore, should be used with caution in old age, for they are then liable to cause mental confusion.

Methylpentynol

Methylpentynol (Oblivon-C) is a drug which has a sedative effect and is particularly useful in allaying apprehension, nervous tension or excitement. It is given in the form of capsules or an elixir.

2. Analgesics
Drugs having analgesic effects (anodynes)

The most important drugs of this type are as follows.

Aspirin (acetylsalicyclic acid; 300 mg–1 g)

When given by mouth this drug is of great value in relieving minor or moderate degrees of pain and discomfort. It also induces sweating and tends to lower the body temperature, i.e. it is also an antipyretic (p. 63).

Aspirin has a slight local anaesthetic action when applied to mucous membranes and so is useful as a gargle to relieve pain after tonsillectomy (600 mg in 30 ml of water).

It is usually given in tablets containing 300 mg.

Calcium aspirin, known also as Soluble Aspirin Tablets (BP) and Disprin, is more soluble than ordinary aspirin. It is therefore more readily absorbed and acts more quickly. It has less tendency to cause gastric irritation. Where a rapid effect is required for acute pain, such as that of a headache or toothache, soluble aspirin, plain or buffered, may be the preparation of choice. For rheumatic disorders, a rapid effect is not the main aim and one of the other preparations may be better tolerated for regular medication.

A variety of other preparations of aspirin have been developed in an attempt to reduce gastric irritation. Among these are buffered soluble aspirin (e.g. Bufferin), enteric coated aspirin (e.g. Safapryn) which is intended to release the drug only in the small intestine, preparations in which the aspirin particles are individually encapsulated in ethylcellulose (as in Levius) so that they are slowly released in the stomach, and aluminium-aspirin compounds (e.g. aloxiprin) which release aspirin only slowly in the stomach but rapidly in the small intestine. Benorylate (Benoral) is a compound of aspirin and paracetamol which is often well tolerated.

Anadin contains aspirin, salicylamide, caffeine and quinine sulphate.

There are many analgesic preparations, including Paynocil Veganin, Anadin, Zactirin and Doloxene Compound containing aspirin in various forms and mixed with other drugs.

Aspirin poisoning

Accidental and suicidal aspirin poisoning is not uncommon. The symptoms include nausea, vomiting, noises in the head, rashes, and a weak, rapid pulse. Large doses cause coma and death.

Treatment

The stomach should be washed out, preferably with 5 per cent sodium bicarbonate solution or an emetic may be given. Milk or water containing bicarbonate by mouth, and intravenous fluids (e.g. sodium lactate solution, saline, dextran or Hartmann's solution) may be needed. Forced alkaline diuresis, using bicarbonate infusions, will increase the rate of urinary excretion of aspirin. An 'artificial kidney' (haemodialysis) may save severely poisoned patients, during the treatment of whom estimations of the plasma salicylate should be made. In infants, the poison can be removed by peritoneal dialysis or by exchange transfusion. The latter is not feasible in adults because of the large volumes of donor blood required.

Vitamin K_1, 10 mg intramuscularly, is given to correct the defect in blood coagulation caused by salicylates.

Aspirin in ordinary doses sometimes causes gastric bleeding and haematemesis, owing to its irritant action on the gastric mucosa, and some asthmatics are sensitive to aspirin.

Diflunisal (Dolobid, 250 mg)

One of the main advantages of this drug is its long duration of action, often relieving pain for 12 hours, so that twice-daily dosage is usually sufficient.

Phenacetin (600 mg)

This is an analgesic drug, obtainable only on prescription, especially used to relieve headache and minor degrees of pain. It is often combined with aspirin and caffeine and given in tablet form. Used regularly for long periods, it may lead to serious kidney damage and it has largely been replaced by the safer paracetamol.

Paracetamol (500 mg to 1 g)

This is a safe analgesic in normal therapeutic doses but massive overdosage, as in a suicidal bid, causes acute hepatic necrosis which is usually fatal. If the patient reaches hospital before liver damage occurs, it can be largely prevented with cysteamine or methionine. One or other of these drugs is given if liver damage is predicted from the plasma concentrations of paracetamol.

Nefopam (Acupan, 30 mg)

This is a strong analgesic, unrelated to any other. It is not narcotic. Oral and injectable (iv or im) forms are available.

Other pain-relieving drugs include mefenamic acid (Ponstan) and the analgesic, anti-inflammatory agents used in the treatment of rhematoid arthritis (see p. 256)

Drugs having both hypnotic and analgesic properties

There are a number of drugs of this type of which opium and its alkaloid morphine are the most important. Their use is controlled by the Misuse of Drugs Act.

Opium

Opium is the dried juice of certain poppy heads which are grown mainly in China, India and Persia. It is one of the oldest of drugs and its use was known to the Egyptians, Romans and Greeks. Its activity is due to a number of alkaloids, of which the most important is morphine. Opium contains about 10 per cent of morphine and its important pharmacological actions can be attributed to this alkaloid.

Morphine (8–20 mg)

Morphine acts on the central nervous system, depressing the important centres and has a special effect on the sensory nerve cells, which explains its value in the relief of pain.

(a) Action on the higher centres

In some persons there is at first a period of well-being or excitement after its administration due to the removal of the control of the highest centres of nervous activity (cf. anaesthetics). This is soon followed by a general dulling of perception so that the patient assumes a drowsy state with diminished power of attention. While this is going on the sensory centres are depressed and the appreciation of pain and discomfort are markedly diminished. Movements tend to become clumsy and the patient passes into a sleep from which he can be easily roused but which returns when he is left undisturbed.

(b) Action on the medulla

The *respiratory centre* is depressed so that respiration becomes slower and shallower—a most important action of morphine. It is helpful in the treatment of dyspnoea in cases of left ventricular heart failure with pulmonary oedema.

The *cough reflex centre* is depressed and this makes opium and morphine of value in allaying irritating and useless cough.

The *vomiting centre* is affected in some persons. In such a case, small doses of morphine appear to have a contradictory action and the centre is stimulated so that the patient vomits. In larger doses the centre is depressed by morphine.

The *vasomotor centre* is somewhat depressed, but to a relatively less extent than the respiratory centre.

Eye reflexes: the pupils are contracted.

(c) Action on the alimentary system

The nerve plexuses in the walls of the bowel are depressed by the action of opium and morphine. This slows down peristalsis, so that constipation results and the faeces tend to become hard and dry from their prolonged stay in the gut, during which additional water is absorbed by the colon. Advantage is taken of this constipating effect in the treatment of some cases of diarrhoea, e.g. kaolin and morphine mixture.

Morphine poisoning

The depth of sleep and other effects produced are dependent on the dose of morphine or opium given. The description so far given would apply to the ordinary therapeutic doses, e.g. not exceeding 20 mg of morphine. In larger and therefore poisonous doses sleep develops into coma from which it is very difficult to rouse the patient. Reflexes are lost. The depression of the respiratory centre is marked and the rate of breathing may be very slow. The contracted pupil becomes pin-point in size. The pulse is weak.

Treatment of morphine poisoning

Until an antidote can be given, the general principle is to stimulate the patient in every way. Also, the stomach may be washed out with a solution of potassium permanganate, 4 g in 8 litres of water, even if the drug has been given by injection, as it is probable that some of the drug given in this way is excreted into the stomach. This may be followed by giving strong black coffee. Sometimes gastric aspiration followed by lavage with not more than 1 litre of water is preferred.

If possible, the patient should be kept awake by walking him about, flicking with wet towels, etc. If breathing has ceased, life must be maintained by some form of artifical ventilation. In other cases, administration of oxygen is necessary. Injections of nikethamide have been used to stimulate the respiratory centre.

Antidotes to morphine poisoning are levallorphan (Lorfan), 0.2–2 mg intravenously, and naloxone (Narcan) initially 0.4 mg by intravenous injection. Naloxone is superior to the other two antagonists in having no central respiratory depressant effect of its own.

Idiosyncrasy

Children do not tolerate morphine or opium well, and doses very small in proportion to the age should be given. This is especially important in infants.

Some adults also are sensitive to morphine, showing profound slowing of breathing or hypotension. Some individuals tend to show a degree of restlessness after the injection of morphine. In others, vomiting may be severe.

Tolerance

The continued use of morphine fairly soon leads to tolerance of the drug and larger and larger doses are required in order to produce effective results. This is probably due to the fact that the tissues acquire the ability of destroying morphine more quickly. It is, therefore, not uncommon to find cases (e.g. those suffering from inoperable carcinoma) receiving 120 mg several times a day. This amount has been reached by increasing the dose gradually over a period of weeks or months. A dose of this size given to anyone unaccustomed to the drug would, of course, have very serious or fatal results.

Undesirable effects of morphine

(1) *On the alimentary system.* Vomiting and constipation have already been mentioned.
(2) *On the respiratory system.* Although useful in allaying cough, the fact that morphine depresses the respiratory centre necessitates great care in its employment in cases of respiratory disease, such as pneumonia (later stages), bronchitis and bronchial asthma. It should never be used in the treatment of an asthmatic attack since it can produce fatal results.
(3) *Psychological and general physical effects.* Morphine is one of the most important substances responsible for drug dependence. While in the Western Hemisphere the habit of opium smoking is rare, it has not been eradicated in the East in spite of attempts to control the evil. This habit ultimately renders the addict a nervous wreck, weak in character, with little moral sense and poor in physique.

The craving for the drug is most commonly produced in the West by its prolonged administration during a painful illness. It is, therefore, most important that it should only be used for very limited periods in acute disease. Only in conditions such as inoperable carcinoma, which are likely to prove rapidly fatal, is its use justifiable in chronic disease.

Drug dependence of the morphine type is characterized by:
(1) an overpowering need to continue taking the drug and to obtain it by any means;
(2) a tendency to increase the dose owing to the development of tolerance;

(3) a psychic dependence on the drug, and
(4) a physical dependence on the drug resulting in an abstinence syndrome when it is withdrawn.

The treatment of drug dependence is extremely difficult. The patient must be confined to a special institution, where attempts are made to substitute the offending drug with others in gradually decreasing doses until both have been withdrawn. Relapses after treatment are common.

Legal control of morphine   See p. 9.

Preparations of opium

Tincture of opium (2 ml).
Nepenthe is a proprietary preparation resembling but more pleasant to take than tincture of opium. Adult oral dose, 2·5 ml (equivalent to 20 mg of morphine). It is vital to note that this is the *adult oral dose*. In children, Nepenthe is usually given by injection and the dose is then 0·06 ml per year of age.

Preparations of morphine (CD)

Morphine sulphate injection (BP), 8–20 mg. Ampoules containing 10 mg, 15 mg, 20 mg and 30 mg are available.
Morphine and atropine injection (BPC). Ampoules of 1 ml contain 10 mg of morphine, and atropine (0·6 mg).
Morphine and hyoscine injection. Ampoules of 1 ml contain morphine 10 mg, and hyoscine (0·4 mg approximately).
Morphine is generally given by subcutaneous injection, but can be given by mouth.

Drugs resembling morphine

Papaveretum injection (CD) (dose 10–20 mg)

This contains alkaloids of opium and is the basis for proprietary preparations such as Omnopon. It has the analgesic and narcotic properties of morphine but produces fewer side-effects.

Papaverine hydrochloride (CD) (oral dose 60–300 mg)

This also is an alkaloid of opium, which has an antispasmodic action but little analgesic effect. Eupaverine is a similar synthetic substance which is stated to be less toxic. These two drugs must not be confused with papaveretum, and it will be noted that the doses are different.

Dromoran (levorphanol), 2–3 mg, is a proprietary preparation having a similar action to morphine.

Pethidine (CD)

This synthetic analgesic, although less powerful, may be used instead of morphine in some cases. It is very useful in obstetrics. Its duration of action is rather short and it may be necessary to administer it every 3 hours. The dose is 25–100 mg, either by mouth or subcutaneous injection. The intravenous dose is 25–50 mg.

Addiction is rapidly acquired, and it may produce dizziness, nausea and sweating.

Pethilorfan contains pethidine (100 mg) with levallorphan (1·25 mg) in 2 ml ampoules. The latter drug antagonizes the depressing effect of pethidine on the respiratory centre.

Methadone (Amidone, Physeptone; 5–10 mg) (CD)

This is a powerful synthetic analgesic having no sedative or hypnotic effect which may be given either by mouth or by subcutaneous or intramuscular injection. It may produce minor toxic effects such as nausea, vomiting, dizziness and sweating. These are more likely to occur in ambulant patients, so that patients should remain in bed after it has been given. It is also the basis of a useful cough linctus which usually contains 2 mg of methadone in 5 ml. Children tolerate only very small doses and the linctus should be kept out of their reach.

Diamorphine (heroin; 5–10 mg) (CD)

This is a drug having a similar action to morphine and is even more likely to produce addiction. Its manufacture is therefore forbidden in some countries. It may be given as an injection for the relief of pain, e.g. in myocardial infarction, but its main use is for pain in terminal conditions. It is also used in a linctus for the relief of troublesome coughs, e.g.:

Diamorphine (heroin) linctus (2.5–10 ml).

Buprenorphine (Temgesic; 300–600 micrograms)

This is a derivative of an opium alkaloid related to morphine. It is a strong, long-acting, narcotic analgesic which is unlikely to cause dependence and is not therefore controlled by the Misuse of Drugs Act. It is particularly valuable in relieving postoperative pain. It can cause adverse effects, such as respiratory depression, which are not reversed by naloxone.

Phenazocine (Narphen) (CD)
This is a powerful analgesic of particular value in relieving pain in biliary colic.

Pentazocine (Fortral)
This analgesic has a potency somewhere between that of codeine and morphine. The dose by subcutaneous, intramuscular or intravenous injection is 30–60 mg. The oral dose is 50–100 mg (2–4 tablets).

Codeine (10–60 mg)
This is an alkaloid derived from opium, having little tendency to promote habit formation. It has mild analgesic and hypnotic properties and depresses the cough reflex. It may be used for the latter purpose in the form of a linctus:

Codeine linctus, 5 ml.

It is also included in Veganin tablets for its analgesic and hypnotic effects.

Dihydrocodeine bitartrate (DF 118)
This drug has powerful analgesic with only mild hypnotic properties. Dose: 30 mg orally or up to 50 mg by intramuscular or subcutaneous injection. The injectable form of DF 118 is a Controlled Drug.

Dextropropoxyphene (Depronal SA, Doloxene)
This analgesic is chemically related to the opiates. It is combined with paracetamol in Distalgesic and with aspirin in Doloxene Compound and Napsalgesic. Over-dosage of dextropropoxyphene is treated with the opiate antagonist, naloxone. If the over-dosage is with the combination Distalgesic, treatment may also be required for paracetamol poisoning (see p. 161).

Cannabis (Indian hemp or *Cannabis sativa*) (CD)
This is the basis of hashish, the smoking of which is one of the forms of drug addiction. It is not used for therapeutic purposes and its mere possession, even by doctors and nurses, is an offence under the Misuse of Drugs Act. The following

is a description of its action (Cushny, 1918) which is included here as an illustration of the effects of certain substances of this type on the drug addict.

'Soon after its administration, the patient passes into a dreamy, semi-conscious state, in which the judgement seems to be lost, while the imagination is untrammelled by its usual restraints. The dreams assume the vividness of visions, are of boundless extravagance, and, of course, vary with the character and pursuits of the individual. In the eastern races they seem generally to partake of an amorous nature. The "true believer" sees the gardens of paradise and finds himself surrounded by troops of houris of unspeakable beauty, while the less imaginative European finds himself unaccountably happy and feels constrained to active movement, often of a purposeless and even absurd character. Ideas flash through the mind without apparent continuity, and all measurement of time and space is lost.'

The principal active ingredient of cannabis is tetrahydrocannabinol (THC). A higher concentration of THC is found in the flowers than in the leaves. Marihuana ('pot') is a mixture of cannabis leaves and blossoms. Hashish is the resin from the tips of the female blossoms.

THC stimulates serotonin secretion in the brain and also releases catecholamines into the blood. Effects produced include a sensation of 'time-stretching', intensification of odours, sound and colours and stimulation of appetite. 'Pot' smokers tend to eat voraciously and care little what they eat.

Probably depending on dosage, people may be relaxed or aggressive after smoking cannabis. The eyes are suffused ('pink eye') but the extremities are vasoconstricted, making the hands cold. The pulse and diastolic blood pressure are increased.

At present cannabis has no medical uses, but research may yet reveal some.

It has been argued, mostly in non-medical quarters, that 'pot' is harmless. However, cannabis may be deliberately adulterated with other substances, including opium. It is true that the purity of cannabis could be controlled if its sale were legalized, but there is no guarantee that addicts would not 'graduate' to more harmful drugs as they sought more 'way-out' experiences. The use of the other drugs, not only the 'harder' ones but also 'soft' ones like barbiturates, may result in premature death from starvation, exposure, psychosis, suicide, hepatitis or septicaemia.

Research has shown that cannabis itself is potentially harmful. Tests simulating driving on a road showed serious impairment of reflexes, slow reaction times and wrong reactions under stress in people under the influence of THC.

In cannabis addicts, gonadal function may be impaired, with low levels of circulating testerone and low sperm counts. Cannabis also induces chromosomal abnormalities, which could damage not only the addict but also his offspring.

Hyoscine also acts as a hypnotic and sedative (see p. 194).

3. Psychotropic drugs

In most cases these do not cure but substantially alleviate psychiatric disorders by suppressing symptoms until the condition remits spontaneously. The patient may also require discussion of his problems with a psychiatrist or with others (e.g. in group therapy), alteration of his environment (housing, employment, etc.), and perhaps other therapy.

Drugs used to relieve anxiety (tranquillizers, ataractics, anxiolytic agents)

An anxiety state may be primary or secondary to depression or an organic illness. For acute anxiety (e.g. panic attacks) sedation with a barbiturate, e.g. amylobarbitone sodium 45 mg t.d.s., may be the treatment of choice. Other agents are preferable for the treatment of chronic anxiety.

Tranquillizers include meprobamate (Equanil), and the benzodiazepine derivatives, i.e. chlordiazepoxide (Librium), diazepam (Valium), oxazepam (Serenid-D), medazepam (Nobrium) and lorazepam (Ativan).

Apart from their use in simple anxiety, benzodiazepines are used to treat agitation in patients with depression and tension in patients with schizophrenia.

Phobic anxiety complicated by reactive depression often responds well to combined therapy with chlordiazepoxide and a monoamine oxidase inhibitor, e.g. phenelzine. Chlordiazepoxide in large doses is used in the treatment of alcohol and drug-withdrawal states.

Other tranquillizers are benzoctamine (Tacitin) and oxypertine (Integrin). These are chemically unrelated to the benzodiazepines.

All patients taking tranquillizers should be warned that they may affect skilled performance, such as driving, and that alcohol may intensify the effect.

The major tranquillizers (neuroleptics)

These are phenothiazines and butyrophenones, e.g. haloperidol (Serenace). Chlorpromazine (Largactil), promazine (Sparine) and trifluoperazine (Stelazine) are examples of phenothiazines and they are used for the treatment of schizophrenia, maniacal and confusional states. In schizophrenia they are taken for about 2 years after recovery. They can be combined with antidepressants to treat a depressed patient who is also tense and agitated. Phenothiazines are used in the treatment of a number of other conditions including vomiting, vertigo and pruritus. The dose of chlorpromazine is 25–100 mg orally or intramuscularly as a single dose or 3 or 4 times a day. Phenothiazines may cause extrapyramidal side-effects (e.g. abnormal movements and postures of the limbs), and with the high doses required for schizophrenia it is usually necessary to prescribe anti-Parkinsonian drugs, e.g. orphenadrine. Phenothiazines may also cause depression, jaundice, agranulocytosis and rashes.

Other drugs used in schizophrenia are fluphenazine and pimozide.

Haloperidol is used for the control of over-activity, especially in mania (1·5–6·0 mg b.d. orally, or 5–10 mg parenterally). As a tranquillizer, it is used in a dose of 0·5 mg twice daily.

Drugs used to treat depression

Depression may be *reactive* (to environmental stress) or *endogenous* (without obvious external cause). Amphetamines are now obsolete in the treatment of depression, and the commonly used antidepressant drugs fall into two main groups, the MAO inhibitors and the tricyclic compounds.

(1) *The monoamine oxidase (MAO) inhibitors*

Monoamine oxidase is an enzyme which destroys serotonin, adrenaline and noradrenaline. Depression may sometimes be caused by a deficiency of serotonin and noradrenaline in the brain. Some drugs inhibit the enzyme which destroys these hormones. Such drugs are called MAO inhibitors and examples are:

iproniazid (Marsilid)	nialamide (Niamid)
isocarboxazid (Marplan)	phenelzine (Nardil)
mebanazine (Actomol)	tranylcypromine (Parnate).

If the patient is also anxious, chlordiazepoxide may be given at the same time.

Warning

Dangerous or even fatal idiosyncratic reactions to MAO inhibitors include jaundice and hypertensive crises, possibly causing a subarachnoid haemorrhage, when the patient eats foods containing tyramine, e.g. cheese, yoghourt, Bovril, Marmite and broad beans. Alcoholic drinks, particularly Chianti wine, may also be dangerous. Ephedrine, amphetamines and levodopa may similarly cause hypertensive crises and should not be administered to patients under treatment with MAO inhibitors. They should also be warned against taking 'Cold cures' which may contain phenyl-propanolamine. Pethidine is also contraindicated in these patients, but for a different reason—it may cause hypotension, coma and convulsions.

(2) *The tricyclic antidepressants*

Examples of these are:

    imipramine (Tofranil)   nortriptyline (Aventyl)
    amitriptyline (Tryptizol)   trimipramine (Surmontil).

The maintenance dose of all these four is 25–50 mg t.d.s. Imipramine is useful when retardation (i.e. inertia) is prominent. The other three drugs have sedating effects and are used when agitation is prominent. Lentizol is a sustained release tablet of amitriptyline and is given in a single nightly dose of 50 mg. Other antidepressants may be given in a single nightly dose, e.g. dothiepin (Prothiaden) 75 mg. Nightly administration takes advantage of the sedative effect of the drug and minimizes unwanted effects such as a dry mouth and blurred vision.

Protiptyline (Concordin) and iprindole (Prondol) act more rapidly than the above-mentioned drugs and have a more stimulating effect.

The side-effects of these drugs are a dry mouth, sweating, constipation and drowsiness. Rarely, ileus may occur.

Reactive depression tends to respond better to a MAO inhibitor, and endogenous depression tends to respond better to a tricyclic antidepressant. A tetracyclic antidepressant, e.g. mainserin (Bolvidon), may be preferable in cardiac cases.

Antidepressant drug therapy may take up to a fortnight to become effective, and if this time-lag is unacceptable (e.g. in severe depression) electroconvulsive therapy (ECT) may be required. Antidepressant drugs potentiate one another and alarming reactions may occur if a MAO inhibitor is given together with a tricyclic antidepressant.

Tricyclic antidepressants are often effective in the treatment of enuresis (bed-wetting). A single dose is given each night for this purpose. Clomipramine (Anafranil) is also used in the treatment of obsessional-phobic states.

(3) *L-tryptophan*

There is evidence of reduced levels of serotonin in the brains of people with depression. This deficiency cannot be corrected by administering serotonin to patients because it does not cross the blood-brain barrier. However, if the patient is given extra l-tryptophan, an essential amino acid normally present in the diet, it can be converted to serotonin in the brain. A daily dose of 3 g of l-tryptophan (Optimax, Pacitron) is given in divided dosage. The amount present in the normal daily diet is 1–2 g.

(4) *Lithium salts*

Lithium salts are useful in the management of manic-depressive illness. They calm manic patients and help to maintain them in a normal mood. Lithium is usually given as the carbonate (e.g. Priadel). The usual dose is 800–1600 mg daily, adjusted to keep plasma levels within the therapeutic range of 0·6–1·2 mmol/l. If toxic levels occur, the most serious effect is on the kidneys, resulting in a water-losing nephritis.

4. Drugs which stimulate the nervous system

It has already been mentioned that certain drugs stimulate the respiratory and vasomotor centres in the medulla (e.g. nikethamide, leptazol, strychnine, caffeine). Strychnine and caffeine also have a stimulating effect on others parts of the nervous system and must be considered further, although their use in modern medicine is very limited. Cocaine also has a stimulating effect.

Caffeine (300 mg)

This drug has a number of actions:
(1) Diuretic (p. 140).
(2) Respiratory stimulant (p. 126).
(3) Central nervous system stimulant. Caffeine excites the higher centres of the cerebrum, increasing mental activity and sensory impressions.

It is often combined with analgesics in a variety of tablets, e.g. Antidol, Antoin, Cafadol, Doloxene Compound-65, Hypon, Myolgin, Paralgin, Pardale, Saridone and Solpadeine.

It is also included in certain migraine remedies (e.g. Cafergot and Migril) to make the patient feel brighter.

Cocaine (16 mg) (CD)

This drug has two important and opposite actions. It stimulates the higher centres of the brain but depresses or paralyses the sensory endings of the peripheral nerves when applied locally (i.e. it acts as a local anaesthetic) (p. 180). The former action outweighs much of its value as a local anaesthetic and cocaine itself is only used occasionally. There are, however, many alternative local anaesthetics with a lesser effect on the higher centres.

Action on the higher centres

Cocaine stimulates the mental processes, producing hilarity and loquacity. In larger doses, it results in depression and finally coma. It is very prone to cause drug addiction and gives rise to serious results, with rapid mental and moral deterioration. For this reason its supply is most carefully guarded by the Misuse of Drugs Regulations.

Strychnine (2–8 mg)

This is the alkaloid of nux vomica and was used as a constituent of some arrow poisons. The main points about its action are:
(1) The highest centres of the brain are not markedly affected by therapeutic doses, although possibly the senses do become more acute after its administration.
(2) It stimulates the spinal cord so that reflexes are increased and become brisker.
(3) Both strychnine and nux vomica are very bitter and act as 'bitters' which improve the appetite and increase the tone of the stomach. They are used as 'tonics.

Strychnine poisoning

The main symptom is the occurrence of muscular spasms which, with larger doses, become generalized convulsions. They are due to stimulation of the spinal cord and resemble those occurring in tetanus. Consciousness remains unclouded.
Treatment:
(a) gastric lavage;
(b) intravenous injection of thiopentone to control convulsions;
(c) barbiturate or other sedative drugs by mouth.

Preparations of nux vomica and strychnine

Tincture of nux vomica, 2 ml.
Strychnine mixture BPC 1963. Dose: 15–30 ml.
Strychnine and iron mixture BPC, 1963. Dose: 15–30 ml.

Amphetamine sulphate (Benzedrine (2·5–10 mg) (CD))

The following drugs have a similar action and uses:

dexamphetamine (Dexedrine)
methyl amphetamine (Methedrine).

These synthetic drugs stimulate the higher centres, produce increased mental alertness and temporarily abolish fatigue. They are strongly habit-forming, i.e. addictive, and have been superseded by other drugs in the treatment of mental depression. Care should be taken not to give them near bedtime as they may result in insomnia. Locally they have an effect on the nasal mucous membrane like adrenaline and ephedrine (i.e. they are vasoconstrictors) but are not now used for this purpose because of the danger of addiction. For the same reason, they are no longer recommended for the treatment of obesity.

Almost the only indication for amphetamines now is narcolepsy.

Methylphenidate (Ritalin) (CD) is an alternative drug for the treatment of narcolepsy.

Dexamphetamine and methylphenidate are, paradoxically, also used in the treatment of the hyperkinetic syndrome in childhood. Sedatives and tranquillizers are generally disappointing in this condition.

5. Anticonvulsants

While it is not possible to state the cause of idiopathic epilepsy it is clear that the seizures are associated with some local increase in the irritability of the cerebral cortex and that by reducing this irritability by means of anticonvulsant drugs which have a sedative action on the cortex, the fits are controlled or even abolished. The drugs used may either be given alone or two may be combined.

Drugs used for major epilepsies
Phenobarbitone (Luminal)

Dose: 30–120 mg, 2 or 3 times daily.

Methylphenobarbitone (Prominal)

A drug similar in action to phenobarbitone which is said to produce less drowsiness and less mental depression.

Phenytoin (*Epanutin*)

This is the drug of first choice in the control of grand mal. Toxic symptoms are common and include swelling of gums, rashes, tremor and unsteadiness of movement. Occasionally megaloblastic anaemia occurs.
   Dose: 50–100 mg 2 to 3 times daily.

Sulthiame (*Ospolot*)

This drug is advocated for temporal lobe epilepsy.
   Dose: 10–15 mg/kg in divided doses.

Methoin (*Mesontoin*)

Dose: initially 50–100 mg daily.

Primidone (*Mysoline*)

Dose: 250–500 mg twice daily.

Pheneturide (*Benuride*)

Dose: 200 mg 3 times a day.

Beclamide (*Nydrane*)

Dose: up to eight 500-mg tablets daily.

Carbamazepine (*Tegretol*)

This drug is useful in temporal lobe epilepsy and grand mal. It is also useful in the treatment of trigeminal neuralgia.
   Dose: initially 100–200 mg once or twice daily.

Drugs used in petit mal
Phensuximide (*Milontin*)

Dose: 1–3 g daily.

Ethosuximide (Emeside, Zarontin)

This is usually considered the drug of choice in petit mal.
  Dose: 250–1500 mg daily.

Troxidone (Tridione, Trimethadione)

This drug, 600–1800 mg daily in divided doses, is sometimes employed in petit mal. Cases of agranulocytosis have followed its use which is, therefore, limited by its toxicity. Paramethadione (Paradione) is also used for petit mal.

Drugs suitable for all forms of epilepsy
Clonazapam (Rivotril)

Dose: 4–8 mg daily in divided doses.

Sodium valproate (Epilim)

Dose: initially 200 mg t.d.s.
  It should be given with water and food because it is otherwise likely to cause heartburn and vomiting. In this context, it is well to remember that antacids absorb anticonvulsants and prevent their absorption.
  Sodium valproate may be the drug of choice in petit mal and is useful in all forms of epilepsy. Its interaction with clonazepam may, however, cause a severe reaction and these two drugs should not be given together.

Status epilepticus

Intramuscular injection of (*a*) soluble phenobarbitone (200 mg) or (*b*) paraldehyde (5 ml) may be given, or intravenous injection of (*a*) diazepam (Valium; 0·15–0·25 mg/kg), (*b*) clonazepam (Rivotril; 1 mg), or (*c*) chlormethiazole (Heminevrin) infusion.

6. Drugs used in Parkinsonism

There are three particular facets of Parkinsonism which require treatment. They are:
(*a*) tremor

(b) rigidity

(c) hypokinesia (diminished mobility).

In general, drugs are more effective against rigidity than against tremor. Only levodopa and amantadine relieve hypokinesia.

Antiparkinson drugs fall into several groups as follows:

(1) Anticholinergic drugs (e.g. atropine, belladonna and stramonium)

Synthetic anticholinergic drugs are usually used and they include benzhexol (Artane), ethopropazine (Lysivane), orphenadrine hydrochloride (Disipal), procyclidine (Kemadrin), benztropine (Cogentin) and benapryzine (Brizin).

(2) Antihistamines

Drugs such as diphenhydramine (Benadryl) and phenindamine (Thephorin) may occasionally be of value.

(3) Levodopa (L-dopa, Larodopa, Brocadopa)

This compound repletes the depleted dopamine levels in the brains of patients with Parkinsonism. Results are often dramatic and sometimes spectacular; patients who have long been chair-bound may walk again. Improvement occurs early but does not usually reach its maximum for 6 weeks or more. The starting dose is 250 mg daily and dosage is increased by steps of 250 mg at intervals of 3–4 days until the optimum dosage level is reached. Too rapid an increase or too high a dosage is liable to cause side-effects. The average daily maintenance dose is 3 g and the usual maximum is 8 g. The drug is given in divided doses, three or four times a day. The principal side-effect, nausea, may be abolished or lessened by giving the drug with or after food. Other side-effects are vomiting, anorexia, hypotension, cardiac dysrhythmias, flushing, mental changes (especially agitation and paranoia), and involuntary movements such as facial grimacing and jerking of the limbs. Reduction of dosage is often all that is needed to abolish these side-effects.

Sinemet and Madopar are combinations of levodopa with an enzyme inhibitor (carbidopa or benzerazide). The latter inhibits the conversion of levodopa to dopamine in tissues other than the brain. Therapeutic levels of dopamine may therefore be achieved more quickly and with lower doses of levodopa. The side-effects of levodopa may at the same time be reduced.

(4) Amantadine (Symmetrel)

This compound has similar therapeutic effects to levodopa, to which, however, it is chemically unrelated. Side-effects (e.g. nervousness, insomnia, dizziness and psychiatric symptoms) are minimal and no elaborate build-up of dosage is necessary. The dose is 100 mg once daily for a week and thereafter 100 mg twice daily. Amantadine is also an antiviral agent (see p. 287).

Levodopa or amantidine is usually used in combination with an anticholinergic agent such as benzhexol in the treatment of Parkinsonism.

(5) Bromocriptine (Parlodel)

This is a semi-synthetic ergot alkaloid which stimulates dopamine receptors in the central nervous system and is therefore useful in Parkinsonism. The usual dose is 40–100 mg daily.

The drug is also used in the treatment of acromegaly and for the suppression of lactation.

Nausea is the most common side-effect and is less likely to occur if the drug is taken with food.

7. Drugs used in migraine
Treatment of the attack

The patient may experience relief from mild analgesics such as aspirin, paracetamol or Veganin. Other patients require **ergotamine.** This acts by constricting the painfully dilated extracranial arteries. It constricts other arteries at the same time and is therefore contraindicated in patients with serious vascular disease, e.g. coronary disease and hypertension. It is also contraindicated in pregnancy, because it stimulates the uterus to contract.

Ergotamine, to be effective, must be given very early in the attack. The most effective mode of administration is by subcutaneous or intramuscular injection (e.g. Femergin) 0·25–0·5 mg. Suppositories (2–6 mg) act quickly for patients who overcome the aesthetic objection to using them. Sublingual administration (e.g.

Lingraine) 2 mg, or inhalation of a measured dose (0·36 mg) from an aerosol (e.g. Medihaler-Ergotamine) is, however, usually adequate and is certainly more convenient. Oral administration, of tablets to be swallowed, is the least effective but is adequate for some patients. The dose is 1–2 mg ergotamine, repeated half-hourly (to a maximum of 6 mg) until relief is obtained. Caffeine is often used to enhance the action of ergotamine, as in Cafergot tablets and suppositories. In addition, in Migril tablets, cyclizine is used to counteract nausea and vomiting due either to the disease or the ergotamine.

Prevention of attacks (prophylaxis)

Prochlorperazine (Stemetil) and clonidine (Dixarit) may reduce the frequency of attacks of migraine. Clonidine (25–75 micrograms twice daily) acts directly on the blood vessels to diminish their responsiveness to constrictor and dilator stimuli. Pizotifen (Sanomigran) also has a prophylactic effect and is usually given in a dose of 725 micrograms three times a day. Methysergide (Deseril) is sometimes used when other drugs have failed. Its use is limited by occasional serious adverse reactions, e.g. retroperitoneal fibrosis which obstructs the ureters and causes hydronephrosis.

8. Drugs used in some other conditions
Subacute combined degeneration of the cord

Vitamin B_{12} is necessary (p. 110).

Multiple Sclerosis

Acute episodes may remit more quickly with intramuscular injections of ACTH or Synacthen Depot.

Chronic spasticity may be treated with baclofen (Lioresal), which acts at spinal level, or dantrolene (Dantrium) which acts directly on the muscle fibres. In both cases, a regime of gradually increasing dosage is used.

Myasthenia gravis

Neostigmine (p. 191), pyridostigmine (Mestinon) and distigmine (Ubretid).

Trigeminal neuralgia

Carbamazepine (Tegretol), 200 mg, 6-hourly.

Sydenham's Chorea (St Vitus' Dance)

Aspirin is given.

Syphillis of the nervous system

The usual antisyphilitic measures are employed.

Meningitis

Sulphonamide drugs are used for meningococcal meningitis and penicillin is used against pneumococcal meningitis. Meningitis due to *Haemophilus influenzae* is treated with chloramphenicol or ampicillin.

Toxic substances acting on nerves

Lead, arsenic, mercury and alcohol may all have a toxic action on the peripheral nerves resulting in peripheral neuritis. Various forms of paralysis ensue. The toxins of the diphtheria bacillus also have a special affinity for nervous tissue.

Local Anaesthetics (see also p. 208)

1. Local (topical) applications to mucous membranes

Because of the thinness of the epithelium of mucous membranes, some drugs are absorbed and can easily reach and paralyse the sensory nerve endings in the vicinity.

(a) Cocaine

This can be used as a solution (5–10 per cent) or ointment (4–10 per cent), especially in operations on the nose. The dangers of excessive absorption with toxic symptoms must always be remembered when cocaine is being used (see also p. 173). Cocaine drops (4 per cent) are of value in anaesthetizing the conjunctiva prior to the removal of foreign bodies and eye operations. It also dilates the pupil. Amethocaine eye-drops are usually preferable because they neither dilate the pupil nor damage the corneal epithelium which cocaine does. Solutions of these strengths must never be injected.

(b) Amethocaine (1–2 per cent)

This may be used in the same way as cocaine. It is also employed as a spray to anaesthetize the pharynx and larynx before the passage of a gastroscope and prior to bronchoscopy. It is less toxic than cocaine and, therefore, safer to use but is considerably more toxic than procaine.

(c) Benzocaine (Anaesthesin)

This has a similar action and is employed as a lozenge or ointment. It is useful for painful or irritating lesions of the mouth and anus, viz.:

compound benzocaine lozenge.
compound benzocaine ointment.

2. Drugs given by injection (see also p. 208)

These may be injected locally into the operation area (infiltration) or in the vicinity of the nerves which supply the area at some distance from the site of the operation (nerve-block). They should not be injected into inflamed or infected tissue. The most important are as follows.

Lignocaine (Xylocaine)

This is a local anaesthetic of low toxicity injected in strengths up to 2 per cent. It is a very stable substance, rapid in action, which can be stored indefinitely. The maximum dose is 200 mg or 500 mg with adrenaline. It may be used as a topical application to mucous membranes (2–4 per cent solution). An ointment (5 per cent) is also available.

It is interesting to note that lignocaine may be used intravenously in the treatment of some disorders of cardiac rhythm, especially those following myocardial infarction.

Procaine

Procaine is used as a 2 per cent solution (Novutox Plain) or in 2 per cent, 3 per cent and 4 per cent solutions with adrenaline (Novutox).

Cinchocaine (Nupercaine)

Formerly known as Percaine, and also used as a spinal anaesthetic, this must not be confused with procaine. It may be used locally but is very much stronger and more toxic than procaine and, therefore, weaker solutions are employed. It is also made in the form of an ointment.

Adrenaline (0·5 ml of 1 in 1000 solution) is often added to injected local anaesthetics in a dose not exceeding 0·5 mg or a greater concentration than 1 in 25 000. It should not be used when a digit is being anaesthetized. It acts on the blood vessels in the vicinity of the injection and constricts them, thereby diminishing the amount of local anaesthetic which can be carried away in the blood stream so that the duration of the anaesthesia is prolonged. In addition, the amount of bleeding is diminished.

3. Freezing the skin

Ethyl chloride spray is sometimes employed and, by its rapid evaporation, freezes the area to which it is applied. The duration of the effect is very short and it is only suitable for incising superficial abscesses. Complete anaesthesia is not always obtained and the process of thawing may be painful.

A most important warning must be given in connection with the use of all local and spinal anaesthetics. The names of the substances employed are often similar and may be confused. Further, they are used in strengths varying from 0·5 per cent to 10 per cent. Fatal accidents have occurred from the substitution of Percaine for procaine (hence the advantage of the name Nupercaine, or better still, cinchocaine for the former). Also mistakes can be made in reading the strengths on the labels by not observing the exact position of the decimal point. The nurse must therefore be most careful in handling these drugs and be quite sure that the one being put out for use is the correct one and in the strength in which it is ordered. The nurse must also check with the doctor whether a plain local anaesthetic solution or one containing adrenaline is required.

Spinal anaesthesia (Epidural block)

1·5 per cent lignocaine is introduced by means of lumbar puncture into the epidural (extradural) space of the spinal canal, where it surrounds the nerve roots in the neighbourhood of the injection. Here it paralyses the nervous tissue in the nerve roots so that impulses, both sensory and motor, are unable to pass. It follows that the motor impulses will not be able to pass from the anterior horn cells via the anterior nerve roots to the muscles which are, therefore, paralysed and completely relaxed. Likewise, sensory impulses coming from the periphery will not be able to enter the cord via the posterior nerve roots and pass up the sensory tracts to the brain. Therefore pain is not felt.

The paralysis also involves the nerves to the blood vessels of the limbs and abdominal organs which dilate and so accommodate more blood. There is thus less blood in the general circulation and the blood pressure tends to fall.

One of the most serious consequences of a fall in blood pressure is lack of blood to the brain. Lowering of the head of the operating table, an appropriate time after the spinal anaesthetic has been given, counteracts this effect of a fall in blood pressure.

If there are any signs of collapse during the operation, the head should be lowered in order to increase the blood supply to the brain, and a pressor drug such as metaraminol may be given by intravenous infusion.

Epidural injection has superseded subarachnoid injection because it is safer.

Epidural analgesia may be used to relieve pain in labour but it increases the number of forceps deliveries.

12 Drugs acting on the involuntary nervous system

It will be recalled that the involuntary nervous system consists of the sympathetic system together with the cranial and sacral autonomic systems (parasympathetic), viz.:

Sympathetic system supplies
{
pupils
heart
lungs, trachea, bronchi
stomach and intestines
adrenal glands
bladder
uterus.
}

Cranial autonomic supplies
{
pupils
heart
lungs, trachea, bronchi
stomach.
}

Sacral autonomic supplies
{
rectum
bladder
uterus.
}

The nerve fibres pass mainly to involuntary, unstriped muscle in the walls of the various organs and also to the muscle in the walls of the arteries, i.e. the autonomic system supplies the viscera as distinct from the skeletal muscles, which are supplied by the central nervous system.

A number of organs have both sympathetic and parasympathetic nerve-supplies which have opposite actions. Thus, the parasympathetic fibres which reach the heart carry impulses which slow the heart rate (inhibitors), whilse those from the sympathetic increase its rate (accelerators). The normal rate of the heart is maintained by a balance between the opposing impulses.

Further, the involuntary system is greatly influenced by the activities of the ductless glands. In particular the secretion from the adrenal gland, adrenaline, stimulates the sympathetic system and acts as a vasoconstrictor.

Just as reflex action in the central nervous system takes place in the spinal cord, which receives afferent impulses and sends out

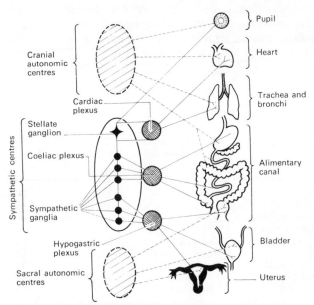

Fig. 12.1 Illustrating distribution of involuntary nervous system

efferent impulses, so reflex action occurs in the autonomic system through collections of nerve cells called ganglia. These ganglia also have connections with the spinal cord and brain. The sympathetic ganglia are situated in chains on either side of the vertebral column. The parasympathetic ganglia tend to be in or near the organ which they supply and are mainly grouped in the cranial and sacral autonomic centres.

Physiology

When an autonomic nerve is stimulated chemical substances are liberated which transmit the impulse at the nerve endings in the organ concerned. Other substances are also formed at the same time which antagonize the action of these stimulators and so prevent their effect being too powerful or too prolonged. These various substances differ in the sympathetic and parasympathetic nerve endings.

Parasympathetic stimulation liberates acetylcholine at the nerve endings. This is antagonized by cholinesterase.

Sympathetic stimulation liberates noradrenaline and adrenaline in addition to acetylcholine. At the same time adrenaline and noradrenaline may be secreted from the adrenal glands. Monoamine oxidase (MAO) antagonizes their action.

Table 12.1. Summary of autonomic effects

Organ	Effect of sympathetic stimulation (adrenaline)	Effect of parasympathetic stimulation (carbachol pilocarpine: eserine)	Action of atropine
Pupils	Dilated	Contracted	Dilated
Heart rate	Increased	Decreased	Increased
Bronchial muscle	Relaxed	Contracted	Relaxed
Stomach movements and secretion	Decreased	Increased	Decreased
Saliva	Slight increase	Increased	Decreased
Bladder muscle	Relaxed	Contracted	Relaxed
Bladder sphincter	Contracted	Relaxed	Nil
Blood vessels	Contracted	Nil	Nil

The involuntary system is somewhat complicated and classification of the drugs which affect it is made more difficult by the fact that they all differ in their mode of action. As a matter of convenience they may be divided into four main groups:
(1) Those which produce results similar to stimulation of the sympathetic (sympathomimetic).
(2) Those which 'block' the action of adrenaline and noradrenaline on the sympathetic receptors in the tissues.
(3) Those which produce results similar to stimulation of the parasympathetic (parasympathomimetic).
(4) The drugs of the atropine group (acetylcholine inhibitors), which 'block the action of acetylcholine.

Drugs acting on the involuntary nervous system may do so in a number of ways. Among the most important are:
(1) General stimulants.
(2) Ganglion-blocking agents which prevent reflex action taking place.
(3) Drugs suppressing the action of:
   (a) cholinesterase, thus increasing the action of acetylcholine. Such drugs are called anticholinesterases, an example being neostigmine;
   (b) monoamine oxidase, thus increasing the action of adrenaline and noradrenaline. Such drugs are called MAO inhibitors and they are used in the treatment of depression. An example is tranylcypromine (Parnate).

Cheese contains tyramine which is normally destroyed by monoamine oxidase in the gut wall and liver and so causes no harm. MAO inhibitors allow the tyramine to enter the general circulation and to cause the release of noradrenaline from local stores. This results in acute severe hypertension which may cause a subarachnoid haemorrhage.

(4) Drugs inhibiting the action of acetylcholine. Examples are atropine and belladonna.

Drugs acting as sympathetic stimulants
Adrenaline

Adrenaline or epinephrine is the active principle extracted from the medulla of the adrenal glands, and normally small amounts are continually passing from the glands into the blood stream. It is produced synthetically for therapeutic purposes.

If it is remembered that adrenaline stimulates the sympathetic system and that the symptoms of sympathetic stimulation are those which occur in fight or fright, i.e. those which are most necessary to the individual for self-preservation, it will not be difficult to understand some of its actions. Thus:

(1) The maximum amount of blood is required for the muscles of the body, therefore there is a vasoconstriction of the blood vessels in the skin and alimentary organs. This also leads to a rise in blood pressure.

(2) Glucose is needed in order to supply energy to the muscles, and so the liver liberates glucose from its store of glycogen into the blood.

(3) The plain muscle of the bronchi is relaxed, thus allowing the maximum amount of air to enter the lungs.

Uses

(i) Relaxation of spasm of the bronchial muscles in asthma (p. 133). Small doses of adrenaline 0·05 to 0·5 ml of a 1 in 1000 solution, which is the strength in which adrenaline is generally used, are injected subcutaneously as soon as the attack starts and are more efficacious than larger ones given when it is fully established. If the responsibility of administering the drug is left to the nurse, she should, therefore, give it as soon as possible. It is not uncommon to be summoned to a patient who has had an attack of asthma which has been in progress for a considerable period, for whom an injection of adrenaline has been ordered 'p.r.n.' (whenever required) and which could have been given by the nurse at its onset. An intelligent patient may be taught to give the injection to himself.

(ii) As a cardiac stimulant. By stimulating the heart and constricting the peripheral arteries and those of the abdominal organs the blood pressure is raised, so that adrenaline is sometimes used in the treatment of shock and collapse. The injection of adrenaline directly into the heart will sometimes re-start the heart beating when it has stopped (cardiac arrest, e.g. in anaesthesia, asphyxia, drowning or carbon monoxide poisoning).

(iii) Adrenaline has a powerful local action in constricting the blood vessels when injected or applied to an open surface, i.e. it is a local haemostatic. Thus, it may be used as a spray or on gauze soaked in the solution for epistaxis, and for plugging a bleeding tooth socket (p. 61). Its value in delaying the absorption and so prolonging the action of a local anaesthetic has also been mentioned (p. 182).

(iv) It is sometimes used in allergic conditions such as urticaria and angioneurotic oedema, and in anaphylaxis.

Adrenaline is destroyed by the digestive juices and so is inactive when given by mouth.

Preparations

Injection of adrenaline tartrate is issued in ampoules of 0·5 ml and 1·0 ml. The dose is 0·05 to 0·5 ml subcutaneously, depending on age. Doses of 1 ml are, however, sometimes given.

Solution of adrenaline hydrochloride (1 in 1000) is not given by injection.

Other preparations include sprays, ointments and suppositories (in which it is sometimes combined with cocaine).

Isoprenaline (5–20 mg)

This has a similar action to adrenaline and may be given either by inhalation or in the form of tablets which are allowed to dissolve under the tongue. It is frequently used in the treatment of asthma. Intravenous isoprenaline (5 mg in 500 ml of 5 per cent dextrose) and Saventrine, a long-acting oral form of isoprenaline, are of value in the treatment of heart block.

Noradrenaline

Noradrenaline (dose 2–8 micrograms per minute by intravenous infusion) is a hormone secreted by sympathetic nerve endings and by the adrenal medulla, and also produced synthetically, which raises blood pressure by acting as a vasoconstrictor. It is sometimes used in the treatment of shock (p. 99).

Levophed is a suitable preparation.

(N.B.—One ampoule contains either 2 ml or 4 ml of 1 in 1000 solution. One ml contains the equivalent of 1 mg of noradrenaline. One ampoule, 4 ml, is added to 1000 ml of saline or dextrose which is infused at the rate of 0·5 to 2 ml per minute by intravenous drip.)

Ephedrine (16–60 mg)

This is an alkaloid obtained from a Chinese plant, but can also be prepared by chemical means. Its action and uses are very similar to those of adrenaline. It is, however, slower and more prolonged in action and has advantages when used in some conditions. Unlike adrenaline, it can be given by mouth and is employed in regular doses between attacks of asthma in order to reduce their frequency.

Ergotamine tartrate

This is an alkaloid which is extracted from ergot (a drug used for its effect on the uterus, p. 244). Although it has some actions which are similar to those of adenaline, it is not used for the same purposes but may be conveniently mentioned here. Its most important action is to constrict the blood vessels (vasoconstriction). This may be so marked that if used in excessive doses or over a long period it may lead to gangrene of the extremities. It is sometimes used in the treatment of migraine (p. 178).

It may be given (*a*) by injection (0·25–0·5 mg), (*b*) by mouth (1 to 2 mg), when tablets should be placed under the tongue. A proprietary preparation is known as Femergin.

Sympathetic (adrenergic) receptors

The sympathetic nervous system exerts its effects via receptors which are present in various tissues. The receptors are of two kinds—alpha (α) and beta (β). The α-receptors are generally *excitatory* (stimulating) and the β-receptors are generally *inhibitory*: an important exception is in the heart, where the β-receptors are excitatory.

Stimulation of α-receptors causes contraction of smooth muscle in the walls of blood vessels, and hence *vasoconstriction*, contraction of the iris, with consequent *dilation of the pupil*, contraction of the sphincter of the urinary bladder and contraction of the pilomotor muscles—the little muscles which make hairs stand up. One substance which stimulates α-receptors is **noradrenaline.** The action of noradrenaline is inhibited by drugs, such as phentolamine (Rogitine), which block the α-receptors

Stimulation of the β-receptors results in relaxation of smooth muscle in the walls of blood vessels, and hence *vasodilatation*, especially in skeletal muscles, relaxation of smooth muscle in the walls of bronchi, with consequent *bronchodilatation*, relaxation of smooth muscle in the walls of the intestines, relaxation of the muscular wall of the urinary bladder and stimulation of the heart so that it beats more rapidly and more forcibly. **Isoprenaline** is a drug which stimulates β-receptors and thereby produces these effects. Salbutamol (Ventolin) is a beta-adrenergic stimulator with selective action on bronchial muscle. **Adrenaline** stimulates both α- and β-receptors, the result being the sum of all the effects mentioned. The effect of adrenaline on a tissue depends on the affinity of the substance for the receptors and on the proportions of the two types of receptor present in the tissue. **Propranolol** is a β-receptor blocking agent and prevents the stimulation of β-receptors by noradrenaline. It is of value in cases of angina pectoris because it inhibits sympathomimetic influences and consequently slows the heart, reduces its force of contraction and decreases its oxygen consumption. It is also effective against certain disturbances of cardiac rhythm.

Propanolol is contraindicated in patients with asthma since it inhibits the bronchodilating effects of adrenaline and may result in bronchospasm. Some more recently introduced β-receptor blocking agents, e.g. acebutalol and metoprolol, are more selective in their action on the heart and may often be used in asthmatic patients.

Drugs acting as parasympathetic stimulants

There are a number of drugs which have an action similar to that of the parasympathetic system. Their main actions are:
(1) To stimulate the muscular movements of the bowel, i.e. to increase peristalsis. They are therefore used in conditions in

which the gut is distended, e.g. postoperative distension, paralytic ileus, acute dilation of the stomach, certain types of constipation.
(2) To dilate the blood vessels in the limbs in conditions such as Raynaud's syndrome.
(3) To relax the sphincter of the bladder, e.g. postoperative retention of urine.

Group I. Acetylcholine type

Carbachol, 0·25 mg.

Group II. Anticholinesterase drugs
Physostigmine (*Eserine*) (0·6–1·2 mg)

This is an alkaloid which has two main uses:
(i) to relieve paralytic conditions of the bowel, e.g. postoperative distension, but drugs such as carbachol have tended to replace it;
(ii) to contract the pupil of the eye, e.g. in the treatment of glaucoma (p. 247).

Neostigmine (*Prostigmin*)

This is a similar drug used especially in the treatment of myasthenia gravis. It may also be used in paralytic ileus and atony of the bladder. The dose given by mouth is 15 mg, or by injection, 1 mg.

Pyridostigmine (*Mestinon*)

Pyridostigmine, which has a more prolonged action than neostigmine, is also used in myasthenia gravis. Five to twenty 60-mg tablets are given daily.

Distigmine (*Ubretid*)

Distigmine has a much longer duration of action than pyridostigmine. The dose in myasthenia gravis is 5–10 mg twice daily by mouth.

Ambenonium (Mytelase)

This is another long-acting anticholinesterase drug used in myasthenia gravis. The dose is usually 5–25 mg three or four times a day.

Pilocarpine (3–12 mg)

This is an alkaloid obtained from a plant. It has two main actions:
(i) It stimulates the secretion of sweat and saliva.
(ii) It contracts the pupil of the eye.

Drugs inhibiting the action of acetylcholine (atropine group)

Atropine (250 micrograms to 1 mg)

Atropine is an alkaloid obtained from the belladonna plant (Deadly Nightshade), and the effects of belladonna preparations in the body are mainly due to the atropine which they contain. Atropine has many actions and is used for a number of therapeutic purposes.

Action on plain muscle

Atropine relaxes plain muscle. Thus it helps to relax the spasm of the bronchial muscle in asthma and is included in some inhalants (e.g. Brovon, Rybarvin). It relaxes spasm in the muscle of the bile duct and ureter and so is of value in the treatment of biliary and renal colic.

Action on secretions

Atropine diminishes the secretion of the salivary glands, the sweat glands and the glands in the mucous membrane of the respiratory tract.

Its power of diminishing the secretion of mucus from the respiratory tract is made use of in the pre-anaesthetic injection of atropine.

It may be given with morphine to prevent the accumulation of bronchial secretion in the lungs, because morphine depresses the cough reflex and if an excess of mucus is present it may accumulate in the smaller bronchioles.

Action on the stomach

Atropine diminishes the movements of the stomach and also the amount of gastric juice secreted. Related compounds (e.g. Pro-

Banthine) are therefore sometimes used in the treatment of peptic ulcer. It also tends to diminish intestinal movements and spasms and so may be given in cases of colic.

Action on the eye (p. 247)

Atropine when given by hypodermic injection or instilled into the conjunctival sac, dilates the pupils. Atropine drops are therefore employed to dilate the pupils in cases of iritis and eye injury.

Action on the heart

Atropine blocks the inhibitory effect of the vagus nerve and so causes an increase in heart rate and contractility. This action may be of value when bradycardia and hypotension complicate acute myocardial infarction.

Poisoning

Poisoning by atropine or belladonna produces the following symptoms:
(1) Dryness of the mouth and throat with hoarseness of the voice.
(2) Wide dilatation of the pupils.
(3) Stimulation of the higher centres of the nervous system which is not apparent when therapeutic doses are used, viz. restlessness, talkativeness, delirium and often violent maniacal excitement. With large doses this stage of excitement soon passes off and is followed by depression developing into coma.
(4) Skin eruptions, e.g. generalized erythema, may be present.

Treatment
(1) Gastric lavage.
(2) Artificial ventilation and oxygen.
(3) Neostigmine 2-hourly until skin becomes moist.

Preparations of belladonna

For external application:
    Glycerin of belladonna
    Belladonna plaster.
    These preparations are applied externally for the relief of pain, and possibly act as counter-irritants.

Preparations of atropine

Atropine sulphate injection, BP (0·25–2 mg)
Atropine sulphate tablets, BP (0·25–2 mg).

Most of the other preparations, e.g. ointments and drops, are used for eye conditions (p. 247).

Substances like atropine

Homatropine (p. 247). Used in eye work to dilate the pupil.

Atropine methonitrate (Eumydrin) (p. 71). Used in congenital pyloric stenosis, whooping cough, and in aerosol inhalations for asthma.

Hyoscine hydrobromide (*Scopolamine*) (0·3–0·6 mg)

This is one of the alkaloids obtained from hyoscyamus. Some of its actions resemble those of atropine but it does not cause tachycardia. In addition, it depresses the central nervous system and so has an hypnotic action. It has the following uses:

(1) As an hypnotic, by injection, in the treatment of mania and acute delirium, including delirium tremens, etc., although in some cases it appears to increase excitement.

(2) To relieve the spasm and muscular rigidity in paralysis agitans.

Like atropine, it inhibits the secretion of saliva and dryness of the mouth may be produced. This is counteracted by giving pilocarpine (6 mg) at the same time. In this instance hyoscine is given by mouth in the form of a tablet.

(3) To prevent travel sickness.

Hyoscyamus

This is the dried leaf of a plant. It is mainly used for the treatment of bladder conditions. Preparations include a tincture (dose 2–4 ml).

Synthetic anticholinergic drugs

These drugs, such as propantheline (Pro-Banthine), reduce secretion and motility in the gastro-intestinal tract, and are therefore used in the treatment of peptic ulcers.

13 Drugs used in general anaesthesia

Although chloroform, introduced by Simpson in 1847, was the first anaesthetic to come into general use, the anaesthetic properties of nitrous oxide were observed by Davy in 1788 and Long used ether in 1842. In more recent years many new substances have been discovered and employed in addition to those substances given by intravenous injection and as local, spinal and nerve-blocking injections. Chloroform, in particular, has largely fallen into disuse. The fact that it is non-inflammable has been an advantage when diathermy has been employed or when there has been a possibility of the development of static electricity in the operating theatre—a spark from which may ignite an explosive mixture.

General anaesthesia

Drugs used in the production of general anaesthesia fall into three main classes:

(1) Volatile substances the vapour of which is inhaled, e.g.:

chloroform trichlorethylene (Trilene)
ether halothane (Fluothane).
ethyl chloride

(2) Gases such as:

nitrous oxide cyclopropane.

(3) Substances given by:

intravenous injection, e.g. thiopentone sodium (Pentothal)
rectal injection, e.g. bromethol (Avertin).

Preoperative preparation

(a) General.
(b) Immediate (premedication).

(a) *General*

Most patients about to undergo an operation have some degree of apprehension. Therefore, reassurance reinforced, if necessary, by some sedative drug is usually required. Breathing exercises are desirable especially in patients with chronic chest disease and suitable antibiotics to control any infection may be necessary. Special conditions such as diabetes may need careful adjustment of diet and drugs; any anaemia should be corrected by blood transfusion before and during operation or treated with anti-anaemic drugs if time permits. Patients on steroids require special consideration and additional doses may be required. Patients being treated with the monoamine oxidase inhibitors (MAOI), e.g. iproniazid (Marsilid), phenelzine (Nardil), isocarboxazid (Marplan), tranylcypromine (Parnate), should not receive pethidine as they greatly enhance its effect.

In other words, before anaesthesia an enquiry should always be made into the general health of the patient and any drugs which he or she may be taking.

(b) Premedication before general anaesthesia

(i) A sedative the night before operation is usually desirable.

(ii) Immediate premedication $1–1\frac{1}{2}$ hours before with papaveretum (Omnopon), 10–20 mg, and hyoscine (Scopolamine), 0·2–0·4 mg, is usually employed. Atropine, which helps to dry secretions, may be used instead of hyoscine.

NB.—Morphine and allied substances (papaveretum) should be used with the greatest caution, if ever, in young children. Atropine may be all that is required; it may produce tachycardia but it is usually well tolerated by young children. Rectal thiopentone may be used as a preoperative sedative if it is desired to avoid injections.

Postoperative management

With the use of muscle relaxants modern anaesthetic techniques are generally directed to light anaesthesia. Restlessness and vomiting may therefore occur early and even during the transfer of the patient from the operating theatre to the ward. At all times one of the most important things is to keep a clear airway and to ensure that the tongue does not fall backwards, by pulling the tongue forwards with the finger if necessary and then turning the head or body to one side and holding the jaw forwards. If vomiting occurs the head should be lowered and a suction apparatus employed.

In many severe cases the patient is moved directly into a recovery ward or intensive care unit before return to a general ward. Intravenous drips, blood transfusion and oxygen administration must be continued as required. Solid food is generally withheld for 12–24 hours but sips of fluid are permitted when consciousness has returned.

Stages of anaesthesia

Basically there are three stages during the induction of general anaesthesia, especially with ether, but with modern premedication or the use of intravenous anaesthetics these are not usually observed.

Stage 1. Mental dullness and analgesia.
Stage 2. Excitement.
Stage 3. Surgical anaesthesia.

1. The stage of mental dullness

The first effect is a sensation of slight suffocation and warmth of the body due to dilation of the blood vessels in the skin. The senses become less acute, voices appear distant and may be replaced by ringing sounds and other noises. The patient has a 'far away' feeling and to some extent the appreciation of pain becomes dulled though not necessarily abolished.

2. The stage of excitement

This is variable. In children it is often nonexistent; in some, scarcely evident; in others, slight movements may become violent struggles, secrets may become common property, bad language in one person may have its counterpart in prayer in another, abuse may alternate with protestations of affection, while the vocal efforts may be ecclesiastical in character, operatic or reminiscent of the music hall.

3. The stage of anaesthesia

The third stage of complete anaesthesia is ushered in as the muscles relax and the struggles cease. Vocal refrains give place to regular breathing, which tends to become slower and more shallow as the depth of anaesthesia increases. The pupils contract somewhat, only to dilate again if the anaesthesia becomes dangerously deep, the corneal reflex is lost and finally there is no longer any pupillary reaction to light. The cough reflex is abolished and unless the jaw is supported, the tongue tends to fall back and impede respiration.

The pulse generally remains steady in rate and regular in rhythm, unless the patient is gravely ill or the operation is very prolonged, when it may become more rapid, weaker and, sometimes, irregular. Blood pressure tends to fall a little, except with ether anaesthesia, during which it is generally maintained. In some instances the fall may be considerable and cause grave anxiety.

During recovery, the patient returns to consciousness through the same stages, although they may be less obvious. Reflexes return, there is often some degree of restlessness and, finally, a period of drowsiness and dulled mental state before full recovery is attained.

Summary

(i) Anaesthetics given by inhalation reach the lungs in the inspired air. They pass through the alveoli into the blood, by which they are carried to the cells of the brain. Here they act by depressing the activity of the cells to such an extent that consciousness is lost.

(ii) The tendon, pupillary and corneal reflexes are lost.

(iii) The cough and vomiting reflexes are lost.

(iv) The muscles are relaxed.

(v) The blood pressure falls progressively with increasing depth of anaesthesia in the cases of chloroform and halothane.

(vi) The blood vessels of the skin are dilated. Therefore, there is a tendency to considerable loss of heat from the body. This is minimized by clothing the patient suitably in a flannel gown and woollen stockings, and by maintaining the temperature of the operating theatre.

(vii) Volatile anaesthetics are excreted from the body mainly by the lungs. Therefore the inhalation of carbon dioxide and oxygen mixture after the administration has ceased stimulates the respiratory centre so that the increased rate and depth of breathing hastens their excretion (p. 126).

NB.—There are three important questions which a nurse should ask, and verify, of every patient about to have a general anaesthetic:

(1) Have you any false teeth?

(2) Have you had any food or drink during the last four hours?

(3) Is the bladder empty?

1. Volatile substances

Chloroform

This is a heavy volatile liquid having a characteristic sweetish odour and is a very powerful anaesthetic. Its only advantage is that it is non-inflammable and non-explosive. On the other hand, it is very dangerous because it causes severe depression of the vaso-motor centre and myocardial depression with cardiac arrest. In the presence of adrenaline it may lead to ventricular fibrillation and may later have a fatal toxic effect on the liver (delayed chloroform poisoning). Therefore, it is now rarely, if ever, used.

Ether (diethyl ether)

This is a light, colourless, highly volatile liquid which evaporates very quickly and produces a marked cooling of the body surface to which it is applied. It dissolves fat and oil and is sometimes used for cleaning the skin, especially when an injured area is contaminated with oil or grease. It undergoes chemical change if exposed to strong light and is therefore kept in amber-coloured bottles.

It may be administered by the 'open method' on a mask or by a 'closed method' using a special anaesthetic apparatus. The endotracheal (intratracheal) route may also be used.

It has the following advantages as an anaesthetic:

(i) It does not depress the respiratory centre or the heart except in large doses and, therefore, there is a considerable margin of safety in its administration. Chloroform is 25 times more toxic to the heart.

(ii) It does not tend seriously to lower the blood pressure and so is useful in cases of shock.

Disadvantages include:

(i) It tends to irritate the bronchial mucous membrane.

(ii) It is highly inflammable and, when mixed with air or oxygen, forms a highly explosive mixture. Under no circumstances must there be a naked light or any apparatus liable to produce a spark, e.g. diathermy, or high temperature, e.g. the electric cautery, in the room while ether is being used.

Metal anaesthetic trolleys and operating tables, etc., with rubber castors are liable to carry a charge of electricity which may produce a small spark, and this has been sufficient to cause explosions and fires, having fatal results. It is therefore customary to 'earth' such apparatus by means of a metal chain which makes contact with the ground and to use trolleys with special wheels. 'Antistatic' wheels are coloured yellow.

Ethyl chloride

This is a very volatile liquid which evaporates so rapidly that it produces a freezing effect on the skin. Advantage is taken of this to produce local anaesthesia. It has an unpleasant smell and, for purposes of general anaesthesia, is often mixed with eau-de-Cologne. Ethyl chloride has a powerful action and induces anaesthesia rapidly. For general anaesthesia it is only suitable for short operations lasting a few minutes, e.g. incision of abscesses, etc., and for inducing anaesthesia which is continued by the administration of ether. It is usually given on an open mask.

Trichlorethylene (Trilene)

This is a useful, non-inflammable anaesthetic which is less toxic than chloroform. It is non-irritant to the respiratory passages but does not produce the complete muscular relaxation necessary for some major operations. It may be used in obstetrics. An added blue colour distinguishes it from other liquids.

Halothane (Fluothane)

The vapour of this colourless volatile liquid is a potent anaesthetic which is non-irritant to the bronchial tree. As ordinarily used it is neither explosive nor inflammable. It may be used for induction (mixed with an oxygen/nitrous oxide mixture if desired) and for maintenance. It induces anaesthesia easily and rapidly. Maintenance is straightforward and recovery is rapid and smooth, usually without nausea or vomiting. It causes a moderate fall in blood pressure, which is desirable in some cases and undesirable in others. Very rarely, hepatitis has occurred after operations performed under halothane anaesthesia (especially after repeated exposure to the drug), and is possibly due to a hypersensitivity (immunological) reaction.

Adrenaline injections may precipitate cardiac dysrhythmias in patients anaesthetized with halothane. The dose of adrenaline is therefore restricted and a β-receptor blocker is administered if necessary.

Methoxyflurane (Penthrane)

This is a clear, almost colourless liquid with a vapour which has a characteristic fruity odour. For general anaesthesia it is usually used together with nitrous oxide and oxygen, following induction by an intravenous agent such as thiopentone.

As with halothane (another halogenated anaesthetic agent), methoxyflurane anaesthesia has on rare occasions been followed by jaundice or other evidence of hepatic damage. An excessive dosage of methoxyflurane may have a toxic effect on the kidneys (nephrotoxicity), associated with a high serum level of inorganic fluoride. The use of methoxyflurane is avoided in patients with impaired renal function. All patients who receive methoxyflurane should have their fluid intake and output carefully charted in order to detect polyuria or oliguria.

Apart from its use in the maintenance of general anaesthesia, methoxyflurane is used alone (0·35 per cent in air) or with nitrous oxide for obstetrical analgesia. It is approved for use with the Cardiff Inhaler by midwives for analgesia during labour. The total dosage of methoxyflurane used in this way should not exceed 15 ml of the liquid.

Enflurane and isoflurane

These are newer halogenated compounds (containing fluoride and chloride radicals) used as inhalational anaesthetic agents. They are non-flammable volatile liquids. They are very potent anaesthetic agents but are poor analgesics, unsuitable for obstetrical analgesia.

2. Gaseous substances
Nitrous oxide (N_2O)

Nitrous oxide is a colourless gas having a very faint odour and sweetish taste. It is the oldest anaesthetic and its early name 'laughing gas' is indicative of the hilarity which may be produced during the excitement stage of induction or recovery. It is stored in cylinders and administered via a bag and rubber face-piece, either directly from the cylinders for short anaesthesia, or by means of more elaborate apparatus for prolonged administration.

Advantages:

(i) It is a very safe anaesthetic if administered with 20 to 40 per cent oxygen;

(ii) it does not lower blood pressure or increase shock;

(iii) it rarely produces vomiting;

(iv) it may be given by the endotracheal method or nasally.

Disadvantages:

(i) cumbersome and expensive apparatus is necessary for its administration;

(ii) it is not always possible to obtain full muscular relaxation without adequate premedication with a hypnotic or basal anaesthetic, and the addition of ether may be necessary. The quantity of ether required, however, is much less than when ether is used alone and, in this respect, nitrous oxide is one of the most useful anaesthetics available.

Use in midwifery

Inhalations of nitrous oxide and oxygen are supplied pre-mixed (50 per cent of each) in a cylinder and administered by the patient herself with an Entonox apparatus. This apparatus may also be used, in ambulances for example, for the relief of pain due to myocardial infarction.

Cyclopropane

This is a non-irritating gas which has powerful anaesthetic properties. It can be given with large amounts of oxygen, with which it may form an explosive mixture. It is only used with safety by experts, but has advantages which render it especially valuable in thoracic surgery.

3. Substances given by injection

A. Substances given by intravenous injection

(a) Barbiturates

(i) As general anaesthetics for short operations.

(ii) For longer operations if repeated doses are given or a continuous drip method employed.

(iii) For induction of anaesthesia followed by ether or nitrous oxide.

(iv) As basal anaesthetics.

(v) To control the spasms of tetanus.

They are all extremely quick in action and if given rapidly the patient passes into unconsciousness in less than 30 seconds. The effect of a full single dose of Pentothal lasts about 15 minutes; that of Brietal for 5 to 7 minutes. This may be prolonged, as stated above, by repeated injections of smaller doses or by a continuous drip method.

Great care must be taken to maintain an efficient airway. The jaw, which always tends to fall back even before the injection has been completed, must be properly supported until recovery from the anaesthetic is in sight.

The patient must be lying flat during the administration as a fall in blood pressure is produced and, if the patient were allowed to sit up, e.g. in a dental chair, the lack of blood supply to the brain might be sufficient to produce dangerous symptoms. Twitching of the muscles, which may be violent, is sometimes observed.

> The solutions are strong irritants and it is most important that none should get into the tissues surrounding the vein. The immediate injection of Hyalase in normal saline into the area is helpful. Accidental injection into an artery is even more serious and may lead to gangrene.

Thiopentone sodium, BP (Pentothal)

This drug, 250–500 mg, is dissolved in 10 ml of sterile distilled water (Water for Injection, BP) before injection. About 5 to 10 ml are generally required to induce anaesthesia.

Methohexitone sodium (Brietal sodium)

50–120 mg intravenously, gives a short period of anaesthesia with quick recovery. It is also useful for induction of more prolonged anaesthesia.

(b) Eugenol derivatives, e.g. propanidid (Epontal)

This group of drugs is derived from oil of cloves (eugenol). Their action is brief and they are useful in cases where an extremely rapid recovery of consciousness is required. Unlike barbiturates they do not cause a hangover and they are therefore useful for minor operations on out-patients. Propanidid is, however, more likely to cause postoperative vomiting and this is a definite drawback to the use of the drug.

(c) Etomidate

This drug is chemically related to propanidid. It very rapidly produces unconsciousness of brief duration and is used for induction of anaesthesia. It has few side-effects but may induce uncoordinated movements.

(d) Ketamine (Ketalar)

This is a rapidly acting agent which produces an anaesthetic state with profound analgesia. Anaesthesia lasts for 5 to 10 minutes and the drug is best suited to short procedures. It is used intravenously for induction of anaesthesia, for supplementing weaker anaesthetic agents such as nitrous oxide, and as the sole agent for anaesthesia in some cases. It is also used intramuscularly, mainly in children.

It produces a temporary elevation of pulse rate and blood pressure and is contraindicated in patients with a history of a cerebrovascular accident and in patients with hypertension. Tonic and clonic movements occur in a few patients receiving ketamine.

(e) Steroid agents, e.g. Althesin

Althesin is a mixture of alphaxalone and alphadolone. It gives a pleasant induction and recovery. Postoperative nausea is infrequent. An occasional adverse reaction consists of hypotension, bronchospasm and flushing, which may recur, in milder form, after an intermission of 12 hours.

(f) Flunitrazepam

This is related to nitrazepam. The injectable preparation may be used as an intravenous induction agent.

B. Substances given by rectal injection

These are now rarely used as 'basal anaesthetics' with the object of rendering the patient drowsy or unconscious before reaching the operating theatre. Their disadvantages are that respiration may be depressed and that once the dose has been given and absorbed it is slowly excreted so that should the patient collapse little can be done to hasten the recovery from the anaesthetic. They include:

Bromethol (Avertin)

This still has a use in the treatment of some cases of eclampsia but may be contraindicated in some associated diseases, e.g. acute renal insufficiency.

The patient must be closely supervised by a nurse from the time bromethol is given until consciousness is regained.

Paraldehyde

This drug, which is described under hypnotics (p. 158), is sometimes given in appropriate doses per rectum as a basal anaesthetic. Up to 0·6 ml/kg body weight is given in saline as a 10 per cent solution. It is less powerful than bromethol.

Aids to anaesthesia
Muscle relaxants
1. Tubocurarine (Tubarine)

Preparations of curare and similar substances, e.g. gallamine (Flaxedil), and pancuronium are given by injection in order to increase muscular relaxation, thus diminishing the amount of general anaesthetic necessary. These drugs act by competing with acetylcholine, the normal chemical transmitter, at the neuromuscular junction. Their action is potentiated by diazepam, ether, and certain antibiotics. A test dose of 5 mg of tubocurarine is often given intravenously to detect unusually sensitive individuals. If after 4 minutes there is no indication of unusual sensitivity, another 10–25 mg are given. Repeated doses are given as necessary during the course of the operation. If recovery of respiration is delayed after tubocurarine, its action can be antagonized with neostigmine, 1–5 mg intravenously, preceded by atropine 1 mg.

Apart from its use in anaesthesia, tubocurarine may be used in the treatment of tetanus and in a diagnostic test for myasthenia gravis.

2. Pancuronium (Pavulon)

This is a potent neuromuscular blocking agent with an onset of action sufficiently rapid to permit endotracheal intubation without using a depolarizing agent. The normal adult dose range is 4–6 mg intravenously. The duration of effect is about 45 minutes and supplementary doses of 2 mg can be given as required. The effects of the drug are easily reversed with neostigmine and atropine. Cardiovascular side-effects, if any, are minimal and hypotension is not induced.

3. Suxamethonium

The usual dose is 25–100 mg intravenously. Suxamethonium produces neuromuscular block by depolarizing the motor end plates in muscle. It rapidly produces profound muscular relaxation of brief duration (less than 5 minutes). It facilitates endotracheal intubation and is also useful in electroconvulsive therapy (ECT). There is no specific antagonist to suxamethonium. Neostigmine prolongs its action. Normal individuals possess an enzyme (cholinesterase) which destroys suxamethonium. Some individuals exist who have a hereditary abnormality or deficiency of the enzyme and cannot therefore destroy the drug. These patients fail to resume spontaneous breathing after suxamethonium administration. They have to be maintained on a mechanical ventilator until the relaxant has been excreted or until sufficient cholinesterase has been given by way of fresh blood transfusion.

4. Mephenesin (Myanesin)

This is a synthetic substance which produces some muscular relaxation, but generally insufficient for surgery. It appears to act on the spinal cord and has been used in strychnine poisoning and tetanus.

It is now used only by mouth as a general muscle relaxant in spastic conditions.

Induced hypotension

Reducing the blood pressure will diminish bleeding during an operation which may thereby be conducted in a relatively bloodless field. This may be important when fine structures may have to be identified, as in neurosurgery and ENT surgery. There are various means of inducing a controlled fall in blood pressure and the easiest is to administer hypotensive drugs, e.g. ganglion-blocking agents, intravenously. Postoperatively the patient must be left lying supine unless express orders are given to the contrary. If the patient is sat up before the effect of the drug has fully worn off, his blood pressure may drop dangerously. A suitable ganglion-blocker is trimetaphan (Arfonad) which is short-acting and is usually given as a continuous intravenous infusion.

Halothane by itself may produce a surgically adequate degree of hypotension and ganglion-blockers are used less frequently than they were.

Vasopressors

Vasopressors have little place in anaesthesia but it is important to know about them. In shock the emphasis is on restoring the blood volume with suitable intravenous fluids, usually blood or dextran preparations. Hypotension due to adrenal insufficiency is treated with hydrocortisone intravenously.

Vasopressors which may be used include methoxamine (Vasoxine) 2 mg intravenously, metaraminol (Aramine) 2–10 mg intramuscularly or intravenously, or, as a last resort, noradrenaline (Levophed). Adrenaline or adrenaline-like drugs, such as metaraminol (sympathomimetic amines), must not be administered to patients receiving chloroform, cyclopropane or trichlorethylene, as dangerous disorders of cardiac rhythm and even ventricular fibrillation may result. Methoxamine is particularly useful in anaesthesia because it is compatible with cyclopropane and halothane. Any vasopressor must be used only with the greatest of caution in patients with cardiovascular disease or thyrotoxicosis.

Hypothermia

In some operations it may be necessary or desirable to stop or restrict the blood flow to the heart or brain (or other organs). Neither organ could normally tolerate this for long because each has a great need for oxygen which, of course, is carried in the blood. The need for oxygen is however, governed by the metabolic rate which may be reduced by cooling the patient. This gives more time, although for many cardiac operations it is not enough and a pump-oxygenator (heart–lung machine) is necessary.

Cooling may be achieved by immersing the body in cold water, or by passing the blood through a heat exchanger. Whichever method is adopted, drugs may be used to facilitate cooling. These drugs prevent shivering which would increase oxygen consumption and would also retard the process of cooling. Chlorpromazine (given as a premedication) acts centrally to abolish shivering and the vasoconstrictor response to cold, and acts peripherally as a vasodilator, both of which actions facilitate cooling. Muscular relaxants and also anaesthetics themselves prevent shivering, and the latter have a vasodilator effect which increases heat loss from the skin.

Neurolept–analgesia

This is a technique in which a tranquillizer is combined with an analgesic to produce a state in which there is drowsiness and analgesia, but consciousness and co-operatives are retained. The tranquillizer (the neuroleptic component) is usually a butyrophenone derivative such as **haloperidol** or **droperidol.** The analgesic is usually **fentanyl, phenoperidone** or **dextromoramide.**

The technique is used for patients on prolonged artificial ventilation and for procedures in which general anaesthesia is merited but is unavailable, inadvisable or impracticable.

When an inhalational anaesthetic such as nitrous oxide is added, to produce loss of consciousness, the term 'neurolept-anaesthesia' is sometimes used.

Dissociative anaesthesia

This is a preferable technique for infants and small children. It is an altered state of consciousness accompanied by profound analgesia permitting, for example, painful dressings and skin grafting in children with severe burns. The effect is produced by ketamine in a dose of 10 mg/kg. The nurse must not attempt to awaken the patient prematurely after ketamine anaesthesia for fear of inducing vivid and disturbing dreams.

Local anaesthetics (see also p. 180)

Local anaesthetics are drugs which paralyse the sensory nerves in the region of their application, so that the passage of painful stimuli towards the spinal cord becomes impossible. Motor nerves in the vicinity are also affected. They may be used in the following ways:

(1) Direct local applications to mucous membranes, e.g. cocaine.
(2) By injection, the same drugs being used for all the following;
　(*a*) injection into the skin and tissues at the site of the operation;
　(*b*) injection around nerves at some distance from the site of the operation so that the area which they supply is anaesthetized, i.e. 'regional anaesthesia' produced by nerve-block;
　(*c*) 'Splanchnic nerve-block', i.e. injection of the nerve ganglia on the posterior abdominal wall which receive the nervous impulses from the abdominal viscera such as the stomach and gall bladder. This is combined with local anaesthesia of the abdominal wall for some operations.
(3) Freezing the skin with ethyl chloride spray.

The ideal requirements of a local anaesthetic are:
(1) To paralyse the sensory nerves without damaging them or the surrounding tissues.
(2) To be easily sterilized.
(3) To be devoid of toxic effects after absorption.
(4) To produce anaesthesia of sufficient duration for the operation to be performed and to leave no after-effects.

14 Vitamins and drugs used in disorders of metabolism

The vitamins

Vitamins or accessory food factors are substances the presence of which in the food is essential for normal health and growth.

They are found in many natural foodstuffs but, in order to maintain health, only minute quantities, compared with the bulk of other articles of diet, are required.

Our knowledge of their composition and nature has increased rapidly in recent years and it is now possible to manufacture a number of them in the laboratory. In many instances it is these synthetic products which are used in Therapeutics.

Deficiencies may be serious in underdeveloped countries and in times of war and famine. It should be made clear, however, that vitamin deficiency is rare in this country and that their addition to a normal diet is rarely necessary, except perhaps in the case of infants, nursing mothers, and elderly persons who may not look after themselves properly. In other words, quantities are prescribed and consumed unnecessarily and it must be remembered that prolonged over-dosage (especially of vitamin D) may be dangerous.

But some special diets may be deficient in vitamins and in some diseases their absorption may not be adequate.

Vitamin A (Axerophthol)

Sources

This fat-soluble vitamin is found especially in milk, butter, egg-yolk, cream, margarine and fish-liver oils. It is formed in the walls of the small intestine from carotene, a yellow pigment found in certain vegetables, e.g. tomatoes, carrots and spinach.

Effects

Its deficiency, which is rare, produces:
(i) a dry condition of the eyes called xerophthalmia.

(ii) Night-blindness or difficulty experienced by some people in seeing in the dark.

(iii) Roughness and dryness of the skin ('toad skin') resulting from changes in the epithelium which may lead to diminished resistance to infection both of the skin and mucous membranes.

Vitamin A is necessary for health and growth of the young.

Vitamin B

A number of separate substances having different actions are distinguishable in this group of water-soluble vitamins.

Sources

Most of the members of this complicated family of vitamins occur together in nature. For example they are present in the cells of both animal and vegetable tissues and are essential to the metabolic needs of the body. They are found especially in yeast, seeds (pea, bean and lentil), in eggs, and in cereals such as wheat and rice. Some of the members of the group can also be prepared synthetically.

The most important are:

vitamin B_1 or thiamine, aneurine
vitamin B_2 or riboflavine
vitamin B_3 or nicotinic acid amide, nicotinamide (niacin)
vitamin B_6 or pyridoxine
vitamin B_{12} or cyanocobalamin (the extrinsic anti-anaemic factor).

Other substances in this group include pantothenic acid, folic acid and biotin (vitamin H).

Thiamine (aneurine, vitamin B₁)

Severe deficiency results in beri-beri, a disease affecting the nerves (peripheral neuritis) and heart. This mainly occurs among the rice-eating populations of the East where the staple diet is polished rice.

Minor degrees of deficiency may occur either due to lack of intake or to poor absorption. The latter may take place when the normal bacterial content of the intestines is altered by the pro-

Table 14.1. Vitamins

Vitamins	Names	Sources	Effects	Notes
A	*Axerophthol*	Milk butter cream egg-yolk cod-liver oil spinach tomato carrots	Raises resistance to infection Prevents night-blindness Prevents eye disease (xerophthalmia)	Found in vegetables as carotene, converted into vitamin A in wall of small intestine
B	*Thiamine* or *Aneurine* Antineuritic vitamin	Peas beans lentils wholemeal bread husks of cereals (rice, wheat, oats, barley) yeast raw carrot cabbage	Prevents beri-beri Helps in treatment of alcoholic neuritis	—
	Riboflavine	Milk, yeast	Energy	—
	Nicotinamide	Meat, cereals	Prevents pellagra	—
	Cyanocobalamin	Meat liver	Prevents anaemia	—
C	*Ascorbic acid* Antiscorbutic vitamin	Most fresh fruit and vegetables	Prevents scurvy	Easily destroyed by heat and alkalis
D	*Calciferol* Antirachitic vitamin	Cod-liver-oil eggs butter milk cream	Prevents rickets Necessary for calcium absorption	Also manufactured in the body by the action of sunlight (ultraviolet rays) on the skin
E	*Tocopheryl* *acetate*	Wheat germ oil	?	—
K	*Menaphthone*	Liver spinach other vegetables	Necessary for production of prothrombin	Antidote to Dindevan over-dosage (K_1)
P	*Hesperidin* *Rutin*	Rose hips lemon juice	Affects permeability of capillaries	—

longed administration of antibiotics by mouth and inadequate intake may occur in chronic alcoholism.

NB.—Broad-spectrum antibiotics, e.g. tetracycline, may interfere with the absorption of vitamin B_1 from the gut.

In treatment the vitamin may be administered either by mouth or by intramuscular injection. The prophylactic dose is 2–5 mg daily and the therapeutic dose is 25–100 mg daily.

Riboflavine (vitamin B_2)

Deficiency of this vitamin is associated with soreness of the lips and tongue and the development of fissures at the angle of the mouth. The average dose is 5–15 mg daily.

Nicotinamide

Pellagra, a disease causing intestinal upset, skin eruptions, nervous symptoms and mental changes is due to lack of this vitamin. This is a tropical disease not seen in this country in its fully developed form. Nicotinic acid is sometimes used as a vasodilator in a number of conditions but its effect is uncertain. It is also sometimes used to reduce serum cholesterol levels when they are abnormally high. Doses vary from 50 to 500 mg daily.

Cyanocobalamin (vitamin B_{12})

This is the extrinsic anti-anaemic factor used in the treatment of pernicious anaemia (p. 110).

Folic acid

Folic acid is used in the treatment of tropical sprue, coeliac disease and certain types of macrocytic anaemia. Dose 5–20 mg daily.

Vitamin C (ascorbic acid—the antiscorbutic vitamin)
Sources

This is found in fresh foodstuffs, especially fruits such as oranges, lemons, black currants, rose hips, tomatoes and green vegetables, and is therefore present in salads. It is rapidly destroyed by heat and is consequently lacking in boiled or dried milk.

Effects

Deficiency results in scurvy, a disease which may affect either infants or adults. It is characterized by haemorrhages into the tissues under the skin and from the gums.

Ascorbic acid may also be a factor in the formation of haemoglobin and is sometimes given at the same time as iron in the treatment of anaemia. It can also act as a diuretic in heart failure. It is given by mouth in doses of 50–100 mg 3 times daily.

Vitamin D (the antirachitic vitamin—calciferol)
Sources

This very important vitamin is more complicated than some of the others because it has two distinct sources:
(a) Its natural distribution especially in cod-liver oil and, to a lesser extent, in butter and eggs.
(b) The human body is able to manufacture it by the action of sunlight on a steroid substance in the skin called 7-dehydrocholesterol.

It is the ultraviolet rays of sunlight which have this action and 'artificial sunlight' has the same effect.

Effects

Lack of vitamin D causes rickets, a disease of young children characterized by deformities of the bones which are deficient in calcium. It plays an important part in the intestinal absorption and metabolism of calcium.

Prolonged high dosage is dangerous and may lead to the deposition of calcium in the kidneys and other organs.

The therapeutic dosage varies from 1000 to 100 000 units daily. The prophylactic dose is much less; about 400IU (10 micrograms) is the daily requirement of infants, young children, and lactating women.

1-alpha hydroxyvitamin D_3 (alphacalcidol, One-alpha) is used for the treatment of conditions (e.g. renal bone disease) resistant to ordinary vitamin D.

Vitamin E (tocopheryl acetate)

This fat-soluble substance is present in the germ of wheat, in cereals, in vegetable oils, and in eggs. One of its actions is anti-oxidant. For example, it prevents the oxidation of vitamin A. The precise requirement for vitamin E is unknown but 8–16 mg daily is probably adequate. There is no scientific justification for self-medication with vitamin E. Deficiency of vitamin E causes sterility in rats. It has no established use in general medicine.

Vitamin K (menaphthone)

This vitamin complex, which has been further subdivided into K_1 and K_2, is present in liver, spinach and other green vegetables. It is necessary for the production of prothrombin (p. 121) in the body and, therefore, its deficiency results in a tendency to increased bleeding. It is given in some cases of jaundice, especially before operations and in neo-natal haemorrhage. Bile salts, which aid its absorption, are given at the same time in cases of obstructive jaundice. Synthetic preparations having the same action include menaphthone (1–10 mg by intramuscular injection) and aceto-menaphthone (5–20 mg by mouth).

Vitamin K_1 (phytamenadione)

Vitamin K_1 acts especially as an antidote to over-dosage with the oral anticoagulant drugs, such as Dindevan, but not heparin. (1–10 mg are given by mouth, subcutaneously or intravenously.)

Vitamin P

Little is known about this vitamin group, but the resistance of the capillaries appears to be influenced by it. Rutin and hesperidin have vitamin P activity.

Vitamin preparations

There are a number of 'official' and even more proprietary vitamin preparations available. In many instances, more than one vitamin may be included in a preparation. The doses of the vitamins may be prescribed in units or by weight.

A: strong tablets of vitamin A (Ro-A-Vit) 50 000 units.
B: thiamine, 25–100 mg, available as tablets or an injection
   nicotinamide up to 500 mg
   riboflavine up to 15 mg

Bemax, Marmite, Benerva and Becosym are proprietary preparations containing the vitamin B complex.

C: ascorbic acid, up to 1 g or more
syrups of black currant and rose hips are rich sources of vitamin C, especially useful for children.

D: calciferol.
prophylactic: 10 micrograms (400 units)
therapeutic: 25 micrograms to 2·5 mg (1000–100 000 units).

E: tocopheryl acetate, up to 200 mg. Ephynal.

K: menaphthone (Synkavit), vitamin K_1, phytomenadione (Konakion).

Substances and preparations containing mixed vitamins include:

A and D: cod-liver oil emulsion, 8–30 ml daily in divided doses. In addition to the oil various emulsions are available which are designed to obscure its fishy taste:

halibut liver oil capsules, 1 capsule daily
vitamins A and D capsules (BNF) (A = 4500, D = 450 units). Vitamins A, B, C and D are contained in Vitamins Capsules (BNF), Multivite.

Many proprietary vitamin preparations are available but only a few can be mentioned here.

Massive doses of mixed vitamin B complex with vitamin C are sometimes used in the treatment of confusional states and alcoholic psychoses. Preparations for intravenous and intramuscular injection are available, e.g. Parentrovite.

Drugs used in metabolic disorders
Diabetes

Diabetes is a disease due to a relative or absolute deficiency of insulin, which is secreted by the islets of Langerhans in the pancreas. It might therefore be regarded as an endocrine disorder, but its main feature is a disturbance of carbohydrate and, to some extent, fat metabolism. Normally, glucose can only be utilized and fully oxidized by the tissues in the presence of insulin. If this is deficient, then glucose will accumulate in the blood and some of the excess will be excreted by the kidneys in the urine (glycosuria).

Further, it is only when glucose is being oxidized in the body that an equivalent amount of fat can be fully broken down into carbon dioxide and water. If glucose is not being properly used by the tissues owing to lack of insulin, the breaking down of fat ceases at the fatty acid stage and acetoacetic acid and acetone (ketones) appear in the urine. The accumulation of ketones in the blood is called ketosis and ultimately leads to diabetic coma. There is also a form of diabetic coma in which the blood glucose concentration is high but there is no ketosis; this is called hyperosmolar coma.

Diabetes may be controlled (*a*) by diet, (*b*) by insulin, (*c*) by oral hypoglycaemic agents or (*d*) by some combination of these.

Insulin

The discovery of insulin has enabled the majority of diabetics to lead a normal life and to enjoy an interesting even though restricted diet. In many cases the patient can learn to give his own injections, test his own urine, and adjust his diet to his daily requirements. The risk of diabetic coma has been very greatly reduced, but the possibilities of insulin over-dosage must not be forgotten.

Three main types of insulin are employed:
(1) Those with rapid action of short duration, e.g. Soluble insulin (insulin injection), Actrapid.
(2) Those with an intermediate duration of action, e.g. insulin zinc suspension (Insulin Lente) and isophane insulin injection.
(3) Those with an action of slow onset and long duration, e.g. protamine zinc insulin (PZI) and globin insulin, which is now rarely used.

Each of these may be used alone or a dose of soluble insulin may be added to protamine zinc or globin insulin, but not to insulin zinc suspension

Soluble insulin

This is rapidly absorbed and has its maximum effect in about 2 to 4 hours. The effect lasts for 6 to 8 hours. Soluble insulin or Actrapid may be given subcutaneously, intramuscularly or intravenously. Other insulins are given subcutaneously or intramuscularly but never intravenously.

Insulin zinc suspension (lente)

This is a mixture of special types of short-acting (semilente or amorphous) and long-acting (ultralente or crystalline) insulins which is administered in a single morning dose and exerts its influ-

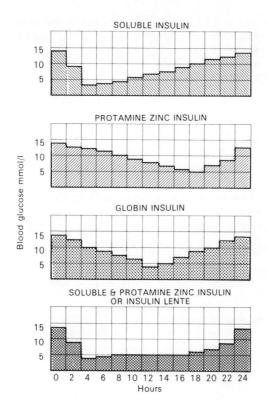

Fig. 14.1. The effect of a dose of the various types of insulin on the blood sugar of a diabetic patient

ence over the whole 24 hours in a manner similar to a mixture of soluble and protamine zinc insulin. Insulin zinc suspension must not be mixed with other types of insulin and should not be used if the total dose required is high or if the patient shows a marked tendency to ketosis.

Soluble insulin and Insulin zinc suspension cannot be mixed in the same syringe because of their differing pH values.

Protamine zinc insulin

This acts more slowly. It has little action immediately after injection, but has its greatest effect in 16 to 18 hours, and continues to act for over 24 hours.

Soluble insulin and PZI must not be mixed in the same syringe or injected at the same site because some of the soluble insulin will be converted to PZI.

Globin insulin
Globin insulin has a maximum effect at 12 hours.

Neutral insulin
Two preparations, Actrapid MC and Nuso, are neutral in reaction and may produce less discomfort at the injection site than soluble insulin, which is acid. Actrapid is of porcine origin (obtained from pigs) and Nuso is a beef insulin. One of them may suit a patient who develops hypersensitivity to insulin from the other source. Porcine insulin is much less likely than bovine insulin to induce an allergic reaction. Some insulins are of mixed animal origin.

Biphasic insulin (Rapitard MC)
This consists of beef insulin crystals, giving a rapid action, suspended in a neutral solution of pig insulin, which acts for 18 to 22 hours.

Table 14.2. Insulins: duration of action

Type of insulin	Duration of action (hours)
Short-acting	
Soluble	6–8
Neutral	7
(Actrapid & Nuso)	
Medium-acting	
Semilente	16
Semitard MC	16
Long-acting	
Globin	18
Rapitard MC	22
Isophane	24
Lentard	24
Monotard MC	24
Lente	24–30
Ultralente	36
Ultratard MC	36
Protamine Zinc (PZI)	36–48

Monocomponent (MC) insulins

These are highly purified porcine insulins from which impurities of pancreatic origin have been removed. Because of their purity they have little or no tendency to induce immunogenic reactions. They are therefore described as 'non-antigenic'. They may be advantageous in patients who are allergic or resistant to other insulins or who have insulin fat atrophy. The range includes Actrapid MC (rapidly-acting), Semitard MC (an intermediate-acting insulin) and Monotard MC (long-acting insulin). These insulins may be intermixed in the syringe.

The various types of insulin are supplied in vials containing 40 or 80 units/ml. Soluble insulin is also supplied in a concentration of 20 units/ml. It is most important for both the nurse and the patient to be quite sure which strength is being used. In the case of protamine zinc and globin insulin the bottle must be shaken gently so that the suspended matter is evenly diffused throughout the mixture before any is withdrawn.

A patient ordered 20 units of soluble insulin would be given 1 ml of ordinary strength insulin, or 0.5 ml of double strength, or 0.25 ml of quadruple strength, and so on. The appropriate strength should be chosen to give a convenient volume for injection.

Table 14.3. Soluble insulin, 20 units/ml

Units	Single strength ml	Double strength ml	Quadruple strength ml
10	0.5	0·25	—
20	1	0·5	0·25
30	1·5	0·75	0·38
40	2	1	0·5
50	2·5	1·25	0·63
100	5	2·5	1·25

The above table gives the amounts to be injected when different strengths of insulin are employed.

Insulin keeps well if stored in a cool, dark place, but soluble insulin should not be used if it becomes cloudy. It may be administered with an ordinary hypodermic syringe or one specially graduated in units. This is kept in a metal case filled with spirit and is rinsed in boiled water before use. It is wise to keep one needle for piercing the rubber cap and a separate one for injecting the insulin as the rubber is apt to cause blunting. The top of the rubber cap having been cleansed with spirit the requisite amount of insulin is drawn into the syringe. The patient is taught that a small amount of air injected into the insulin bottle facilitates the removal of the liquid. The skin is cleaned with spirit, and the injection is given subcutaneously. It may be made into the arms, thighs or abdomen—the latter sites being chosen if the patient is administering it himself.

Soluble insulin or Actrapid is given $\frac{1}{2}$ hour before a meal, which must contain some carbohydrate food. The other types are given before breakfast.

While the best dose of insulin for the individual is being found, the urine must be tested for sugar and acetone before each meal. When the regular dose of insulin has been determined, daily tests should be carried out on the morning specimen.

Usually the dose of insulin must be increased if the patient is suffering from any infection (e.g. a boil, severe cold, bronchitis, etc.).

It must be clearly understood that insulin is not a cure for the disease and, once being necessary, it is probable that the patient will have to continue taking it for the rest of his life, adjustments in the dosage being required from time to time.

Because of their delayed action, the medium and long-acting insulins are not suitable for use in diabetic coma.

Unless the dose is carefully adjusted, protamine zinc and globin insulin are very liable to produce hypoglycaemia.

Other uses of insulin

(a) Small doses of insulin are sometimes given in order to increase the appetite in under-nourished patients.

(b) Large doses are used to produce a state of shock associated with hypoglycaemia in the treatment of certain mental illnesses (schizophrenia).

(c) Insulin and glucose are given together intravenously in the emergency treatment of hyperkalaemia. Insulin stimulates the transport of glucose across the cell wall and this is accompanied by a movement of potassium ions into the cell.

Oral hypoglycaemic agents

Patients on these agents should adhere to a strict diet calculated to maintain the normal weight for their height, sex and age. They are unsuitable for juvenile diabetics, with a tendency to ketosis, and for patients presenting in hyperglycaemic coma. They are generally used to treat patients with maturity-onset, non-ketotic diabetes which cannot be adequately controlled by diet alone.

(a) The sulphonylureas

These have been thought to act by stimulating the islet cells of the pancreas to produce insulin.

Tolbutamide (Rastinon)

Dosage: 500 mg to 1·5 g daily in 2 or 3 divided doses.

Chlorpropamide (Diabinese)

This has a similar action and use but is given in smaller doses, viz. 100 mg up to a maximum of 500 mg once daily with breakfast.

Side-effects such as nausea, vomiting and headache may occur and intolerance of alcohol may develop. Rarely jaundice or a skin rash is seen and indicates that the drug must be stopped at once.

Other sulphonylureas include **tolazamide** (Tolanase) 100–500 mg, **acetohexamide** (Dimelor) 250–750 mg, **glymidine** (Gondafon) 500 mg, **glibenclamide** (Daonil) 5 mg and **glipizide** (Glibenese) 2·5–30 mg daily.

> *Equivalent dosages* 1·5 g tolbutamide = 500 mg chlorpropamide = 5 mg glibenclamide.

Certain drugs may potentiate the hypoglycaemic action of the sulphonylureas and result in a dangerously low level of plasma glucose. These drugs include beta-blockers, chloramphenicol, coumarin anticoagulants, MAO inhibitors, phenylbutazone, probenecid, salicylates and sulphonamides.

(b) The biguanides

These compounds differ from the sulphonylureas in their mode of action, which is incompletely known. They reduce the absorption of glucose from the intestine, decrease the formation of new glucose in the liver (gluconeogenesis), and increase the uptake of glucose by muscle. They may be used alone (in maturity-onset diabetes) or in conjunction with insulin or a sulphonylurea. Used as sole therapy for diabetes, high doses cause gastrointestinal upsets. Occasionally, a serious acidosis (lactic acidosis) without hyperglycaemia results from biguanide-therapy especially with phenformin. Because of this, biguanides are best avoided in patients with renal failure, impaired liver function or cardiac failure. In patients with serious intercurrent illnesses, especially those such as myocardial infarction which are liable to cause shock, diguanides should be withdrawn and hyperglycaemia treated with insulin.

Phenformin (Dibotin)
Dose: 50–150 mg daily.

Metformin (Glucophage)
Dose: 1–3 g daily.

These drugs are taken in divided dosage, 2–3 times a day, after meals.

Obesity

Obesity, an excess of body fat, is the commonest form of malnutrition in the Western world. It predisposes to some diseases (e.g. diabetes mellitus) and makes others worse (e.g. heart disease and osteoarthritis).

The first approach to the treatment of obesity should be dietary. If the patient can be persuaded to eat less food than he requires for his daily energy expenditure, he will lose weight. The essence of a reducing diet is that it is low in calorific value. As most of a person's calories normally come from carbohydrates (sugar, flour products, potatoes, rice, etc.) it is these which have to be reduced particularly. Few people eat too much protein or fat, partly because these are more expensive and partly because they are less palatable.

A number of drugs (anorectics) have been used to suppress appetite. The amphetamines were used for this purpose but many people became addicted to them because they had a stimulant effect on the central nervous system. They have therefore fallen into disfavour. Related drugs are phenmetrazine, phentermine and diethylpropion.

One drug which does not excite the central nervous system, and is not addictive, is **fenfluramine** (Ponderax). It causes an increase in the muscle uptake of glucose and has a fat-mobilizing action. The dose is 2–6 20 mg tablets or 1 or 2 Pacaps 60 mg capsules daily. The drug is contraindicated in patients taking MAO inhibitors. Patients taking sedatives, antihypertensive drugs or hypoglycaemic agents may have to have the doses of these reduced when fenfluramine is administered. **Mazindole** (Teronac) is a newer appetite suppressant. One tablet (2 mg) is given 1 hour before lunch. It potentiates the effects of catecholamines (adrenaline and noradrenaline) and should not be given in conjunction with MAO inhibitors, methyldopa, guanethidine, debrisoquine, or bethanidine.

This section may be appropriately concluded by quoting from the British National Formulary 1976–78: 'Appetite suppressant drugs have little place in the management of the obese patient and there is no substitute for willpower.'

Gout

Gout is a disorder of metabolism which results in the accumulation of uric acid in the blood and its deposition in the form of salts (urates) in and around joints, producing recurrent attacks of acute arthritis.

(a) Drugs used during acute attack

An acute attack of gout is quickly suppressed by phenylbutazone, 200 mg 3 times daily, or indomethacin 25 mg 4 times a day. Corticosteroids are effective but are not recommended for routine use. Colchicine is now rarely used for acute attacks. It has an irritating effect on the alimentary tract, causing vomiting and purgation. One mg is given, followed by 0·5 mg every 2 hours by mouth until the acute pain subsides or diarrhoea occurs.

(b) Drugs used between attacks

Uricosuric drugs

A number of compounds increase the urinary excretion of uric acid. They are called uricosuric agents and are used (for the remainder of the patient's life) to reduce the number of acute attacks of gout, to reduce the size of tophi and to minimize renal damage. Drugs used are **salicylates, probenecid** (Benemid) 0·5–2 g daily, **ethebenecid** (Urelim) 0·5–1·5 g daily and **sulphinpyrazone** (Anturan) 200–400 mg daily. Ample fluids, and often alkalis, should be taken to prevent urate deposition in the kidneys. These drugs are contraindicated in the presence of existing renal calculi.

Salicylates antagonize the action of probenecid and sulphinpyrazone and should not, therefore, be administered concurrently with them.

Allopurinol

Allopurinol is not a uricosuric agent. It inhibits the enzyme xanthine oxidase and thereby interferes with the oxidation of xanthine to uric acid. In this way, allopurinol **blocks the production of uric acid** and restores serum uric acid levels to normal. Less uric acid passes through the kidneys and the drug therefore helps to prevent renal damage and uric acid stone formation. Dose: 200–600 mg daily in divided doses.

During the early weeks or months of treatment with uricosuric drugs or allopurinol, there is an increased tendency for acute attacks of gout to occur. Colchicine (0·5–1 mg daily) is therefore often administered prophylactically during this period.

15 The ductless glands and their products

The ductless glands or endocrine organs are those glandular structures which pour their secretions (containing hormones) directly into the blood. A number of hormones have been isolated and some can be prepared in the laboratory. The functions of all the ductless glands are intimately connected with each other and also with the nervous system. The pituitary gland, in particular, exercises control over the adrenal, thyroid and sex glands. They play an important part in the metabolic processes of the body and in growth. Because of the balance which exists between the activities of the various glands, a disorder of one may upset the functions of others.

In a broad sense, disordered function of a ductless gland may result either in an increase or a decrease in the amount of its secretion. The various ductless gland products employed in therapeutics may be used either to substitute for a deficiency due to under-secretion of the gland, or in order to influence the activity of other glands or organs.

The substances used may be:

(i) The actual gland substance itself (rarely nowadays).
(ii) Specially prepared extracts from the gland.
(iii) Chemically prepared substances identical with or closely resembling the natural hormone.
(iv) In certain instances, some hormones can be extracted from the urine.

The thyroid gland

The internal secretion of the thyroid is found in the colloid material secreted by the epithelium lining the vesicles of the gland. Its active principles are thyroxine and triiodothyronine (liothyronine), hormones with high iodine contents.

Over-secretion of the thyroid gland produces thyrotoxicosis (exophthalmic goitre or Graves' disease). Among the effects of this disease is a general increase in metabolism so that the individual eats more but tends to lose weight. Under-secretion results in myxoedema in the adult, and cretinism in the infant.

Thyroid hormones are used for the following purposes:

(1) In myxoedema and cretinism, because the secretion is defective. In such cases, the patient must continue to take appropriate doses for the rest of his life.

(2) In some cases of non-toxic (simple) goitre.

Excessive dosage produces symptoms resembling thyrotoxicosis, the most important being marked loss of weight, sweating and a rapid pulse.

Preparations
Thyroxine sodium (Eltroxin)

This very powerful synthetic substance, resembling the natural hormone, has superseded dried thyroid extract. Dose: 50–300 micrograms daily.

Liothyronine sodium (Tertroxin)

This is more potent than thyroxine and its greater rapidity of action renders it useful for certain cases, e.g. hypothyroid coma.

Dose: 5–60 micrograms daily. Twenty micrograms is equivalent to 100 micrograms of thyroxine.

Antithyroid substances

In cases of thyrotoxicosis it is necessary to diminish the activity of the thyroid gland. This may be done either by surgical removal of a considerable proportion of the gland or by the administration of a drug which suppresses its activity. In any event it is usual to give some medical treatment to patients before an operation is performed.

Iodine

This will temporarily depress the function of the thyroid but its maximum effect is reached after 2 weeks of administration, after which it may be given for a further period of 3 weeks, when it ceases to be effective. It is, therefore, only suitable as a preoperative and immediate postoperative measure. Lugol's iodine, 0·3–1 ml, a watery solution of potassium iodide, may be employed, commencing with 2 drops and increasing to 5 or 10 drops 3 times a day. Potassium iodide in doses of 60–100 mg thrice daily may be used instead.

Radioactive iodine (^{131}I)

This may be used in the treatment of thyrotoxicosis in patients over the age of 45, and in carcinoma of the thyroid. Cases are carefully selected and an appropriate dose is required for each of the uses mentioned.

Carbimazole (Neomercazole)

Dose: initially 30–45 mg daily in divided doses (maintenance 5–15 mg).

This is a drug which depresses the activity of the gland and can effect a medical cure of thyrotoxicosis in suitable cases. Symptoms may be controlled in 1 to 3 months but it is usually necessary to continue with a maintenance dose for 1 to 2 years. It may be 2 or 3 weeks before a therapeutic response is apparent.

It is less toxic than thiouracil but may also cause serious agranulocytosis and skin rashes.

Thiouracil

This is a sulphur-containing drug which has been used in the treatment of thyrotoxicosis in the form of methyl- or propyl-thiouracil. Like carbimazole it restores the increased metabolism to normal and many patients are able to return to work after 1 to 3 months of treatment.

Toxic symptoms are sometimes produced. The most serious is diminution of the white blood cells (agranulocytosis): others include pyrexia, gland enlargement and rashes. Iodine should not be used at the same time.

Potassium perchlorate (Peroidin)

This has been used as an antithyroid drug in doses of 200 mg 4 times daily when others are contraindicated. As a rule this dose may be halved after 3 or 4 weeks. Iodine-containing drugs should not be given at the same time. Aplastic anaemia is a rare, but usually fatal, complication of therapy with this drug which is best avoided.

The parathyroid glands

The parathyroid glands secrete a hormone, parathormone, the function of which is to control calcium metabolism in the body. An excess of it causes an increase in the serum calcium level. Another hormone, calcitonin, reduces the serum calcium level.

Calcitonin originates in the C cells of the thyroid gland and in the parathyroids.

Deficiency of parathyroid secretion results in tetany, which is characterized by muscular spasms and increased irritability of the nervous system. The blood calcium is low. Tetany may occur, (a) after removal of the parathyroids, (b) in some cases of rickets, (c) after very large doses of alkali, (d) in sprue.

Increased activity of the parathyroids gives rise to a rare disease (hyperparathyroidism) in which there is loss of calcium from the bones. The calcium is lost into the urine where it may cause stone formation in the urinary tract.

Preparation
Parathyroid (Parathormone)

This must be given by injection. It is used for diagnostic purposes but is not now generally used for the treatment of parathyroid deficiency. The main reasons for this are:

(a) It acts too slowly to be of use in acute tetany.

(b) The body becomes refractory to its action if it is used for long-term treatment.

Calcium gluconate (10 ml of 10 per cent solution) given intravenously is the immediate treatment for tetany. In the long-term management of parathyroid deficiency, a diet low in phosphorus is recommended. This is supplemented by calcium salts, e.g. calcium lactate or gluconate (up to 20 g daily). Such treatment is adequate for mild cases but in more severe cases it is also necessary to give calciferol (vitamin D_2) usually in a dose of 100 000 units daily, by mouth, or alfacalcidol (One-alpha), initially 1 microgram daily. Alternatively, a chemically related substance, dihydrotachysterol (AT 10) may be given in a dose of 1–10 ml daily, by mouth. This substance resembles parathyroid hormone in causing increased urinary excretion of phosphate.

The adrenal (or suprarenal) glands

The two adrenal glands consist of an outer cortex and central medulla each of which produces hormones differing in chemical character and function. The glands are plentifully supplied with blood and also with sympathetic nerve fibres from the coeliac (solar) plexus.

The functions of the cortex

The adrenal cortex is essential to life and secretes a number of hormones, each having different functions. Some of these have been extracted from the gland and some can be made in the laboratory.

Chemically they belong to a class of fatty or wax-like substances called steroids or corticoids. The most important ones fall into three main groups:

(1) The **mineral corticoids** of which deoxycortone (DOCA) and aldosterone are examples. These act on the tubules of the kidney in such a way that:

(a) sodium and chloride are retained in the body,

(b) excess of potassium is excreted.

They therefore help to maintain the water and electrolyte balance of the body. Any excess or over-dosage will tend to cause water retention (oedema) and hypertension.

(2) The **glucocorticoids** or **corticosteroids.** This group includes cortisol (hydrocortisone) and its derivatives. For brevity the term 'steroid' may be employed. These hormones have a number of actions, one of the main ones being to influence carbohydrate metabolism.

(a) They increase the blood sugar.

(b) They increase serum lipids.

(c) They cause water and electrolyte disturbances.

(d) They decrease the number of lymphocytes and eosinophils in the blood.

(e) They reduce the rate at which certain connective tissue cells multiply and so tend to suppress the natural reaction to infection and to delay healing.

(f) They increase the secretion of hydrochloric acid in the stomach and reduce gastric mucus, thus tending to cause peptic ulcers or to delay their healing.

(g) In large doses cortisone produces symptoms similar to Cushing's syndrome, viz. a swollen, round 'moon face', excess of hair and a tendency to acne.

(3) **Sex hormones** similar to those produced by the ovary and testis (oestrogens and androgens). These influence growth and sex development.

The output of hormones from the cortex of the adrenal is controlled by another hormone secreted by the pituitary gland known as the adrenocorticotrophic hormone (ACTH) or corticotrophin.

Unlike the medulla of the adrenal the secretions of the cortex are not regulated by nervous impulses.

Cortisone, hydrocortisone and many similar synthetic substances (e.g. prednisone and prednisolone) are all used in clinical medicine. When cortisone is administered in large doses, among the complications observed is a disturbance of salt and water balance, due to the fact that it has some mineralocorticoid effect in addition to its glucocorticoid action.

It must be remembered that although the individual hormones mentioned each have separate effects on metabolism, in health, normal adrenal cortical secretion represents the sum of all these individual actions.

In disease, if the adrenal cortex is destroyed or if the secretion of corticotrophin (ACTH) fails there will be no adrenal cortical hormones produced.

Mineral corticoids

(1) **Deoxycortone.** This mineral corticoid which causes water and sodium retention may be used in conjunction with cortisone in the treatment of Addison's disease. Over-dosage produces oedema and hypertension.

(a) Deoxycortone acetate (DOCA) is given by intramuscular injection in doses of 2–5 mg daily.

(b) Pellets (100–400 mg) may be implanted under the skin whence it is slowly absorbed over a period of about 6 months.

(c) Deoxycortone pivalate (Percorten M) is given by intramuscular injection only once every 4 weeks.

(2) **Fludrocortisone** (Florinef). This synthetic salt-retaining steroid has now largely replaced deoxycortone in the treatment of Addison's disease. Its great advantage is that it is an oral medication. Dose: 0·1–0·3 mg daily.

Deoxycortone remains of value in patients who are vomiting or cannot, for some reason, take tablets.

(3) **Aldosterone,** the main natural salt-retaining steroid, is commercially available as Aldocorten. Dose: 0·5 mg intramuscularly or intravenously, repeated as necessary.

Glucocorticoids (corticosteroids)

Since **cortisone** was discovered a number of other substances having a similar general action have been made by varying slightly its chemical composition. By means of these variations it has been possible to minimize some of the side-effects so that prednisone and prednisolone cause less salt and water retention particularly as they can be given in one-fifth of the dose of cortisone. The more recent synthetic steroids, methyl prednisolone, triamcinolone, dexamethasone and betamethasone, have minimal salt-retaining effect. The latter two have 35 times the anti-inflammatory effect of cortisone. Prednisone and prednisolone are, however, generally the steroids of choice for systemic administration.

Hydrocortisone (cortisol) is the form in which the hormone is actually secreted in the body by the adrenal glands and its action is identical with that of cortisone.

There are a large number of proprietary preparations of these substances each having different names and too numerous to mention here.

The cortisone group of drugs may be used as tablets, injections, ointments and eye-drops.

(a) Cortisone, prednisone and prednisolone are used mainly for internal administration.

(b) Hydrocortisone is used (a) for local application and local injection into and around joints, (b) intravenously for life-threatening conditions.

Cortisone (50–400 mg), prednisone and prednisolone (5–100 mg daily) etc.

These substances may be used either as direct replacement therapy, i.e. to replace the natural hormone when the secretion of the adrenal gland is defective as in Addison's disease or after removal of both glands (which may be performed for certain cases of carcinoma, e.g. of the breast) or empirically, where increase of the cortical steroid hormones has been shown by experience to be beneficial.

Among the many conditions in which they may be used are:

(1) *Rheumatic and connective tissue disorders*
   rheumatic fever   polyarteritis nodosa
   rheumatoid arthritis   lupus erythematosus

(2) *Allergic disorders*
   severe asthma   drug sensitivity   status asthmaticus
                                                      serum sickness

(3) *Skin diseases*
   pemphigus vulgaris   dermatitis   erythema
                                                      multiforme

(4) *Endocrine disorders*
   Addison's disease   pituitary disorders   adrenalectomy
(5) *Blood diseases*
   haemolytic anaemia   purpura
(6) *Other disorders*
   ulcerative colitis   temporal arteritis   nephrotic
   burns   sarcoidosis   syndrome
                                                               delirium tremens

There are a number of other uncommon conditions in which the use of cortisone may be considered desirable. It must be understood, however, that it is only used in selected cases and is not necessarily employed in every case of the diseases listed.

Contraindications

Being a very powerful drug cortisone must be used with great caution and under careful supervision. It is usually contraindicated in the presence of peptic ulcer, hypertension and cardiac insufficiency, and in most cases of active or old tuberculosis although there are special indications for its use in some cases of tuberculosis.

Precautions

When cortisone is given in large doses the following measures may be desirable:
(*a*) Daily weight, urinary output and blood pressure records.
(*b*) Observation for oedema, 'moon face' and thrombophlebitis of legs.
(*c*) Diet: high protein, restricted fat and carbohydrate.
(*d*) Drugs:
   potassium chloride to prevent potassium depletion;
   aluminium hydroxide to prevent peptic ulcer;
   antibiotics in the presence of infection;
   sedatives to minimize mental disturbances.

These precautions are less necessary when prednisone and prednisolone are used unless large doses are employed.

In view of the fact that the administration of corticosteroids tends to inhibit the natural secretion from the adrenal gland, they should be withdrawn gradually over a period of several weeks when therapy has been completed otherwise serious withdrawal symptoms may occur.

During steroid therapy and for up to 2 years afterwards, the patient may not be able to cope with such emergencies as trauma, surgery, or severe infection, because of suppression of pituitary–adrenal function and hence diminished resistance to stress. At such times, supplementary steroid therapy is necessary and without it death may occur.

Table 15.1. Side effects of corticosteroid therapy

Acne
Cushing's Syndrome
Delayed tissue repair (exacerbation of
    peptic ulceration and tuberculosis)
Osteoporosis
Retardation of growth in children
Retention of salt and water (oedema and
    hypertension)
Suppression of pituitary–adrenal
    function, causing diminished resistance
    to stress

Hydrocortisone

This may be injected with strict aseptic precautions into or around joints. Doses of 0·25–1 ml (25 mg/ml) are used according to the size of the joint or area to be infiltrated.

Among the conditions for which it may be employed are:

rheumatoid arthritis	traumatic arthritis
osteoarthritis	'tennis elbow'
periarthritis	acute gout
bursitis	keloid scars.

Retention enemas may be given in ulcerative colitis, e.g. 50–100 mg in 150 ml of 1 per cent methyl cellulose emulsion or normal saline once or twice daily. Prednisolone (Predsol or Predenema) and betamethasone (Retenema) are also given in retention enemas for ulcerative colitis.

Hydrocortisone lotion and skin ointment

Lotions are generally used for wet surfaces and extensive lesions, ointments for dry localized lesions and those near the eyes. At first applications may be made up to 4 times daily and later reduced to daily or alternate days. Among the indications are:

allergic skin disorders	discoid lupus erythematosus
eczema of various types	dermatitis.

Hydrocortisone eye-drops (1%) and eye ointment (2·5%)

blepharitis   interstitial keratitis
conjunctivitis   iritis.

Their use is contraindicated in acute corneal ulcer.

Many other steroids, synthetic analogues of cortisone and hydrocortisone, are used topically in ointments, creams, lotions, eye-drops and ear-drops. For conditions with an infective element (e.g. infective eczema and intertrigo) an antibacterial agent is incorporated in the preparation; clioquinol is often used for this purpose since it has both antibacterial and antifungal properties.

In some resistant skin conditions, the effect of steroids is enhanced by covering the treated area with Polythene film, thus making what is called an occlusive dressing. Lichenified eczema, hypertrophic lichen planus and some patches of psoriasis are treated in this way. If extensive areas are so treated, however, there is a risk of systemic effects (e.g. adrenal suppression) from absorption of the steroid through the skin into the blood stream.

Functions of the adrenal medulla

The medulla secretes **adrenaline,** the properties of which have already been mentioned (p. 187); they include:

(i) it is a general stimulant of the sympathetic system;
(ii) it is a vasoconstrictor;
(iii) it raises blood pressure;
(iv) it causes the liver to liberate glucose from glycogen.

The medulla also secretes **noradrenaline** (p. 189), a natural hormone closely related to adrenaline which can also be prepared synthetically. It also raises blood pressure by vasoconstriction but has little effect on the bronchial muscle.

A rare tumour of the adrenal medulla (phaeochromocytoma) is a cause of hypertension, because of the noradrenaline and adrenaline which it secretes.

The pituitary gland

This consists of two parts which have different modes of development and entirely different functions.

Anterior lobe

This secretes a number of hormones:

(a) The growth hormone (somatotrophin).

(b) The thyrotropic or thyroid stimulating hormone (TSH). This stimulates the growth and activity of the thyroid gland.

(c) The adrenocorticotrophic hormone (ACTH). This hormone is a protein substance which stimulates the cortex of the adrenal gland to secrete its own hormones.

(d) The gonadotrophic hormones. These are essential for the normal development of the sex organs and stimulate the production of the various sex gland hormones. They are:

   (i) the folicle stimulating hormone (FSH). In the female this stimulates the ripening of the ovarian follicles. In the male it stimulates the production of spermatozoa;

   (ii) the luteinizing hormone (LH). In the female this stimulates rupture of the follicles (ovulation) and formation of corpora lutea. Acting with FSH, it stimulates oestrogen production. Acting with prolactin, it stimulates progesterone production in the corpus luteum. In the male, it stimulates the testes to produce testosterone.

(e) Prolactin (luteotrophin, the lactogenic hormone) which helps to control the secretion of milk from the breast. It also maintains the secretory activity of the corpus luteum.

Adrenocorticotrophic hormone (ACTH), corticotrophin

ACTH is a hormone obtained from the anterior lobe of the pituitary gland. Its action is to stimulate the cortex of the adrenal gland to produce various hormones, the most important of which is cortisol (p. 230).

The effect of cortisol or cortisone can, therefore, be produced either by its own direct administration or by giving ACTH which stimulates its production in the body.

They may be used in diseases affecting the respective glands, i.e. ACTH may be given in hypopituitarism and cortisone in Addison's disease. In practice, however, cortisone is prescribed for both conditions. Cortisone and ACTH also have effects in many other conditions.

ACTH is given by intramuscular injection in doses of 10–25

units at 6-hourly intervals. Gelatin preparations which delay absorption are also available so that only a daily injection is necessary.

Tetracosactrin

This is a synthetic substance which stimulates the adrenal cortex as ACTH does. It is available in a short-acting form (Synacthen), used mainly for diagnostic purposes, and in a long-acting form (Synacthen Depot) which acts for up to 48 hours and is therefore used therapeutically. The dose of the long-acting preparation is 0·5–1 mg intramuscularly, perhaps daily at first and later twice a week.

Anterior lobe preparations

ACTH is prepared from the anterior lobe of animal pituitary glands. Human growth hormone (HGH) is available, in short supply, for the treatment of hypopituitary dwarfs. FSH is extracted from human pituitary glands and used in the treatment of infertility. Growth hormone and FSH of animal origin are ineffective in the human subject.

Substances having an action on the gonads or sex glands similar to that produced by the anterior pituitary hormones can be obtained from the placenta and urine of pregnant women and mares. These are called **gonadotrophic hormones** and are sometimes used in the treatment of primary and secondary amenorrhoea with anovulatory infertility. In the male they may be used for undescended testes and to stimulate the production of spermatozoa in certain cases of hypopituitarism. Their effects are variable and uncertain.

(1) Human chorionic gonadotrophin (HCG), from urine of pregnant women. Dose: 500–3000 units intramuscularly at prescribed intervals. Proprietary preparations include Pregnyl and Gonadotraphon LH. The action resembles LH.

(2) Serum gonadotrophin (from serum of pregnant mares). Preparations include Gestyl and Gonadotraphon FSH. Dose: 500–3000 units intramuscularly at prescribed intervals. The action resembles FSH.

The patient's own pituitary gland may often be stimulated to secrete gonadotrophins by administering a synthetic drug known as **clomiphene** (Clomid). This effect may be used to induce ovulation and thereby to make pregnancy possible in some women who are infertile because of ovarian dysfunction (failure to ovulate). Multiple births sometimes result from clomiphene therapy and the treatment should be supervised by a doctor with special experience.

Posterior lobe preparations

Extracts of the posterior lobe contain two active substances:

(1) *Oxytocin* (*Pitocin*)

This is used in obstetrics, to cause contraction of the uterus without increasing the blood pressure:
(i) To induce labour.
(ii) In the second stage of labour, when the os is fully dilated, to overcome uterine inertia.
(iii) In the prophylaxis and treatment of post-partum haemorrhage.
(iv) To aid the expulsion of the placenta or retained products from the uterus after delivery.
(v) To stimulate uterine contraction during the operation of Caesarean section, immediately after the infant and the placenta have been removed. In this instance it is sometimes injected directly into the uterine muscle.

Dose: Injection of oxytocin (BP) 2–5 units. This is given by slow intravenous infusion (in 1 litre of 5 per cent dextrose solution), intramuscularly or subcutaneously. It is also prepared in a tablet (Pitocin Buccal, 200 units) for absorption in the mouth.

For induction of labour, synthetic oxytocins (e.g. Syntocinon) are now often used. They are purer than Pitocin which contains small amounts of other pituitary hormones. They are given by slow intravenous infusion and the dose is titrated against the uterine contractions. Prostaglandins are used for resistant cases.

(2) *Vasopressin* (*Pitressin*)

This has the following actions:
(*a*) To raise blood pressure by acting on the plain muscles of the arteries producing vasoconstriction.
(*b*) To cause contraction of plain muscle, especially of the intestines and bladder.
(*c*) An antidiuretic action causing water retention in the body. Use is made of this property in the treatment of diabetes insipidus,

in which it may be administered by injection or in the form of snuff.

Dose: Injection of vasopressin (BP), 2–20 units. The effect of this aqueous solution lasts only a few hours and it is used mainly for diagnosis. An oily suspension of vasopressin tannate, 0·5–1 ml (2·5–5 units) intramuscularly every 1–3 days, is used for the treatment of diabetes insipidus. A synthetic compound known as **desmopressin** (DDAVP Desmopressin) has greater antidiuretic activity and a longer duration of action than the natural hormone. It also has the advantage of a greatly reduced vasopressor (blood pressure-raising) effect. It is administered intranasally. **Lypressin** (Syntopressin), which is synthetic lysine-vasopressin, is also administered by nasal spray, and is suitable for mild cases of diabetes insipidus.

Pituitrin and **Di-Sipidin** are proprietary preparations containing both substances and therefore have the following actions:
(*a*) Those due to oxytocin—see above.
(*b*) Those due to vasopressin which stimulates plain muscle:
   (i) it increases peristalsis in the intestines and is used in cases of paralytic ileus and postoperative distension;
   (ii) it causes vasoconstriction by acting on the plain muscle in the arteries and so it raises blood pressure. It is not recommended for this purpose, however, because it may cause dangerous constriction of the coronary arteries;
   (iii) on account of other actions it is sometimes used in diabetes insipidus, haemoptysis and herpes zoster.

The sex glands

The hormones used in therapy may be divided into two main groups:
(1) Female sex hormones derived from the ovary.
(2) Male sex hormones derived from the testis.
   Some synthetic preparations are also available.

1. The internal secretions of the ovary

Two main types of preparation are used:
(*a*) Oestrogens.
(*b*) Progesterone and synthetic progestational compounds (progestogens).

(a) Oestrogens

These are substances which produce the effects of the hormone of the ovarian follicle including:
(i) development of the female secondary sexual characteristics, i.e. growth of pubic and axillary hair, the breasts and external genitalia;
(ii) rhythmic contraction of the Fallopian tube and its fimbriae which collect the ovum at the time of ovulation;
(iii) growth of the uterine muscle and endometrium;
(iv) secretion from the glands of the cervix;
(v) the smoothness of the female skin in comparison with the greasy skin of the male.

The main uses are:
(i) in a minority of women, to diminish some of the unpleasant symptoms occurring at the menopause (hormone replacement therapy, HRT). In most menopausal women, however, there are either no symptoms or symptoms which respond to non-hormonal therapy;
(ii) in the treatment of post-menopausal osteoporosis;
(iii) to suppress lactation on weaning or after a stillbirth, but bromocriptine is preferable, if a drug is required;
(iv) in certain cases of excessive uterine bleeding (metropathia haemorrhagica);
(v) in some cases of amenorrhoea;
(vi) in senile vaginitis and kraurosis vulvae;
(vii) in some cases of carcinoma of the prostate in males and of the breast in females;
(viii) in some cases of acne both in the male and female.

Toxic effects include:
(i) nausea and vomiting;
(ii) excessive uterine bleeding especially after the drug is withdrawn.

There are two main types of oestrogen:
(i) natural: obtained from human sources or from the urine of pregnant mares: e.g. oestrone, oestradiol, Premarin.
(ii) synthetic: e.g. stilboestrol, dienoestrol, ethinyloestradiol, methallenoestril.

Generally speaking the former are expensive and the latter relatively cheap (especially stilboestrol).

The doses vary according to the preparation and the purpose for which it is given. Oral administration is usually effective but preparations for intramuscular injection are available. Many proprietary preparations are on the market. Menopax cream, used locally for pruritus vulvae, contains stilboestrol, testosterone, amethocaine and benzocaine.

(b) Progesterone

This is a hormone formed mainly by the cells of the corpus leteum which develop in the ovarian follicle after the ovum has been extruded. Its main action is to sensitize the endometrium and prepare it for the reception of the fertilized ovum. It also relaxes plain muscle, which may contribute to the occurrence of varicose veins, constipation and dilatation of the ureters during pregnancy.

Its main use is when combined with oestrogen in the treatment of menstrual disorders and in the treatment of excessive uterine bleeding. Its effects in the treatment of abortion and sterility are uncertain. Preparations are given by intramuscular injection in the form of an oily solution.

Ethisterone and other synthetic preparations are given by mouth. Progestogen/oestrogen mixtures (e.g. Anovlar 21, Conovid, Norlestrin, Ortho-Novin) are used for fertility control. Side-effects include amenorrhoea, nausea, headaches and thromboembolic complications.

2. The male sex hormones (androgens)
Testosterone

This is an active substance which is obtained from the testes and which can also be prepared chemically.

Various compounds of testosterone may be given by intramuscular injection (e.g. Primoteston Depot) or by implantation under the skin. Methyltestosterone is given by mouth.

Main uses:
(1) Male hypogonadism and after castration.
(2) In disseminated carcinoma of the breast in post-menopausal women.

Testosterone may produce excessive growth of facial hair in the female and salt and water retention leading to oedema.

Major side-effects

Fortunately these are rare but blood coagulability is increased and there is a slight increase in the incidence of venous thrombosis which may lead to fatal pulmonary embolism. This must, however, be measured against the possible complications of pregnancy.

The number of fatal cases of pulmonary embolism associated with oral contraceptives has fallen substantially since the introduction and general use of 'low-oestrogen' contraceptives, containing not more than 50 micrograms of oestrogen.

Fertility drugs

The use of these drugs is still largely experimental and in the hands of experts. Lack of fertility involves investigation both of the male and female partners in the first instance. At this stage of knowledge little can be done to improve male infertility and lack of spermatogenesis except in a few rare cases where genadotrophin secretion is low and FSH together with HCG (see p. 236) may restore fertility. On the other hand, provided that the ovaries contain the necessary follicles there are preparations (e.g. clomiphene) which readily influence ovulation in the female. They may, however, lead to multiple births.

Other drugs

Danazol (Danol)

This is an antigonadotrophic agent which is used to control the pituitary release of the gonadotrophins, LH and FSH. It is used in the treatment of endometriosis, fibrocystic mastitis, gynaecomastia, and precocious puberty. Dosage is usually within the range of 200 to 800 mg daily in divided doses orally.

Cyproterone (Androcur)

This is used for the treatment of male hypersexuality and sexual deviation (e.g. exhibitionism). It also controls hirsutism in women. It is thought to act by competitive inhibition, the androgens being displaced from their sites of action (effector sites).

Anabolic steroids

One important property of testosterone is its stimulatio
synthesis, i.e. its anabolic effect. Compounds have been
which have the anabolic but only a fraction of the andro
of testosterone. They may therefore be used in wome
risk of inducing virilization. These drugs include noreth
(Nilevar) and nandrolone (Durabolin). They are used to
growth in some types of dwarf. They are also used in d
illnesses and osteoporosis. Their long-term value in the
dition is very doubtful and so is calcium therapy. Oxy
(see p. 112) is effective in the treatment of some cases
anaemia.

Oral contraception

This involves giving healthy women of childbearing age
drugs for social purposes. It avoids the use of mechanical
of contraception, intra-uterine devices, chemical sperm
fertility control by periodic abstinence.

Oral contraceptives generally contain an oestrogen an
gestogen. Most contain 50 micrograms of oestrogen (usu
inyloestradiol). Some contain 30–35 micrograms and or
strin 20) contains only 20 micrograms of oestrogen. All
also contain a progestogen, e.g. norethisterone 1 mg.

If oral contraceptives are taken according to direction
practically 100 per cent effective in preventing pregnancy a
the advantage that aesthetic considerations are not in
There may be, however, a few minor and even major side
There are two main types of preparation in use:
(1) Preparations containing oestrogen and progestogen, ta
21 consecutive days in each 28-day cycle (e.g. Minovla
(2) Two sets of tablets (e.g. Serial 28), (a) those contair
oestrogen taken for the first 16 days of the cycle; (b) thos
for the next 5 days, containing both progestogen and oest
There are also preparations containing only a proge
(such as norethisterone) which are less reliable.

Minor side-effects

These include headache, temporary nausea, breast tende
weight gain, hypertension and depression.

Anabolic steroids

One important property of testosterone is its stimulation of protein synthesis, i.e. its anabolic effect. Compounds have been developed which have the anabolic but only a fraction of the androgenic effect of testosterone. They may therefore be used in women with less risk of inducing virilization. These drugs include norethandrolone (Nilevar) and nandrolone (Durabolin). They are used to accelerate growth in some types of dwarf. They are also used in debilitating illnesses and osteoporosis. Their long-term value in the latter condition is very doubtful and so is calcium therapy. Oxymetholone (see p. 112) is effective in the treatment of some cases of aplastic anaemia.

Oral contraception

This involves giving healthy women of childbearing age powerful drugs for social purposes. It avoids the use of mechanical methods of contraception, intra-uterine devices, chemical spermicides or fertility control by periodic abstinence.

Oral contraceptives generally contain an oestrogen and a progestogen. Most contain 50 micrograms of oestrogen (usually ethinyloestradiol). Some contain 30–35 micrograms and one (Loestrin 20) contains only 20 micrograms of oestrogen. All of these also contain a progestogen, e.g. norethisterone 1 mg.

If oral contraceptives are taken according to direction they are practically 100 per cent effective in preventing pregnancy and have the advantage that aesthetic considerations are not involved. There may be, however, a few minor and even major side-effects.

There are two main types of preparation in use:

(1) Preparations containing oestrogen and progestogen, taken for 21 consecutive days in each 28-day cycle (e.g. Minovlar).
(2) Two sets of tablets (e.g. Serial 28), (a) those containing an oestrogen taken for the first 16 days of the cycle; (b) those taken for the next 5 days, containing both progestogen and oestrogen.

There are also preparations containing only a progestogen (such as norethisterone) which are less reliable.

Minor side-effects

These include headache, temporary nausea, breast tenderness, weight gain, hypertension and depression.

Major side-effects

Fortunately these are rare but blood coagulability is increased and there is a slight increase in the incidence of venous thrombosis which may lead to fatal pulmonary embolism. This must, however, be measured against the possible complications of pregnancy.

The number of fatal cases of pulmonary embolism associated with oral contraceptives has fallen substantially since the introduction and general use of 'low-oestrogen' contraceptives, containing not more than 50 micrograms of oestrogen.

Fertility drugs

The use of these drugs is still largely experimental and in the hands of experts. Lack of fertility involves investigation both of the male and female partners in the first instance. At this stage of knowledge little can be done to improve male infertility and lack of spermatogenesis except in a few rare cases where genadotrophin secretion is low and FSH together with HCG (see p. 236) may restore fertility. On the other hand, provided that the ovaries contain the necessary follicles there are preparations (e.g. clomiphene) which readily influence ovulation in the female. They may, however, lead to multiple births.

Other drugs

Danazol (*Danol*)

This is an antigonadotrophic agent which is used to control the pituitary release of the gonadotrophins, LH and FSH. It is used in the treatment of endometriosis, fibrocystic mastitis, gynaecomastia, and precocious puberty. Dosage is usually within the range of 200 to 800 mg daily in divided doses orally.

Cyproterone (*Androcur*)

This is used for the treatment of male hypersexuality and sexual deviation (e.g. exhibitionism). It also controls hirsutism in women. It is thought to act by competitive inhibition, the androgens being displaced from their sites of action (effector sites).

16 Miscellaneous drugs

Drugs acting on the uterus

The uterus is an organ composed of plain muscle fibres and lined by a special type of mucous membrane, the endometrium. Its functions are (i) to receive the fertilized ovum and to retain the developing fetus throughout pregnancy, (ii) to expel the fetus and placenta at the end of pregnancy.

After puberty the endometrium undergoes a series of periodic changes by which it is prepared to receive a fertilized ovum at regular intervals of about a month. Menstruation is the process by which the specially prepared endometrium is shed when no fertilized ovum has been received.

When the end of pregnancy is reached, the greatly hypertrophied muscle of the body of the uterus commences to contract in a succession of recurring spasms which gradually increase in frequency. At the same time the muscle of the cervix dilates, and when fully dilated the head of the fetus can descend to the perineum, whence the child is finally delivered. Some minutes later this is followed by the placenta and the membranes which surround the fetus during its development in the uterus.

Apart from the female sex hormones which may influence ovarian and uterine function, comparatively few drugs have any important action on the non-pregnant uterus.

On the other hand it must be remembered that some modern drugs may affect fetal development, and careful consideration must be given before they are administered, e.g. cytotoxic drugs. Drugs which cause fetal malformations are said to be **teratogenic**. All new drugs are tested for teratogenicity in animals. Unfortunately, absence of teratogenicity in animals does not guarantee safety for the human fetus. All new drugs are therefore used with great caution in women who may be in the early stages of pregnancy. In prescribing *any* drug for a pregnant woman the doctor has to be sure that it is essential.

Drugs which increase uterine contraction

The drugs which increase uterine contraction once labour is due or has commenced are called **ecbolics.**

Until the introduction of the prostaglandins, there were no drugs which acted on the uterus in the early stages of pregnancy to cause it to expel its contents without producing poisonous symptoms dangerous to the life of the mother.

Ergot

This is a fungus which grows on rye and sometimes on other kinds of grain. Its action is due to the various alkaloids which it contains. It causes contraction of the muscle of the pregnant uterus during and after labour, and is, therefore, especially valuable:

(i)   In the treatment of post-partum haemorrhage, when the contraction of the uterine muscle closes the bleeding vessels.

(ii)   In aiding the expulsion of the placenta and any retained products of conception.

(iii)   To keep the muscle firmly contracted during the first few days of the puerperium.

The following preparations may be employed:

ergometrine maleate
ergot capsules and tablets, 150–500 mg.

Ergometrine maleate

This is an alkaloid which is given in the following doses:

by mouth (tablets): 500 micrograms to 1 mg
by intramuscular injection: 250 micrograms to 1 mg
by intravenous injection: 125 to 500 micrograms
Syntometrine contains ergometrine and synthetic oxytocin.

Pituitary (posterior lobe)

It has already been noted (p. 237) that the extract of the posterior lobe of the pituitary contains **oxytocin** (Pitocin) which causes the plain muscle of the pregnant uterus to contract without producing a rise in blood pressure. Subcutaneous or intramuscular dose, 2–5 units.

Pituitary (posterior lobe) (Injection, BPC 1968, 0·2–0·5 ml, subcutaneously or intramuscularly) is now less often used than the pure hormone oxytocin (which may be prepared synthetically).

Quinine

Quinine is a drug having a number of actions (p. 255). Among them is the ability to cause labour to commence during the last weeks of pregnancy. It has been used in the 'medical induction' of labour, but oxytocin (Pitocin, Syntocinon) is now preferred for this purpose.

Prostaglandins

These are highly potent physiological compounds with a wide spectrum of activity including stimulation of smooth muscle, inhibition of gastric secretion and dilatation of the bronchi. They are present in minute quantities in all mammalian tissues but the highest concentration is in seminal fluid. The total synthesis of prostaglandins has made them available for clinical use.

All prostaglandins have the same basic chemical skeleton—prostanoic acid—but their remaining structural differences enables them to be divided into six groups: E, F, A, B, C and D.

The E and F groups are active in the sphere of obstetrics and gynaecology, especially as **oxytocics** in the induction of labour. For this purpose, prostaglandins E_2 and $F_{2\ alpha}$ are respectively available as dinoprostone (Prostin E2) and dinoprost (Prostin F2 alpha). Uterine hypertonus, unduly severe uterine contractions and fetal distress may result from over-dosage, and the uterus, cervix and fetus must be carefully monitored throughout labour. The prostaglandins potentiate the effect of oxytocin, which should not be used simultaneously.

Side-effects of prostaglandins E_2 and F_2 are dose-related. Nausea, vomiting and diarrhoea are common with the high doses used intravenously for the therapeutic termination of pregnancy.

Uterine sedatives

These are substances which diminish the force and frequency of the muscular contractions of the pregnant uterus, e.g. morphine, chloral hydrate. Halothane effectively relaxes the uterus during the time that it is being administered.

Salbutamol (Ventolin) inhibits uterine contractions by its action on the beta$_2$–adrenoreceptors of the uterus (see p. 189 for discussion of adrenoreceptors). It is given by intravenous infusion to prevent premature labour but is contraindicated if there is associated toxaemia or antepartum haemorrhage.

Ritodrine (Yutopar) is a uterine relaxant which acts selectively on the uterus. Given intravenously or intramuscularly, it quickly controls premature uterine contractions and thereby stops premature labour. An oral preparation of the drug is available for maintenance therapy.

Diagnosis of uterine conditions

Hypaque may be injected into the uterine cavity. Normally, it fills this cavity and also the Fallopian tubes. An x-ray after the injection shows the outline of the uterus, its size and shape and also the patency of the tubes. This procedure may be of importance in the diagnosis of sterility and is called hystero-salpingography.

Preparations acting on the vagina

(1) *Trichomonas* infection: (*a*) acetarsol pessaries, (*b*) Metronidazole (Flagyl) tablets, taken orally, 1 t.d.s. for 7 days. An alternative is nimorazole (Naxogin 500) in a single oral dose of 2 g. The male consort should concurrently receive the same treatment.

Metronidazole is also used in a number of other conditions, viz. anaerobic infections, amoebiasis, giardiasis and acute ulcerative gingivitis.

(2) *Candida* infections: (*a*) crystal violet pessaries, (*b*) nystatin, (*c*) miconazole (Gyno-Daktarin) pessaries and vaginal cream, clotrimazole (Canesten) pessaries and cream.

(3) Antiseptic application: (*a*) chloroxylenol irrigation, one tablespoonful of solution mixed with one pint of warm water, (*b*) proflavine pessaries, (*c*) Penotrane pessaries.

(4) Astringent lotions: zinc sulphate irrigation, 6 g in 500 ml of warm water.

(5) To alter the acidity of the vagina: lactic acid pessary, lactic acid irrigation; one tablespoonful in one pint of warm water.

(6) For senile vaginitis: stilboestrol pessary.

Drugs acting on the eye

Therapeutic substances may be applied to the eyes in the following types of preparation:

eye lotions (*Collyria*)
eye-drops (*Guttae pro oculis*) ⎫ For details see British National
eye ointments (*Oculenta*). ⎭ Formulary.

1. Drugs which dilate the pupil (mydriatics)

The most important are atropine and homatropine.

Atropine

Atropine dilates the pupil and paralyses the power of accommodation when given internally and when applied locally to the eye (p. 193). Locally, it takes several hours to produce its full effect, which lasts for several days. It has the disadvantage of increasing the tension within the eye and is, therefore, contraindicated in cases of glaucoma. It is used for the following purposes:

(i) In the treatment of iritis. By paralysing its power of movement the iris is rested.

(ii) In cases of corneal ulcer.

(iii) In injury to the eyeball.

(iv) For purposes of examination of the retina.

It may be applied in the form of drops, or as an ointment:
Atropine sulphate drops, 1 per cent
Atropine eye ointment, 1 per cent.

These preparations are sometimes combined with cocaine for use in painful conditions.

Homatropine

This has a similar but much more rapid, though less prolonged, action than atropine. The pupils are dilated in 5 to 15 minutes and the effect passes off in a few hours.

Homatropine is especially useful for rapid dilatation of the pupils prior to examination of the optic fundi.

Drops (2 per cent) may be employed. Ointments are also available, and cocaine may be added for the treatment of painful conditions.

It must be remembered that patients may not be able to see properly until the effects of atropine and homatropine have worn off. Reading will be impossible and they may find it very difficult to get about out of doors in bright light.

Adrenaline

Neutral adrenaline (Eppy) Eye-Drops consist of 1 per cent adrenaline in a stable isotonic, neutral solution. They are used in the treatment of open-angle glaucoma. Adrenaline acts partly by decreasing the rate of production of aqueous humor.

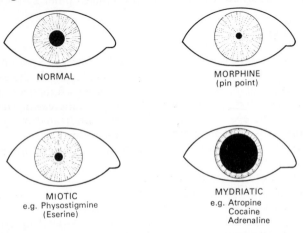

Fig. 16.1. Diagram illustrating the action of drugs on the pupil

2. Drugs which contract the pupil (miotics)

Physostigmine (Eserine)

This is the most important miotic drug. It is used especially in the treatment of acute glaucoma ('closed-angle' glaucoma) and may be employed to counteract the effect of atropine and homatropine when eye examinations have been completed. In glaucoma, contraction of the iris helps to open up the lymph channels in the ciliary body, thereby facilitating the drainage of fluid from the interior of the eye and lowering intraocular tension (see also p. 191):

drops and ointment may be used

physostigmine (eserine) drops, 0·25–1 per cent
physostigmine (eserine) eye ointment, 0·125 per cent.

Pilocarpine eye-drops (1 per cent)
These have similar uses to physostigmine eye-drops but their action is shorter in duration.

Guanethedine (Ismelin) eye-drops
These are used in the treatment of chronic glaucoma and also in the exophthalmos and eyelid retraction of thyrotoxicosis.

Ecothiopate drops
These also may be used in the treatment of chronic simple glaucoma ('open-angle' glaucoma).

3. Local anaesthetics

Cocaine drops (4 per cent)
These are generally employed (a) for operations on the eye, (b) to anaesthetize the conjunctiva in order that a foreign body may be removed, and (c) in the treatment of painful conditions.

Amethocaine eye-drops (1 per cent)
These are very effective and have a more prolonged effect than cocaine.

4. Anti-infective eye-drops and ointments

These are used in the treatment of various types of conjunctivitis and corneal ulceration:

zinc sulphate, 0·25 per cent
sulphacetamide, Albucid, 10, 20, and 30 per cent eye-drops, and 2·5, 6, and 10 per cent eye ointment
chloramphenicol (Chloromycetin) eye-drops and ointment
framycetin (Soframycin) eye-drops and eye ointment
gentamycin (Genticin) eye-drops
neomycin (Nivemycin) eye-drops and eye ointment
idoxuridine (Dendrid, Kerecid) 0·1 per cent drops, or vidarabine (Vira-A) 3 per cent eye ointment for the treatment of ulcerative herpes simplex infections of the cornea.

5. Anti-inflammatory and anti-allergic eye preparations

Castol oil

This is sometimes instilled into the conjunctiva in cases of corneal abrasion. It is also used after anaesthesia with chloroform or ether, to prevent subsequent inflammation due to the irritation of their vapours.

Hydrocortisone

This is used in drops (1 per cent) or ointment (2·5 per cent) in allergic conjunctivitis.

Prednisolone

Eye-drops (0·5 per cent) are used for the same purpose.

6. Diagnostic agents

Fluorescein

Fluorescein 2 per cent placed in the conjunctival sac stains corneal abrasions and ulcers and makes them clearly visible for inspection.

Rose Bengal eye-drops

These (1 per cent) are used in the diagnosis of keratoconjunctivitis sicca ('dry eye').

7. Special eye-drops

Hypromellose

Hypromellose (Isopto Plain and Isopto Alkaline) 0.5 and 1 per cent lubricant eye-drops are used for 'dry eyes', i.e. in cases where there is reduced tear secretion.

Drugs used in the treatment of syphilis

Syphilis is a disease caused by *Spirochaeta pallida* (*Treponema pallidum*). Its clinical manifestations occur in three stages:

(1) The primary sore or chancre.

(2) The secondary stage, commencing about 6 weeks after infection and lasting up to 2 years, during which skin rashes and various other symptoms may arise.

(3) The tertiary stage in which gummata are found. The cardiovascular system, bones or nervous system may be affected. Congenital syphilis may also occur.

The routine treatment of syphilis is to give a full course of penicillin (e.g. 1·2 mega units of procaine penicillin daily for 10–20 days) or one of the other antibiotics (e.g. tetracycline 2–3 g daily for 10–20 days).

Metallic drugs

1. Arsenic

Organic arsenic compounds were formerly used in cases of vaginal discharge especially that due to infection with *Trichomonas vaginalis*. Acetarsol is still incorporated in at least one medication, viz. Pyorex, a paste for the treatment of gingivitis and pyorrhoea.

Poisoning by inorganic arsenic

This may be suicidal or homicidal. Arsenic is present in some weedkillers, in which form it is most easily obtained. The symptoms depend on the dosage taken. A large dose produces epigastric pain, vomiting, diarrhoea, excessive thirst, muscular cramps and collapse which may soon terminate fatally. Smaller doses given over a longer period result in loss of appetite, intermittent attacks of diarrhoea, thirst, colicky abdominal pains, pigmentation of the skin and symptoms of peripheral neuritis such as wrist-drop, numbness and loss of tendon reflexes. Arsenic remains in the body for some time and can be recovered from the hair, nails, liver and other organs.

2. Mercury

Mercury or quicksilver (having the chemical symbol of Hg) is an element which has the form of bright liquid metal. It is used in thermometers, and also in the sphygmomanometer and other types of pressure gauge. A few mercury compounds are still used in medicine.

(1) *External application*

(a) Antiseptic

Thiomersal (Merthiolate) is an organic mercurial compound used for skin antisepsis before surgery. Hydrargaphen is used in pessaries (Penotrane pessaries) for the treatment of infective vaginitis and, together with a barrier cream as Conotrane for skin protection around ileostomy and colostomy stomata.

(b) Antiseptic and antiparasitic ointments

There are a number of ointments containing mercury used, for example, in the treatment of impetigo and pediculosis pubis, e.g. ammoniated mercury ointment.

Oxide of mercury eye ointment, golden eye ointment, is sometimes used for conjunctivitis and blepharitis.

Some people show skin sensitivity to mercury, and its application in any form may be followed by a rash.

(2) *Internal administration*

(a) On the alimentary tract

With large doses the flow of saliva is increased and, if taken over a long period, the mouth and gums become inflamed (stomatitis). Irritation of the intestine is also caused and it will be recalled that calomel has been used as a purgative.

(b) On the kidneys

Certain mercury preparations increased the flow of urine and were available as diuretics (e.g. Mersalyl and Neptal). They have now been superseded.

Mercurial poisoning

The acute symptoms include stomatitis, with a metallic taste in the mouth, gastro-enteritis (diarrhoea and vomiting) and nephritis (blood and albumin in the urine), followed by collapse in serious cases. In chronic cases, in addition to any of the above, peripheral neuritis may develop.

3. Bismuth

Bismuth is employed therapeutically both in its metallic state and in the form of various salts.

Metallic bismuth

Prepared in the form of finely divided particles, bismuth was formerly given by intramuscular injection of a suspension in glucose solution in the treatment of syphilis.

External application
Bismuth subgallate

This is used together with bismuth oxide and other compounds in Anusol suppositories for the treatment of haemorrhoids.

Bismuth and iodoform paste (BIPP), p. 48

Internal administration
Bismuth carbonate

This (2 g) is sometimes used as a weak antacid and gastric sedative in cases of gastritis and gastric ulcer. It is also used in diarrhoea.
De-Nol is a bismuthate compound used in the treatment of peptic ulcers. It causes blackening of the stool.

Drugs used in the treatment of malaria

Malaria is essentially a disease acquired in the tropics and caused by the malarial parasite which is introduced into the body by the bite of an infected *Anopheles* mosquito.

> The parasite reaches the liver where it develops and divides into many small offspring known as merozoites. These escape into the blood stream and invade the red corpuscles. In these cells they undergo a phase of development and division known as schizogony. The resulting new generation of merozoites is liberated from the red cells into the blood stream. They circulate until each again enters a red corpuscle and the cycle is repeated. Circulating parasites can be destroyed by certain drugs and, in the case of malignant tertian malaria, this is the end of the infection. In all other types of malaria, however, the parasites have a persistent phase in the liver. This is known as the exo-erythrocytic phase and accounts for relapses after successful treatment of acute attacks of malaria. Different drugs are required to destroy the parasites in the liver.

The characteristic feature of the disease is the occurrence of rigors at regular intervals of 48 or 72 hours, according to the species of parasite present. The occurrence of rigors coincides with a fresh generation of young parasites being liberated from the red corpuscles.

Antimalarial drugs

For many years quinine was the only drug used in the prevention and treatment of malaria. It has now been largely replaced by various synthetic products, e.g.:

proguanil (Paludrine)
chloroquine (e.g. Nivaquine)

primaquine
pyrimethamine (Daraprim).

Antimalarial drugs may be given in various ways.

(a) Prophylactically

It is a usual practice for persons living in malaria-infested districts to take regular doses of an antimalarial drug in order to suppress or prevent the disease if they happen to be bitten by an infected mosquito.

Those generally used are:

proguanil 100–300 mg daily
pyrimethamine 25–50 mg once weekly
Chloroquine preparations in weekly doses of 300 mg of the base.
Amodiaquine (Camoquin) in weekly doses of 400 mg of the base.

Travellers to malarious areas should be advised to start taking an appropriate antimalarial drug 24 hours before arrival and to continue taking it for 1 month after departure.

(b) For the treatment of an attack

Chloroquine preparations, 600 mg of the base followed by 300 mg 6 hours later and then 300 mg daily for 2 days or amodiaquine 600 mg base for the first 24 hours, then 400 mg daily for 2 more days.

In cerebral malaria and other serious types chloroquine may be given by intramuscular injection or by intravenous drip. Quinine can also be given intravenously but intramuscular injection is likely to cause abscess formation.

(c) For the treatment of the residual infection in the liver

As explained earlier, infection persists in the liver in all types of malaria excepting the malignant tertian variety. **Primaquine** is used to eradicate the liver infection. It is given orally in a dose of 7·5 mg of the base twice daily for 14 days. It may be given concurrently with or following the treatment of the acute attack with chloroquine, amodiaquine or quinine.

Primaquine may cause cyanosis, nausea, vomiting, diarrhoea and abdominal pain. Haemolysis may occur in the blood vessels resulting in anaemia. This complication is more common in some dark-skinned races, owing to an inherited enzyme deficiency. Patients under treatment with primaquine should be under observation for toxic effects. Pamaquine is more toxic than primaquine and has fallen into disfavour.

Mepacrine (Atebrin)

This was the first synthetic antimalarial drug and was of great value during the Second World War. It is slow in action, however, and stains the skin yellow. It occasionally causes mental disturbances. Its use in malaria is no longer recommended where other drugs are available. The drug is still of value in the treatment of tapeworm infestation.

NB.—The real prophylaxis of malaria is to destroy the breeding grounds of the mosquito by draining stagnant water or preventing the hatching of the larva into the adult mosquito by covering such pools with paraffin. A bed net to prevent bites at night is also essential.

Quinine

Quinine is an alkaloid obtained from cinchona bark which is cultivated in the East Indies, India and Sri Lanka. In addition to its now very limited use in malaria it is also employed occasionally for other purposes in therapeutics.

Other uses of quinine

(1) *Antipyretic*. Quinine has an antipyretic action and is occasionally used in the treatment of coryza and mild febrile illnesses.
(2) As a *bitter*. Quinine has a bitter flavour and helps to improve the appetite. It is therefore sometimes included in tonics and is a constituent of 'Bitter Lemon'.
(3) In *obstetrics*. Its former use for the medical induction of labour has been mentioned (p. 245).
(4) In *surgery*. Quinine and urethane solutions have been used for the injection of varicose veins.
(5) To prevent *muscle cramps* at night, 300–600 mg of any of the quinine salts may be taken before retiring. In *myotonia*, a condition where the patient finds it difficult to relax his grip (for example), the dose is 300 mg t.d.s. Procainamide is more effective in this condition.

Some preparations of quinine

Quinine sulphate.
Quinine bisulphate.
Quinine dihydrochloride.

Quinine poisoning and idiosyncracy, see p. 30

Quinidine (p. 95) is another alkaloid obtained from cinchona and is used to prevent the recurrence of cardiac dysrhythmias (e.g. atrial fibrillation) after DC cardioversion.

Anti-rheumatic drugs

A variety of anti-inflammatory drugs is used in the treatment of the rheumatic diseases, which include rheumatoid arthritis, osteoarthrosis (osteoarthritis) and ankylosing spondylitis. The drugs, which are not curative, are used to suppress pain, reduce joint stiffness and swelling, and increase mobility. They reduce inflammation and minimize joint destruction. Analgesic, anti-inflammatory agents form the first line of treatment.

Analgesic, non-steroidal anti-inflammatory agents

These agents also possess antipyretic activity but this is of little or no importance in their use as antirheumatic drugs, except in the treatment of rheumatic fever with aspirin. In varying degree, these drugs inhibit prostaglandin synthesis. This may be the main basis of their analgesic, anti-inflammatory and antipyretic actions.

Aspirin

In ordinary dosage this is a useful analgesic, but in high dosage it also has a definite anti-inflammatory effect. A total of 4–8 g daily is usually necessary in rheumatoid arthritis and larger doses (10 g or more daily) are given in cases of rheumatic fever. Dyspepsia and gastro-intestinal bleeding (usually oozing) are common unwanted effects. If there is gastro-intestinal intolerance, it may be worth trying enteric-coated aspirin, aloxiprin (Palaprin Forte), or benorylate suspension (Benoral). Benorylate is a compound of aspirin and paracetamol which is absorbed in the small intestine.

Propionic acid derivatives

Although these appear to be no more effective than aspirin, they are often better tolerated and have displaced aspirin as the first-line treatment of rheumatoid arthritis. Examples and dosages are as follows:

ibuprofen (Brufen) 200–400 mg 3 times a day
ketoprofen (Orudis, Alrheumat) 50 mg 2 to 4 times a day
fenoprofen (Fenopron) 600 mg 3 or 4 times a day

flurbiprofen (Froben) 50 mg 3 times a day
naproxen (Naprosyn) 250 mg twice daily.

Of these, naproxen is generally the first choice because it combines the greatest effectiveness with the lowest incidence of side-effects. However, it may be necessary to try one-week courses of several or all of these drugs before finding the best one for any individual patient.

The side-effects of treatment with the proprionic acid derivatives are usually related to the upper gastro-intestinal tract—heartburn, nausea, abdominal pain, flatulence, vomiting and anorexia, in decreasing order of frequency. Gastro-intestinal haemorrhage occurs very infrequently.

Acetic acid derivatives

Alclofenac (Prinalgin) is given in a dose of 1 g 3 times a day. It is at least as effective as high doses of aspirin and is well tolerated in long-term therapy. Skin rashes occur in about 2 per cent of patients but other adverse reactions appear to be rare.

Fenclofenac (Flenac) is long-acting and needs to be given only twice daily (2–4 300-mg tablets daily in divided doses).

Pyrazolones

These are long-acting anti-inflammatory, antipyretic and analgesic agents. The best known is **phenylbutazone** (Butazolidine) which is given in a dose of 200–400 mg daily in divided doses. It should be noted that this is less than the dose used to treat an acute attack of gout (p. 223). Phenylbutazone is useful in a number of rheumatic conditions but is particularly effective in ankylosing spondylitis. Its use may be complicated by oedema, rashes and peptic ulceration or, much more rarely, by serious blood dyscrasias – agranulocytosis, thrombocytopenia or aplastic anaemia. **Oxyphenbutazone** (Tanderil) is similar to phenylbutazone.

Azapropazone (Rheumox) has only one-half of the anti-inflammatory activity of phenylbutazone but apparently none of its serious side-effects.

Indomethacin (Indocid)

This anti-inflammatory analgesic is given in a dose of 25 mg 4 times a day or a 100 mg suppository may be inserted into the rectum at bedtime to reduce early morning joint stiffness. Unfortunately, there are many possible reactions, including peptic ulceration, oedema and purpura. Indomethacin is normally eliminated rapidly by the kidneys and should be used very cautiously, if at all, if there is impairment of renal function.

Tolmetin is chemically related to indomethacin and is given in divided doses to a total of 800–1600 mg daily.

Sulindac (Clinoril) is used in the early stages of arthritis as an alternative to aspirin, because it is better tolerated. It is chemically related to indomethacin but considerably less toxic. It causes less gastro-intestinal disturbance than either indomethacin or aspirin. Dose: 100–200 mg twice daily with fluids or food.

Fenemates

Mefenamic acid (Ponstan) is an analgesic which is used in a dose of 500 mg 3 times daily. *Flufenamic Acid* (Arlef) is taken in a dose of 200 mg 3 times daily with food.

Corticosteroids

Long-term corticosteroid therapy (e.g. with prednisolone) is sometimes used in cases which are unresponsive to non-steroidal anti-inflammatory agents. Side-effects (see p. 233) should be watched for and the maintenance dose should be the smallest dose which will suppress symptoms. The aim is to reduce the dose of prednisolone to 6–7·5 mg or less per day.

Intra-articular injections are sometimes useful for individual joints. Suitable preparations are hydrocortisone acetate, prednisolone pivalate injections (Ultracortenol), and triamcinolone hexacetonide (Lederspan).

Gold

Gold is given intramuscularly as **sodium aurothiomalate** (Myocrisin), in rheumatoid arthritis, in an initial dose of 10 mg. A week later a 20 mg dose may be given and thereafter the weekly dose is 50 mg up to a total of 1 g. Further doses may then be given at less frequent intervals. Before each injection it must be ascertained that there is no rash, no albuminuria and no deficiency of platelets or neutrophils in the blood. An eosinophilia may give early warning of a toxic reaction. Clinical benefit is not observed until after several weeks or months of treatment.

A variety of toxic reactions may occur, including rashes, stomatitis, diarrhoea, nephropathy and hepatic and bone marrow damage (agranulocytosis, thrombocytopenia or aplastic anaemia).

The nurse must remember that
(a) the skin, urine and blood must be examined before each dose;
(b) the drug is given by deep intramuscular injection.

Penicillamine

Penicillamine (Distamine) is administered orally, as tablets or capsules, in cases of severe active rheumatoid disease. The dose is 250 mg of the base daily at first. Increments of 250 mg are added at intervals of 2 weeks or more until a daily maintenance dose of 1000–1500 mg is reached. As with gold, clinical benefit is not observed for several weeks or months after starting treatment.

Adverse reactions to penicillamine are also similar to those induced by gold and the skin, urine and blood must be regularly examined.

Antimalarial drugs

Chloroquine and hydroxychloroquine (Plaquenil) are occasionally used as anti-inflammatory agents in rheumatoid arthritis and lupus erythematosus but prolonged administration may cause retinal damage and loss of vision.

Immunosuppressive drugs

Cyclophosphamide (Endoxana) may be given orally in a dose of 50–200 mg daily in cases of rheumatoid arthritis and systemic lupus erythematosus. The blood count must be watched for evidence of serious bone marrow depression and patients should be warned that some temporary loss of hair may occur. An alternative to cyclophosphamide is azathioprine (Imuran).

Immune enhancement

Levamisole, which enhances immunity, may slowly, over several months, produce improvement in patients with rheumatoid arthritis.

It should be noted that the response is similarly delayed with gold, penicillamine, antimalarials and immunosuppressive drugs.

The drugs which a physician uses in the treatment of an individual patient with one of the rheumatic diseases depends on the diagnosis, the stage and severity of the disease, the patient's idiosyncrasies, the presence or absence of dyspepsia, the side-effects of the drugs in question, and possible interactions with other drugs which the patient is taking.

Alcohol

Alcohol is a substance of wide social usage but it must also be regarded as a potential poison and **a drug of addiction.** Its use as a therapeutic measure has been steadily decreasing in medical practice although it probably has a limited sphere of usefulness.

Its main pharmacological actions may be summarized thus:

(1) It is a central nervous system depressant. The apparent stimulating effect in the first instance is due to abolition of the normal mental control of the higher centres of the brain thereby removing inhibitions and anxiety. Progressively its toxic effects precipitate disturbance of behaviour, incoordination of muscular movements and speech and, finally, coma which may prove fatal.

(2) It acts as a peripheral vasodilator which gives rise to a general feeling of warmth. In the stomach this may temporarily improve the appetite.

(3) It is readily metabolized into carbon dioxide and water, providing a number of calories. It is, therefore, to some extent of food value especially as it is quickly absorbed from the stomach.

(4) Excessive intake has a diuretic action, hence the headache and dry mouth due to dehydration in a 'hangover'.

(5) Continued intake is liable to cause defective absorption of vitamins, in particular those of the B complex.

The clinical effects of alcohol

Although many people consume moderate quantities of alcoholic liquor without any obvious harmful effect the clinical manifestations of excess may be considered as: (a) acute and (b) chronic alcoholism.

Acute alcoholism

The symptoms of progressive drunkenness are too obvious and well known to require further description. Several special points should, however, be remembered.

(*a*) It may precipitate migraine, an epileptic fit, or hypoglycaemia in persons subject to these conditions.

(*b*) Alcohol greatly increases the effect of barbiturates, narcotics and some other drugs.

(*c*) It may obscure cerebral or other injury sustained in the inebriated state, sometimes with fatal results.

(*d*) In any case it is unwise to administer it as 'first aid' treatment as the odour of the breath may cause the false impression that the individual is drunk rather than suffering from some organic lesion.

Treatment

In the early stages, before unconsciousness, the simplest measure is to induce vomiting by tickling the back of the throat followed by drinking at least a pint of water which may be repeated at intervals. In comatose patients gastric lavage may be done after inserting an endotracheal tube to avoid the subsequent inhalation of vomitus. Intravenous glucose, injections of nikethamide and vitamin B may be helpful.

The post-alcoholic syndrome ('hangover') may be helped by further intake of water or fruit juice sweetened with sugar or glucose and moderate doses of paracetamol or aspirin. The associated anorexia is usually self-limiting. Whether further small doses of alcohol ('the hair of the dog') are helpful is a matter of individual experience.

Chronic alcoholism

While it must be admitted that some individuals consume considerable quantities of alcohol over many years without ever being obviously intoxicated and without it having any obvious adverse effects, in others many serious conditions may develop. These include:

(*a*) Effects on the nervous system, e.g. neuritis, muscular incoordination ('the shakes'), progressive mental deterioration (alcoholic dementia), insomnia, hallucinations and delirium tremens.

(*b*) Cirrhosis of the liver and its associated symptoms.

(*c*) Chronic gastritis associated with dyspeptic symptoms, vomiting, anorexia and malnutrition.

(*d*) Vitamin deficiency, particularly B_{12}, which may be associated with optic neuritis and visual defects

(*e*) Degeneration of the heart (alcoholic cardiomyopathy).

Social effects of alcohol abuse

(1) It is estimated that alcohol contributes to at least 40 per cent of fatal motor vehicle accidents in Britain.

(2) Alcoholism results in excessive quarrelling in the family, disturbed behaviour in the alcoholic's children, and even frank mental illness (e.g. suicidal depression) in the family. As a result of alcoholism the family may break up.

(3) Alcoholism causes loss of industrial production as a result of absenteeism, sickness and inefficiency.

Treatment

The management of alcohol dependence is essentially a matter for experts and often requires institutional treatment. Gradual reduction of intake covered by sedative drugs helps to minimize withdrawal symptoms. Aversion therapy employing such drugs as apomorphine or disulfiram (see p. 263), given to produce vomiting every time an alcoholic drink is taken, is sometimes employed.

Alcoholics Anonymous is a worldwide organization which is of value to the reformed, but once an individual has been weaned from the habit a single drink may restart the addiction.

Medical uses and abuses

It is not always wise to cut off the supply of alcohol from a patient suffering from an acute disease who is accustomed to its use. In some cases of bronchopneumonia small doses of brandy may induce sleep and act as an easily absorbed foodstuff. A small drink at night sometimes helps the insomnia of the elderly but appropriate sedatives, if necessary, are less expensive! It is used, in combination with amino acids and fructose, as a source of calories in intravenous nutrition (Aminosol-Fructose-Ethanol).

Its use should be forbidden in cases of infective hepatitis, jaundice and peptic ulcer and when it might potentiate the action of any other drugs which are being taken. On the other hand if it produces a feeling of well-being in the terminal stages of cancer or similar fatal conditions its use is certainly justified.

External uses

It has already been mentioned (p. 42) that alcohol and methylated spirit have antiseptic properties and that they harden the skin. Further, their rapid evaporation makes them a useful basis for cooling lotions in the treatment of sprains and contusions.

The alcohol content of various wines and spirits, etc.

	Percent by volume
Liqueurs	up to 50 per cent or more
Brandy, whisky, rum, gin	40 per cent
Port and sherry	20 per cent
Burgundy	up to 14 per cent
Champagne, claret, hock	10 per cent
Beer and stout	3–7 per cent
Cider (bottled)	4 per cent

Disulfiram (Antabuse)

Disulfiram is used, together with psychiatric treatment, to treat chronic alcoholics. It interferes with the metabolism of alcohol, causing acetaldehyde to accumulate in the body. This causes nausea and vomiting, severe flushing, throbbing headache, palpitations and dyspnoea.

The resulting discomfort discourages the patient from drinking alcohol.

When large quantities of alcohol are consumed the reaction may be severe, with hypotension and collapse. Such a reaction is treated with oxygen, intravenous dextrose and, possibly, antihistamines.

The following dosage is used for disulfiram:

day 1 800 mg	day 4 200 mg
day 2 600 mg	day 5 200 mg
day 3 400 mg	

Subsequently 100–200 mg daily for up to 1 year.

Citrated calcium carbimide (Abstem)

This is another drug which interferes with the metabolism of alcohol. As an adjunct in the treatment of chronic alcoholism it is given in a dose of 50 mg (1 tablet) once or twice daily.

Ion-exchange compounds

In some conditions there is an excess of certain ions in the body fluids. For example, there is often an excess of potassium ion in the serum of patients with renal failure. It may be possible to reduce the quantity of the ion in the body by decreasing its absorption via the alimentary tract. It would be possible in most cases to devise a diet containing a negligible quantity of the unwanted ion but such a diet would generally be intolerable for more than a few days and would lack other essential nutrients.

Ion-exchange compounds are drugs (e.g. resins) which combine with certain ions in the alimentary tract and pass out in the faeces, thereby depriving the body of them, other ions being exchanged for the ones removed. The 'donated' ion is, of course, not always wanted and the prescriber must beware of this. Sodium ions would not be wanted, for example, in cardiac failure.

Table 16.1. Ion-exchange compounds

Compound	Binds	Donates
Katonium	Sodium ions	Ammonium and potassium ions
Resonium-A	Potassium ions	Sodium ions
Cholestyramine (Cuemid, Questran)	Bile acids	Chloride ions
Polidexide (Secholex)	Bile acids	Chloride ions
Sodium Cellulose Phosphate	Calcium ions	Sodium ions

Drugs used in the treatment of psychosexual problems

Patients with sexual problems usually need informed and skilled help and advice rather than drugs. There are no genuine aphrodisiacs. However, drugs may be useful in cases where it is desirable to dampen down the male libido. Such a drug is cypoterone acetate (Androcur, p. 242).

17 Antibiotics

An antibiotic is a chemical substance produced by micro-organisms or moulds which prevents the growth (bacteriostatic) of or kills (bactericidal) other micro-organisms.

The most important are:

the **penicillins;**
the **cephalosporins,** e.g. cephaloridine (Ceporin);
the **cephamycins,** e.g. cefoxitin (Mefoxin);
the **tetracyclines**
(*a*) tetracycline (Tetracyn)
(*b*) chlortetracycline (Aureomycin)
(*c*) oxytetracycline (Terramycin)
(*d*) the newer tetracyclines;
the **macrolides,** e.g. erythromycin, spiramycin, oleandomycin;
the **lincomycin group,** e.g. lincomycin and clindamycin;
aminoglycosides, e.g. streptomycin, kanamycin, gentamycin and neomycin;
novobiocin;
chloramphenicol (Chloromycetin);
fusidic acid (Fucidin);
polymyxin B and colistin (Colomycin);
bacitracin;
nystatin, griseofulvin, amphotericin B.

Each antibiotic has its own sphere of activity against the common bacteria. Some ('broad-spectrum' antibiotics) are effective against a wide range of organisms, to others only a few are sensitive, but fortunately most of the common bacteria are affected by at least one of the antibiotics. Certain other micro-organisms, such as the Chlamydia causing lymphogranuloma venereum, psittacosis and some cases of Reiter's syndrome are sensitive to the tetracycline group. *Coxiella burnetii*, the causative organism of Q fever, is responsive to the tetracyclines. The organism (*Mycoplasma pneumoniae*) causing primary atypical pneumonia (formerly regarded as a virus pneumonia) is also sensitive to tetracyclines. Unfortunately, however, antibiotics are ineffective against viruses.

Disadvantages
(1) *Bacterial resistance*

As with sulphonamides, an important drawback to the use of antibiotics is that many bacteria acquire resistance to them after a period of treatment and continue to breed resistant organisms which can cause further disease. This will no longer respond to treatment with the same antibiotic. For example, the tubercle bacillus quickly develops resistance to streptomycin. Staphylococci also acquire resistance both to penicillin and drugs of the tetracycline group.

(2) *Toxic effects and hypersensitivity*

Gastro-intestinal irritation, nausea, vomiting and diarrhoea may occur when antibiotics are given by mouth.

Skin sensitivity may develop to penicillin or streptomycin causing rashes, not only in patients but also in nurses and others handling the drug. Streptomycin may have a serious toxic effect on the vestibular and auditory nerve causing vertigo and deafness.

Very rarely anaphylactic shock with collapse and even death may follow the administration of penicillin in hypersensitive individuals.

For future reference, it is wise to make a conspicuous note on a patient's record if *any* drug sensitivity is observed and the individual should be warned.

(3) *Super-infection*

This applies especially to the antibiotics given by mouth which by killing off some of the normal bacteria inhabiting the alimentary canal permit the overgrowth of other insensitive ones which can cause serious complications.

In particular, there may be an overgrowth of yeasts and fungi (usually *Candida albicans*, the fungus causing thrush) which cause soreness of the mouth and anal regions, or which may even extend into the bronchi and lungs with fatal results.

Staphylococci may develop resistance to penicillin and the tetracyclines and cause serious gastro-enteritis or other infections. Such resistant staphylococci are likely to be susceptible to erythromycin, methicillin, cloxacillin, flucloxacillin, fusidic acid, cephaloridine, cephalexin, novobiocin, neomycin or chloramphenicol.

(4) *Alterations in vitamin formation and absorption from the bowel*

The vitamin B complex, including riboflavine and nicotinic acid, is particularly affected, so that this is sometimes given at the same time as an oral antibiotic, although this is probably only necessary if the administration is prolonged beyond 5 days and in debilitated patients.

(5) *Aplastic anaemia*

Chloramphenicol may occasionally produce aplastic anaemia or agranulocytosis.

The penicillins

These consist of:
(1) Natural penicillins (G and V).
(2) Semisynthetic penicillins.

Benzylpenicillin (penicillin G)

This substance, which was the first antibiotic to be used, and is often simply referred to as 'penicillin', is the active principle of a mould (*Penicillium notatum*) which has a marked action on many bacteria. In the usual doses it is bactericidal. In many instances it is more effective than the sulphonamide drugs and has practically no toxic effects except in sensitive individuals. Although it has a moderately wide range of action not all bacteria are affected by it and even some of those which are can eventually develop some degree of resistance to it.

It is usually given by intramuscular injection but may be given orally, intravenously and intrathecally (in small doses only).

Indications

The suitability of a case for treatment with penicillin depends not so much on the nature of the disease as on the susceptibility of the micro-organism causing it: some species are highly susceptible and others far too resistant for this treatment to have any effect. It follows that in diseases which may be caused by any of several different bacteria (e.g. meningitis, peritonitis), a bacteriological diagnosis and sensitivity test is usually necessary if treatment is to be undertaken with any assurance of success.

The chief organisms susceptible to benzylpenicillin are:

Gonococcus	Diphtheria bacillus
Meningococcus	Organisms of gas gangrene
Streptococcus	Spirochaetes of syphilis and of Weil's disease
Staphylococcus	Actinomyces
Pneumococcus	Anthrax bacillus

Diseases in which penicillin may be used

Examples are:

septicaemia	actinomycosis	carbuncles
puerperal sepsis	anthrax	suppurative arthritis
cellulitis	gonorrhoea	bacterial endocarditis
osteomyelitis	gas gangrene	syphilis
pneumonia	meningitis	

Penicillin is of no value in the following conditions for which it should *not* be used except when some intercurrent infection is present:

tuberculosis
ulcerative colitis
infections caused by viruses such as influenza, poliomyelitis and encephalitis
all Gram-negative bacillary infections such as whooping cough, typhoid fever, dysentery, undulant fever, and infections with *Escherichia coli*.

Properties of penicillin

(a) Once penicillin has been removed from the ampoule or vial it is likely to deteriorate, particularly if exposed to moisture or heat. Solutions or other preparations of penicillin exposed to air and kept at room temperature will not deteriorate significantly in 24 hours, but should be kept in a refrigerator.

(b) Penicillin passes rapidly from the blood into the tissues, but the serous membranes and meninges present a barrier which penicillin does not readily penetrate. Hence intrathecal and intrapleural injections may be necessary.

(c) Penicillin is rapidly excreted; for this reason it must be given in sufficient dosage to maintain an adequate concentration in the blood. Blood concentrations may be raised by blocking renal excretion of penicillin with probenecid 500 mg 6-hourly.

(d) The diffusion of penicillin into dead tissues is poor; sequestra, large sloughs, or collections of pus, are, therefore, likely to harbour bacteria out of reach of the drug, and these usually have to be removed if treatment is to be effective.

Types of benzylpenicillin

Penicillin is an acid substance which forms salts with sodium, potassium and calcium and can be combined with other substances.

There are therefore several different forms of benzylpenicillin which differ somewhat from each other and are used for special purposes.

(1) **Plain benzylpenicillin** or **soluble penicillin** (known also as crystalline penicillin G) which is commonly employed for repeated intramuscular injections in doses of 500 000 to 1 million units (1 mega unit) every 4–12 hours, according to the severity of the infection. Falapen is a form of benzylpenicillin which may be administered orally in twice daily doses of 500 000 units, preferably before a meal.

(2) **Procaine penicillin,** sometimes prescribed as Distaquaine, which is less soluble and therefore more slowly absorbed. It is given in doses of 300 000–600 000 units daily by intramuscular injection. In order to get a more rapid effect the first injection may be combined with a similar dose of soluble benzylpenicillin. In gonorrhoea, one injection of procaine penicillin, 600 000 units is adequate if the organism is sensitive to penicillin but there are now resistant strains.

(3) **Benzathine penicillin** (Penidural LA) is even less soluble and more slowly absorbed. A single intramuscular injection of 600 000 to 1 million units may give an effective blood level lasting several days. A tender hard lump may develop at the site of injection.

NB.—Penicillin is not administered at the same time as tetracycline because the bactericidal effect of the former is diminished by the bacteriostatic action of the latter.

Modes of administration

Benzylpenicillin may be administered in the following ways:
(1) *Intramuscular injection.*
(2) *Intravenous injection. Soluble* penicillin may be injected intravenously in doses similar to those given by intramuscular injection depending on the nature and severity of the infection.
(3) *Intrathecal injection* may be used in certain cases of meningitis. Only specially prepared *soluble* penicillin well diluted, should be employed. The dose should not exceed 20 000 unit in adults or 5000 units in infants.
(4) *Intrapleural injection* may be used in the treatment of empyema.
(5) *Local application.* Penicillin has been used in the form of a solution, a cream and a powder. In the latter instance it has been mixed with a sulphonamide and blown with an insufflator on to raw surfaces or into wounds twice daily.
Apart from eye-drops, local applications are inadvisable and should be discouraged on account of the liability of producing a sensitization rash which may be worse than the original condition.
(6) *Orally*, as in the prophylaxis of recurrences of rheumatic fever.

The duration of treatment

This varies considerably according to the condition and response of the patient, but should seldom be for less than 5 days or more than 12 days. Treatment is usually continued for about 2 days after a favourable response has been obtained. If no response is obtained within 72 hours another antibiotic will probably be needed.

Toxic reactions

Penicillin is usually non-toxic, but it occasionally gives rise to delayed reactions, such as fever, and urticarial rashes. These may be treated with antihistamine drugs and the local application of calamine lotion.

Rarely, as previously mentioned, an immediate reaction—*anaphylactic shock*—with collapse and even death may occur. In this type of reaction adrenaline 1 ml (1 in 1000) should be injected subcutaneously at once, followed by an intravenous anti-histamine, e.g. chlorpheniramine (Piriton) 10 mg and intravenous hydrocortisone (100 mg). Before giving penicillin, it is wise routinely to enquire about previous sensitivity and also if the patient is subject to asthma or other allergic conditions.

Phenoxymethylpenicillin (penicillin V)

Unlike benzylpenicillin, this is able to resist inactivation by gastric hydrochloric acid. It is therefore used as an oral penicillin. Dose: 125–250 mg every 4–6 hours for adults; 62·5–250 mg every 6 hours for children. It is most rapidly absorbed if given on an empty stomach and should be given about half an hour before meals. Proprietary preparations include Crystapen V and Distaquaine V-K.

The semisynthetic penicillins

These are produced by the addition of side-chains to the penicillin nucleus, which was isolated in 1959. They may be classified into 3 types, examples of which are shown in the following table.

Table 17.1 The semisynthetic penicillins

Acid-resistant	Penicillinase-resistant	Broad-spectrum
phenethicillin (Broxil)	methicillin (Celbenin) cloxacillin (Orbenin) flucloxacillin (Floxapen)	ampicillin (Penbritin) amoxycillin (Amoxil) carbenicillin (Pyopen) mecillinam (Selexid)

The acid-resistant penicillins

These resist inactivation by gastric hydrochloric acid and are, therefore, used as oral penicillins. **Phenoxymethylpenicillin** and **phenethicillin** are highly satisfactory and are given in a dosage of 125–250 mg 4–6-hourly. They are generally indicated in minor infections (e.g. acute tonsillitis) by highly susceptible organisms (e.g. haemolytic streptococci).

The penicillinase-resistant penicillins

Benzylpenicillin is inactivated by the enzyme penicillinase, which some bacteria (e.g. resistant staphylococci) produce. Some of the semisynthetic penicillins are resistant to staphylococcal penicillinase and are therefore used against benzylpenicillin-resistant staphylococci. **Methicillin** (Celbenin) is inactivated by gastric acid and must, therefore, be given parenterally. The dose is 1 g intramuscularly every 4–6 hours. **Cloxacillin** (Orbenin) can be given orally, 500 mg 6-hourly, or intramuscularly, 250 mg 4–6-hourly. **Flucloxacillin** (Floxapen) is absorbed more readily and the usual dose by mouth is 250 mg 6-hourly.

Broad-spectrum penicillins

Ampicillin (Penbritin) is active against a wide range of bacteria, including strains of *Escherichia coli*, *Salmonella*, *Shigella*, *Haemophilus influenzae*, *Proteus mirabilis* (but not other *Proteus* species) and enterococci. Of particular value is the activity against Gram-negative bacilli, an activity which benzylpenicillin lacks. It is used principally in urinary tract infections (500 mg 8-hourly) and in chronic bronchitis (usually 250 mg but up to 1 g 6-hourly). Ampicillin may also be used in the treatment of subacute bacterial endocarditis, the serum level of the drug being increased by concomitant administration of probenecid. Ampicillin is effective, at a dose of 8 g *per diem*, in typhoid fever but chloramphenicol is more rapid in action and is the treatment of choice. Ampicillin is excreted in the urine and bile and, because of the high concentration reached in the latter secretion, it is useful in the treatment of typhoid carriers.

Magnapen is a mixture of ampicillin and flucloxacillin. It might be used in cases where it is not known whether the infecting organism is a Gram-negative bacillus or a penicillin-resistant staphylococus, or where both are known to be present.

Amoxycillin (*Amoxil*)

This has the same spectrum of activity and uses as ampicillin, but is more completely absorbed from the gastro-intestinal tract and the oral dose is only 250 mg 3 times a day.

Carbenicillin (*Pyopen*)

This is active against strains of Proteus, Pseudomonas and coliform organisms. It is ineffective by mouth and is given by injection. The intramuscular dose for urinary tract infections is 2 g 6-hourly. Systemic infections, septicaemia and endocarditis necessitate a higher dosage, i.e. 5 g 4–6-hourly by rapid intravenous infusion. Probenecid may be given concurrently by mouth to block the renal excretion of the antibiotic and thereby to increase its serum concentration.

Carfecillin (*Uticillin*)

This is taken orally in a dose of 500 mg to 1 g 3 times a day. It is rapidly absorbed and is hydrolysed in the body to carbenicillin, which reaches high concentrations in the urine. It is used only for urinary tract infections.

Mecillinam

This penicillin is especially active against Gram-negative bacilli, particularly *Esch. coli*. As it is poorly absorbed from the gastrointestinal tract, it is given as pivmecillinam (Selexid), which is rapidly absorbed and converted into the active substance, mecillinam. The dose for uncomplicated cystitis is 200 mg (1 tablet) 3 to 4 times daily, while a total daily dosage of up to 2·4 grams is used in typhoid fever.

General points about the penicillins

(1) Benzylpenicillin remains the penicillin of choice for pneumococcal pneumonia and many other conditions.
(2) Hypersensitive patients show cross-reactivity to all the penicillins.
(3) Oral penicillins are best given on an empty stomach (or $\frac{1}{2}$ hour a.c.) in order to promote absorption and hence achieve high serum levels.

The cephalosporins

These are derivatives of a fungus isolated from the sea near a sewage outfall in Sardinia. One (cephalosporin N) is a broad-spectrum penicillin (otherwise known as penicillin N). Cephalosporin C has a nucleus similar to that of penicillin.

Cephaloridine (Ceporin)

This is a semisynthetic cephalosporin made by adding a side-chain to the nucleus of cephalosporin C. It is highly bactericidal against Gram-negative organisms and Gram-positive cocci including penicillin-resistant staphylococci. It is a broad-spectrum antibiotic having an even wider range of antibacterial activity than ampicillin. It is usually well tolerated by patients who are hypersensitive to the penicillins but in some patients there is cross-allergenicity. Being excreted unchanged in the urine, high urinary levels of the antibiotic are reached and it is contra-indicated in patients with impaired renal function.

This antibiotic is poorly absorbed from the gastro-intestinal tract and it must, therefore, be given by injection (intramuscularly or intravenously). The same is true of **cephazolin** (Kefzol), which is given intramuscularly, **cephalothin** (Keflin), which is given intravenously, and **cefuroxime** (Zinacef), which is given intramuscularly or intravenously.

Oral cephalosporins

Some cephalosporins are readily absorbed from the gastro-intestinal tract and are therefore administered orally. **Cephalexin** (Ceporex, Keflex) is one of these and is usually given in a dose of 250–500 mg 6-hourly. Up to 1 g 6-hourly may be prescribed for pneumonias, however. **Cephradine** (Velosef, Eskacef) is an alternative cephalosporin which may be given orally or by injection.

In brief, the cephalosporins are bactericidal and have a broad spectrum of activity, low toxicity and little tendency to cause allergic reactions. They are used orally for the treatment of genitourinary and respiratory tract infections and by intramuscular injection for the prevention of bacterial endocarditis, and the treatment of severe infections. They are used intravenously for bacteraemias and septicaemias.

It should be noted that the cephalosporins may cause a false positive reaction for glucose in the urine with Benedict's or Fehling's solutions, or with Clinitest tablets, but not with enzyme tests such as Clinistix or Diastix.

The cephamycins

Cefoxitin (Mefoxin) is a derivative of an antibiotic produced by a bacterium known as *Streptomyces lactamdurans*. It has a broad spectrum of bactericidal activity including anaerobic organisms. It is given by intravenous or intramuscular injection, usually in a dose of 1 g or 2 g every 8 hours.

Chloramphenicol (Chloromycetin)

This is a crystalline substance originally obtained from the mould *Streptomyces venezuelae* and which can also be prepared synthetically. It is bacteriostatic.

It may be indicated in:

(1) Typhoid fever.

(2) *Haemophilus* meningitis and *Klebsiella pneumoniae* infections.

(3) Life-threatening infections in which other antibiotics will not suffice.

Some individuals, especially children, are sensitive to chloramphenicol and the drug may affect the bone marrow causing *aplastic anaemia* or agranulocytosis, which may prove fatal. It may occur after relatively small doses. The danger to adults is very small provided the course of treatment does not exceed 10 days.

It is supplied in capsules each containing 250 mg. It has a bitter taste which is sometimes a disadvantage when given to children unless concealed in honey or given in the form of a special preparation (Chloromycetin Palmitate).

The dose is 250–500 mg every 4 or 6 hours.

Ointments are available, also eye-drops and ear-drops. These local applications are almost entirely free from the danger of producing blood dyscrasias.

The tetracyclines

These include:

(*a*) **tetracycline** (Tetracyn, Achromycin).

(*b*) **chlortetracycline** (Aureomycin).

(*c*) **oxytetracycline** (Terramycin).

(*d*) The newer tetracyclines, e.g. demethylchlortetracycline (Ledermycin), methacycline (Rondomycin), lymecycline (Tetralysal), doxycycline (Vibramycin), clomocycline (Megaclor) and minocycline (Minocin).

Although Aureomycin and Terramycin were the first drugs of this group to be isolated and used, chemically they are both derived from tetracycline which has antibiotic effects similar to the others.

The tetracyclines differ slightly in chemical composition but have a very similar antibiotic range which covers not only those organisms which are generally sensitive to penicillin but also an agent (*Mycoplasma*) causing primary atypical ('virus') pneumonia, rickettsiae, Coxiella (Q fever) and some of the larger 'viruses' (Psittacosis). They are sometimes useful against staphylococci which are resistant to penicillin, but staphylococci and streptococci can also develop resistance to tetracyclines. They may be used in chronic bronchitis, where infective episodes are often due to the influenza bacillus (*Haemophilus influenzae*) and the pneumococcus (*Streptococcus pneumoniae*). They are of value in the treatment of diverticulitis of the colon.

The first 3 tetracyclines are usually given by mouth in doses of 500 mg followed by 250 mg every 4–6 hours for 5 days.

Special preparations are available for intravenous and intramuscular injections and local applications such as drops and ointments are also in use.

The physiochemical properties of **lymecycline** make it eminently suitable for intramuscular or intravenous use. **Doxycycline**, unlike the other tetracyclines, may safely be given to patients in renal failure. In contrast to the other tetracyclines, it is not cumulative, does not accelerate uraemia, and is not leached out by peritoneal dialysis. Otherwise, there seems little reason to prefer the new tetracyclines to the old. All of the tetracyclines have a similar antibacterial spectrum.

Tetracyclines given during pregnancy and the first few years of life may cause permanent discoloration of the developing teeth.

The aminoglycosides

These include streptomycin (see p. 279), neomycin, kanamycin, gentamicin, amikacin and tobramycin.

Neomycin

Neomycin is of value orally in some gastro-intestinal infections and may also be applied locally to the skin. It is too toxic for parenteral administration, which may result in deafness.

Kanamycin (Kantrex, Kannasyn)

This is primarily of value in the treatment of resistant *Proteus* infections and also in gonococcal infections when the patient is sensitive to penicillin or the organism is resistant. It is a toxic drug and, like streptomycin, may cause deafness.

Gentamycin (Genticin, Cidomycin)

This is active against *Pseudomonas aeruginosa*. Gentamycin is a broad-spectrum antibiotic and may be used together with penicillin or erythromycin in serious systemic infections and infective endocarditis before the antibiotic sensitivity of the infecting organism is known. High blood levels of gentamycin may cause vestibular damage (hence vertigo), and the dose of the drug is therefore reduced for patients with impaired renal function.

Amikacin (Amikin)

This is active against a broad spectrum of Gram-negative organisms, including Pseudomonas species, and some Gram-positive organisms. It is used for the treatment of serious infections and is given intramuscularly or, in life-threatening infections, intravenously.

Tobramycin (Nebcin)
This also is given by intramuscular or intravenous injection in the treatment of infections due to Pseudomonas and other Gram-negative organisms.

The aminoglycosides can cause damage to the kidneys (nephrotoxicity) and the 8th cranial nerve (ototoxicity), resulting in hearing loss or vertigo or both.

The Macrolides

Erythromycin (200–500 mg, 6-hourly)

This is an antibiotic having a similar range of action to penicillin. It is used against staphylococci which have become resistant to other antibiotics. Resistance to erythromycin also develops rapidly so that its use against staphylococci should be restricted to selected and urgent cases. One of its principal uses now is in situations where penicillin is indicated but cannot be given because of the patient's hypersensitivity. Proprietary preparations include Erythrocin and Ilotycin. Intravenous injections are available.

Spiramycin (Rovamycin) and **oleandomycin.** These have properties similar to erythromycin.

Other antibiotics

Fusidic acid (Fucidin)

This is bactericidal towards staphylococci, and is reserved for treatment of infections due to staphylococci which are resistant to other antibiotics. Usual dose: 2 capsules (500 mg) 3 times a day with meals.

Lincomycin (Lincocin)

Lincomycin penetrates bone well and is useful for treating staphylococcal osteomyelitis. It is also used against serious Gram-negative anaerobic infections; most Bacteroides species are sensitive to it. It is usually given intramuscularly but is also available in capsules and syrup for oral administration.

Clindamycin (Dalacin C)

Clindamycin, a derivative of lincomycin, is given orally, being well absorbed. It is effective against staphylococci, streptococci and pneumococci.

Acute colitis, which may be life-threatening, is one of the occasional toxic effects of lincomycin and clindamycin and these are not drugs for use against minor infections.

Rifampicin (Rimactane, Rifadin)

This is a semisynthetic derivative of the antibiotic rifamycin. It is active against a wide range of Gram-positive and Gram-negative bacteria, mycobacteria (tuberculosis and leprosy) and the trachoma agent. It also inhibits certain pox viruses, e.g. variola minor (a strain of smallpox virus) and vaccinia virus, but unfortunately the high concentrations of the drug which would be required to treat these virus diseases in man could not be maintained.

Bacitracin

Bacitracin, an antibiotic derived from *Bacillus subtilis*, has a limited use against streptococci, staphylococci and some other organisms. It may have a toxic effect on the kidneys and is only given by injection in selected cases when other antibiotics have failed (dose 20 000 units, 6-hourly). It may safely be applied locally to infected wounds.

Polymyxin B

This is effective against *Pseudomonas aeruginosa* and certain other uncommon organisms. It is given in doses of 250 000 units every

4–6 hours by intramuscular injection. It can be given intrathecally in special cases of meningitis.

Colistin (Colomycin)

This resembles polymyxin B chemically and pharmacologically and is equally toxic. Principal toxic effects are on the nervous system and kidneys.

Tyrothricin and gramicidin

These may be used as local applications.

Fungicides

Nystatin

This is a special antibiotic which has no action on ordinary bacteria but is effective against fungi and yeasts such as *Candida albicans*. It may be applied locally for thrush and pessaries are available for vaginal infections. Doses of 500 000 to 1 million units may be given by mouth for candidiasis of the alimentary tract, which may follow administration of tetracycline or other broad-spectrum antibiotics.

Nystatin is not absorbed from the gastro-intestinal tract and is not suitable for systemic candidal infections.

Griseofulvin

This is used in the treatment of fungous infections of the skin, including ringworm. The usual dose is 500 mg to 1 g daily, orally. Treatment may be prolonged if the nails are affected.

Amphotericin B

This is a fungicidal antibiotic used in sytemic mycotic infections with *Candida*, *Coccidioides*, *Cryptococcus*, *Blastomyces* and *Histoplasma*. It is very toxic and may cause kidney damage and, therefore, must only be used with great caution.

Antituberculous drugs
Streptomycin

This is an antibiotic obtained from a soil organism called *Streptomyces griseus*. It is interesting to note that in the process of its manufacture vitamin B_{12} is formed, a fact which has made the preparation of the latter substance commercially possible.

Although streptomycin is used mainly in the treatment of tuberculosis, it is also active against a number of organisms (especially Gram-negative bacilli, many of which are insensitive to penicillin, e.g. *Escherichia coli*), which accounts for its usefulness in a number of other conditions. These include some types of pneumonia, peritonitis, cholecystitis, infection of the urinary tract and any condition caused by organisms which are shown by bacteriological tests to be insensitive to penicillin or other antibiotics. In these conditions its administration is only continued for a few days. Streptomycin may be combined with penicillin (e.g. Crystamycin) for use in some infections.

Disadvantages

Like other antibiotics it has certain disadvantages which include:
(1) Not only the tubercle bacillus but also other organisms rapidly acquire a tolerance to it and permanently resistant strains of micro-organisms are produced which will no longer respond to treatment with it.
(2) If prolonged or heavy dosage, which may sometimes appear necessary in tuberculosis, is employed there is a risk of causing serious toxic effects which include damage to the 8th cranial nerve and the symptoms of giddiness, deafness and tinnitus. The risk increases after the age of 40 years. These symptoms may gradually clear up but in some cases are permanent.
(3) Persons who handle the drug may become sensitive to it after a few weeks and may develop a dermatitis of the hands, forearm and around the eyes, which is often very intractable to treatment. Rubber gloves should, therefore, always be worn when administering streptomycin.
(4) Hypersensitivity reaction in the patient is usually manifested by fever, often accompanied by a rash.
Streptomycin may be used in the treatment of all forms of tuberculosis, the dosage and duration of treatment depending on the individual case.

In pulmonary tuberculosis the dose is usually 1·0 g daily.

In tuberculous meningitis, intrathecal injections of 100 mg in 5–10 ml of distilled water may be given in addition to intramuscular injections.

It is not absorbed when given by mouth but may be given in this way in certain non-tuberculous intestinal infections. Streptotriad is a mixture of streptomycin and three sulphonomides which may be taken in tablet or suspension form.

Rifampicin (Rimactane, Rifadin)

This has replaced PAS as a first-line drug in the treatment of tuberculosis. Rifampicin and isoniazid are given together as basic therapy and ethambutol or streptomycin is also given for the first 6–8 weeks or until cultures are negative. Rifampicin is given as a single daily dose in the region of 10 mg/kg of body weight, usually 450 or 600 mg daily. It may discolour the urine and other secretions, making them brownish-red.

Isoniazid

Isonicotinic acid hydrazide (INAH), Rimifon, etc.

This is a synthetic antituberculous substance.

The average dose is 200–300 mg of isoniazid daily in divided doses.

It passes through the meninges into the cerebrospinal fluid and given with streptomycin, is of importance in the treatment of tuberculous meningitis.

Rifinah and **Rimactazid** are tablet formulations containing both rifamipicin and isoniazid; two strengths are available.

Inapasade granules contain both PAS and INAH and are a convenient form of administration. The average dose is 1 packet twice daily.

Because the tubercle bacillus quickly develops resistance to drugs when they are given singly, it is usual to give 2 of the drugs together. The usual scheme is to give all three 'standard' drugs together initially (standard triple chemotherapy). If the tubercle bacilli are found, in the laboratory, to be sensitive to two of the three drugs, one is withdrawn after 6–8 weeks.

The total duration of a course of antituberculous treatment is usually about a year.

Ethambutol (initially 25 mg/kg once daily)

This is a powerful antituberculous drug. Occasionally it causes retrobulbar neuritis, an inflammation of the optic nerve, which fortunately resolves completely after the drug is discontinued.

Second-line drugs for the treatment of tuberculosis (reserve drugs)

Certain drugs are reserved for use in cases where the tubercle bacilli are resistant to or the patient is intolerant of standard drugs.

Para-aminosalicylic acid (PAS)

This drug which is usually prescribed in the form of its sodium salt (**sodium aminosalicylate**), is not an antibiotic, but it may be used in conjunction with streptomycin for two reasons:
(1) It has itself an action on the tubercle bacillus.
(2) It delays the development of streptomycin resistance.

The usual dose is 12–15 g daily in divided dosage.

It has a bitter taste and may be taken in water with or without flavouring agents, or in cachets.

In some cases the urine of patients taking PAS reduces Benedict's reagent. PAS is detectable in the urine by testing with Phenistix and this is useful if one suspects that a patient is failing to take his prescribed drugs. It may cause nausea, vomiting and diarrhoea. Hypersensitivity reactions are common and are manifested usually by fever and a rash. Liver damage may occur.

Thiacetazone

This drug, 150 mg orally daily, is often an effective alternative to PAS, for combined therapy with isoniazid, and is cheaper.

Ethionamide (0·75–1 g daily)

This is a powerful antituberculous drug but may have unpleasant side-effects. **Prothionamide** has less gastro-intestinal side-effects and may therefore be preferred.

Pyrazinamide (maximum dose 1·5 g twice daily)

This is another powerful antituberculous drug. Liver damage is the most important adverse reaction to this drug.

Cycloserine (1 g daily in divided doses)

Cycloserine is an antibiotic with a relatively weak action on tubercle bacilli. Side-effects include convulsions and psychotic disturbances.

Other second-line drugs are **viomycin, kanamycin** and **capreomycin.**

Antileprotic agents

The treatment of leprosy is often difficult and usually protracted; drugs commonly have to be taken continuously for 4 years. **Dapsone** is the drug which is most used and is given orally in tablet form, commencing with 25 mg once weekly. Acute exacerbations of lepromatous leprosy (lepra reaction) may be induced by dapsone and require treatment with corticosteroids.

DADDS is in the same group of drugs (sulphones) as dapsone but is long-acting and a single intramuscular injection of DADDS suspended in a special oil provides treatment for 75–90 days. **Clofazimine** (Lamprene), a phenazine dye, is the drug of choice when leprosy is resistant to sulphones or is in a state of severe and persistent exacerbation.

Other drugs used in leprosy are **thiambutosine** (Ciba–1906), **thiacetazone, ethionamide, prothionamide, rifampicin** (a derivative of rifamycin), and some long-acting sulphonamides (e.g. sulfadoxine).

Note: PAS, INAH, ethionamide, thiacetazone, pyrazinamide and ethambutol are not antibiotics but are included in this section for convenience. Of the antileprotic agents only rifampicin is an antibiotic derivative.

18 Other antimicrobial drugs

Antibacterial drugs
Sulphonamides

The sulphonamides were the first major antibacterial drugs for systemic use. Their importance has declined as a result of the discovery of antibiotics but they still provide a useful alternative. They are used principally in the treatment of meningococcal meningitis and infections of the intestinal and urinary tracts. They are also useful against antibiotic-resistant organisms and in patients who are allergic to certain antibiotics.

Sulphonamides do not actually kill bacteria but prevent their growth and multiplication in the body so that the patient's own defence mechansims can eradicate the infection. They act by preventing bacteria from using *para*-aminobenzoic acid (PABA), a substance necessary in their metabolism. They are therefore bacteriostatic in action.

The main principle in their administration is the rapid production of a high concentration in the blood, by giving a loading dose, and the maintenance of this concentration for some days, until pyrexia and symptoms have subsided. Many organisms which were originally sensitive to sulphonamides have become resistant, and bacterial sensitivity tests are important.

Sulphadimidine (Sulphamezathine) is one of the most effective, best tolerated, and least toxic sulphonamides. It reaches high concentrations in all tissues and in the urine. It is given in an initial dose of 2–3 g, and this is followed by 1–1·5 g 6-hourly.

Phthalylsulphathiazole (Thalazole) and succinylsulphathiazole (Sulfasuxidine) are poorly absorbed and consequently pass on into the lumen of the whole length of the colon. They are therefore used in preparation for large bowel surgery.

Sulphasalazine (Salazopyrin) is a sulphonamide which is used exclusively in the treatment of ulcerative colitis and Crohn's disease. The dose is 1–2 g 4 to 6 times daily for 3 weeks, followed by a long-term maintenance dose of 1 g twice daily.

The nurse may encounter many other sulphonamides, including sulphathiazole (Thiazamide), sulphadiazine, sulphafurazole

(Gantrisin), trisulphonamide (Sulphatriad, a mixture of 3 sulphonamides), sulphamethizole (Urolucosil) and sulphaguanidine. Long-acting sulphonamides include sulphaphenazole (Orisulf) and sulphamethoxypyridazine (Lederkyn, Midicel). One dose of 500 mg to 1 g of the latter drug is sufficient for 24 hours. For prevention of streptococcal sore throats and recurrences of rheumatic fever, this drug need be given only once a week.

The toxic effects of sulphonamides are mainly allergic and include headache, nausea and vomiting. Occasionally skin rashes, polyarteritis, Stevens–Johnson syndrome (multiform erythematous skin rash and ulceration of the mouth and often the eyes, nose and genital orifices) and agranulocytosis occur. Some of the older sulphonamides tend to crystallize in the urine, causing haematuria and even suppression of urine. This is particularly likely to occur if dehydration is present as a result of diarrhoea or excessive sweating. In these circumstances, an adequate fluid intake must be maintained and it may be advisable to render the urine alkaline with potassium citrate.

Co-trimoxazole (Bactrim, Septrin)

This is a mixture of a sulphonamide (sulphamethoxazole) and trimethoprim, a drug which blocks bacterial folic acid metabolism. The combination is bactericidal and its spectrum of activity is greater than that of sulphonamides alone. It is effective in the treatment of bronchitis, gonorrhoea and most urinary infections and has been used successfully in brucellosis and typhoid and in infections caused by other members of the salmonella group of bacteria. The usual adult dose is 2 tablets twice daily. An intramuscular injection is available for use when the oral route cannot be used or relied upon. Co-trimoxazole may also be given by infusion (e.g. Septrin for Infusion) in, for example, septicaemia, severe chest infections, and typhoid.

Coptin is a similar preparation, incorporating sulphadiazine instead of sulphamethoxazole. The dose is one tablet night and morning.

Nalidixic acid (Negram)

This antibacterial agent is concentrated in the kidney, where it is bactericidal to many Gram-negative organisms. Dose: 500 mg to 1 g 4 times daily.

Nitrofurantoin (Furadantin)

This a broad-spectrum antibacterial agent which is bactericidal in the kidney and urinary tract. It is used for the treatment of urinary tract infections. Dose: 100 mg 4 times a day. It may cause nausea and vomiting but is less likely to do so if each dose is taken with food or milk.

Hexamine hippurate (Hiprex) (see also p. 147)

The antibacterial activity of this agent is confined to the urinary tract, where it is active against a wide spectrum of bacteria, both Gram-negative and Gram-positive. It is particularly suitable for long-term treatment of chronic or recurrent urinary tract infections. It is taken by mouth, usually in a dose of 1 g twice daily.

Metronidazole (Flagyl)

This is an important drug in the prevention and treatment of Bacteroides and other anaerobic infections. Used to cover elective colonic surgery, it practically eliminates wound infection. It may be given by mouth, by rectum (as suppositories) and by intravenous infusion. It is also effective in the treatment of trichomonal vaginitis, ulcerative gingivitis, giardiasis and amoebiasis.

Antiviral agents

Viral chemotherapy is in its infancy but a few clinically effective agents are available. It is relevant that viruses differ in their nucleic acid content, some containing desoxyribonucleic acid (DNA) and some containing ribonucleic acid (RNA). No virus contains both.

Idoxuridine

This interferes with the DNA molecule and can inhibit the replication (multiplication) of DNA viruses when given in one-tenth of the dose which would inhibit human cell reproduction. It is used against herpes simplex virus locally in herpetic keratitis (Kerecid eye-drops) and systemically in cases of herpes encephalitis. It is also used locally as a solution (Herpid) against herpes zoster virus in cases of shingles.

Methisazone (Marboran)

This is active against the pox group of viruses. It is used for the prophylaxis of smallpox, in unvaccinated contacts of the disease, and in the treatment of vaccinia.

Cytarabine (cytosine arabinoside, Cytosar)

This may be used in the treatment of serious herpes simplex infections (e.g. encephalitis), varicellar pneumonia and generalized varicella.

Amantadine (Symmetrel)

Amantadine, which is used in the treatment of Parkinsonism, will prevent influenza due to influenza virus type A_2 and swine-type influenza virus if given orally in a dose of 200 mg daily before and after virus challenge. It does not prevent influenza due to influenza type B and type C viruses. Amantadine is also used for the treatment of herpes zoster.

Antifungal agents

These are used to treat fungal infections (mycoses). Preparations are available for (a) topical use against surface infections (see also p. 55) and (b) systemic administration.

(a) Topical preparations

nystatin—used for candidiasis of skin, mouth, vagina, bowel and bronchial tree
amphotericin—lozenges for oral candidiasis (thrush)
clotrimazole—1% cream and vaginal tablets for skin and vagina
miconazole—cream for fungal infections of the skin
—cream or pessaries for fungal infections of the vagina.

(b) Systemic agents

griseofulvin—for oral treatment of fungal infections of skin and nails amphotericin (Fungizone)—systemic fungicide for life-threatening fungal infections—given intravenously—nephrotoxic

Flucytosine (Alcobon)—given orally for treatment of systemic infections with *Candida* and *Cryptococcus*.

19 Vaccines, sera and other biological products

The preparation and use of vaccines and sera are closely connected with the subject of **Immunity.**

By immunity is meant the ability of an individual to resist disease, and is dependent on:

(i) The power of leucocytes to destroy bacteria.

(ii) The presence of antibodies in the blood and tissues which kill bacteria or of antitoxins which neutralize their toxins.

Immunity may be:

(1) Natural or inborn.

(2) Acquired
   (a) as a result of recovery from infection.
   (b) artificially produced:
      (i) active immunity stimulated by the use of vaccines and toxoids;
      (ii) passive immunity (by the use of serum containing antibodies obtained from other individuals, e.g. human immunoglobulin, or animals, e.g. horse serum).

Vaccines

Strictly speaking, a vaccine is a suspension of bacteria or viruses which have been killed or rendered harmless. It therefore contains the toxins of the organism which have been rendered innocuous and can no longer produce actual disease in the individual.

The toxins, however, have the power to stimulate the production of antibodies and, in this way, to raise the resistance of the recipient to a particular organism.

The vaccine lymph used in the prevention of smallpox differs from most other vaccines since it contains the living organisms which cause cowpox or vaccinia. The immunity produced by its use depends on the fact that the individual vaccinated contracts cowpox, which is a local lesion at the site of inoculation.

The antibodies to cowpox are apparently the same as those to smallpox and, therefore, an immunity to smallpox remains after the local lesion has healed.

In addition to the above types of vaccine containing organisms, preparations can be made of their toxins, specially made in the form of 'toxoids'.

Generally speaking, viral vaccines are suspensions of living organisms the virulence of which has been so reduced that no active disease can result.

Techniques of administration

Most vaccines are given by subcutaneous injection usually over the deltoid muscle. In most instances further injections (boosting doses) are required at intervals appropriate to each vaccine. Some vaccines can be given by mouth, e.g. poliomyelitis, and possibly by nasal spray.

Reactions

The administration of a vaccine may be followed by a reaction which may be either local or general.

(a) Local reaction, with pain, swelling and redness at the site of infection within 12 to 24 hours.

(b) General reactions. These include a rise in temperature and general lassitude.

Certain persons should, in general, not be vaccinated. They are:

pregnant women and

patients with immune deficiency:

cancer patients

patients taking corticosteroids

patients taking immunosuppressive drugs.

Uses

Vaccines are used to produce an immunity which will prevent the individual from contracting the disease or, at least, modify its severity, if the patient subsequently happens to come in contact with the organism concerned. As already indicated the immunity produced only lasts for a limited period, usually from one to several years, after which 'boosting' doses are needed.

In recent years, in order to reduce the number of injections required, it has been possible to combine several different organisms or their toxoids in one preparation.

Routine immunization

Vaccinations in infancy and childhood, in particular, have been largely responsible for the very marked reduction in the incidence of a number of infectious diseases and their serious results and complications, e.g. whooping cough, measles, smallpox, diphtheria and poliomyelitis and even to their virtual disappearance.

Special time schedules have been worked out in order to give the maximum immunity when the child is most likely to be in contact with or affected by the disease; i.e. infancy, school entry and later in life.

It should be stressed that, overall, vaccines are safe and their acceptance should be encouraged. The risk of paralysis following vaccination with poliomyelitis vaccine is about one case in five million.

Diphtheria prophylactics

Originally there were several individual preparations, e.g.:
  alum precipitated toxoid (APT)
  purified toxoid, aluminium precipitated (PTAP)
  toxoid–antitoxin floccules (Dip/Vac/TAF).

The preparation now in use for primary immunization in early childhood is PTAP which is combined with tetanus toxoid and pertussis vaccine, or with tetanus toxoid and poliomyelitis vaccine. As previously indicated these mixed vaccines reduce the number of injections required.

> Diphtheria vaccines may cause severe reaction if given to older children and adults for the first time. A preliminary Schick Test is desirable to detect such individuals. TAF is often preferable in such cases.

Tetanus vaccine (toxoid)

It is now usual to combine this with diphtheria immunization in childhood, with subsequent boosting doses. If commenced later, 0·5 ml is given by intramuscular injection followed by 1·0 ml in 6 weeks. Further doses are desirable after 1 and 5 years in order to give full protection. If such an immunized individual should happen to sustain a wound likely to be infected with tetanus bacilli a further dose should preferably be given immediately if 5 years or more have elapsed since the last dose.

A non-immunized person, in such circumstances, may require

human tetanus immunoglobulin or tetanus antitoxin (horse serum) and penicillin or tetracycline.

Pertussis (whooping cough) vaccine

This is usually given in combination with the two vaccines previously mentioned. It does not always seem to give complete protection but can be expected to modify the severity of the disease.

Rarely, there are serious neurological complications of vaccination against pertussis. Children in high-risk groups include those with existing disorders of the CNS and those with a personal or family history of convulsions. The vaccination of such children is usually better avoided. Otherwise, the benefits of pertussis vaccination outweigh the risks, especially in babies under the age of one year. Children with acute illnesses, especially with respiratory symptoms, generally should not be vaccinated until they have fully recovered.

Poliomyelitis vaccine

Two types of vaccine have been developed.
(a) Salk-type vaccine which is given by intramuscular injection, repeated in 6 weeks and again after 6 months.
(b) Sabin-type vaccine which has largely replaced the former for routine use because it is given by mouth, e.g. three drops on a piece of sugar repeated after an interval of 6–8 weeks, with a booster dose every 3 years. It can be given at the same time as the diphtheria–tetanus–pertussis vaccine but is avoided during early pregnancy or any intercurrent illness, or diarrhoea. It contains three strains of polio virus.

Measles vaccine

This is a live attentuated viral vaccine, given by intramuscular injection. Its administration is advised for children between 1 and 10 years of age, who have not had measles. If its use became universal, measles might very well disappear in its epidemic form.

It should not be used in the presence of any intercurrent disease such as leukaemia, Hodgkin's disease or in children taking steroids.

A mild febrile reaction commonly occurs 5–12 days after immunization.

Rubella (german measles) vaccine

This is a live attenuated viral vaccine given subcutaneously in a dose of 0·5 ml, to girls at the onset of puberty. About 15 per cent of young married women have no acquired natural immunity. If they are exposed to rubella during the first 4 months of pregnancy, their babies may be born deformed, blind, deaf, mentally retarded or with cardiac defects. Hence the importance of vaccinating non-immune girls before they embark on having a family.

Smallpox vaccination

Historically this was the first adventure into the realms of disease prevention for it was Edward Jenner in 1780 who made use of the fact that human beings who contracted cowpox—a local lesion usually on the hands—as a result of milking infected cows were immune to smallpox. Vaccinia is an acute infection affecting cows and characterized by a pustular eruption which is confined to the udder and teats. It is considered that the condition is due to the infection by the virus of smallpox, the virulence of which is so modified by its passage through the body of the cow that only a localized lesion results. Rarely, vaccinia lesions spread extensively over the body—a condition known as *generalized vaccinia*. It occurs particularly in children who lack gamma globulin (hypo-gammaglobulinaemia) and may be fatal. Smallpox vaccine (a live virus vaccine) would not be given to a person receiving cortico-steroid therapy unless that person had been in actual contact with a smallpox case. The vaccination would then be performed under cover of vaccinial globulin given intramuscularly according to body weight.

The material used for the purpose of smallpox vaccination is prepared in the following way. A healthy calf is inoculated with the virus of vaccinia. Vesicles of cowpox develop on the udder of the calf. The lymph from these vesicles is collected and mixed with glycerin, which acts as a preservative. The final product, after tests to ensure its freedom from other organisms, is placed in small glass or plastic tubes and is known as glycerinated calf lymph.

Technique

The site of inoculation is cleaned with soap and water. Antiseptics are not used as they might destroy the virus.

The lymph is introduced into the skin either (*a*) by making a superficial scratch with a needle or point of a scalpel, not more than 1·5 cm (0·5 in) long without drawing blood, through a drop of lymph placed on the chosen spot, or (*b*) by means of the multiple pressure technique using a triangular pointed needle which is held almost parallel to the skin. Fifteen to 30 applications of fine pressure are made through the drop of lymph which are sufficient to roughen the skin and to permit the entry of the virus.

The lymph is allowed to dry and may then be covered by a small sterile but not antiseptic, preferably waterproof, dressing.

The following sequence of events takes place at the site of a primary inoculation. On the 3rd day a red papule appears, by the 6th day it has become a vesicle which reaches its maximum development on the 8th day and has a central (umbilicated) depression. By the 10th day a pustule is formed with some surrounding redness of the skin and local tenderness. The axillary glands may also be swollen and tender. Slight fever and malaise may occur. In the course of 2 or 3 days the pustule dries up, leaving a scab which separates by the end of 3 weeks.

In successful revaccination, the process is accelerated and the lesion is smaller unless a long interval has elapsed since the primary vaccination.

Recent successful vaccination produces complete immunity to smallpox in 9 days from the time of inoculation. The incubation period of smallpox is approximately 14 days. It follows, therefore, that an individual vaccinated within 3 or 4 days of exposure to smallpox will obtain protection.

Methisazone (Marboran) has been shown to protect smallpox contacts even if given late in the incubation period. It is a synthetic drug which is given by mouth, adult dose: 6 g. The drug is not of any value in the treatment of the disease itself but is useful in generalized vaccinia.

Complications of smallpox vaccination

(a) **Post-vaccinal encephalitis** or inflammation of the brain occasionally occurs. It has a high mortality (30–40 per cent) and those who do not succumb may be left with permanent brain damage.

(b) **Local sepsis** which should not occur if the subject is in a good state of health and proper cleanliness is observed.

(c) **Auto-inoculation.** The vaccinee may scratch the itching lesion and transfer the virus, with his fingers, to other parts of his body. Vaccination lesions then appear at these sites. If the eye happens to be one of these sites, corneal scarring and blindness may result.

(d) Generalized vaccinia. The law no longer demands that vaccination shall be performed on infants before the age of 6 months. In view of the possibility of post-vaccinal encephalitis in older children, if it is to be included in the vaccination schedule, children should be vaccinated during the second year of life.

(e) A generalized erythematous rash due to allergy.

Routine smallpox vaccination is no longer recommended in the UK except for doctors, nurses and others who may come in contact with smallpox.

The immunity conferred by this vaccination lasts about 3 years and revaccination should, therefore, be performed at 3-yearly intervals, in particular in individuals who are likely to come in contact with the disease. A lesser degree of immunity persists for about 7 years.

Special immunization

There are a number of infections to which immunity may be provided by the use of vaccines, but generally speaking they are only needed by travellers abroad or workers in special trades, or according to individual circumstances.

Tuberculosis vaccine

A preparation known as BCG vaccine (Bacille Calmette–Guerin) consisting of live tubercle bacilli, specially cultured so that they have become non-virulent and unable to cause disease, has been used to produce a degree of immunity to tuberculosis in newborn infants of tuberculous parents, some adolescents (all tuberculin negative children from 10 to 13) and those who work in contact with tuberculosis, e.g. nurses, who are found to be tuberculin negative. An intradermal dose of 0.1 ml produces a small papule which persists for some weeks. Although this does not promise complete protection it does increase the resistance to the infection.

Influenza vaccine

A single dose containing inactivated (killed) viruses of types A and B (or variations of them) may be given in the autumn. Each year vaccines are prepared against the influenza virus strains expected to be prevalent in the ensuing winter. It is particularly recommended for individuals who are suffering from conditions in which influenza might have serious effects. Examples are patients with chronic heart or lung disease, renal disorders or diabetes mellitus. There is also a good case for vaccinating elderly people resident in institutions. Vaccination of key personnel (including all hospital staff) is also recommended. Influenza outbreaks in hospitals can have a disastrous effect on staffing and hence on patient care. Vaccination must be performed annually, there being no broad-spectrum once-in-a-lifetime vaccine.

The injection is given subcutaneously; the dose for an adult is 1 ml and for a child (6–12 years old) it is 0·5 ml. Some vaccines should not be administered to anyone who is allergic to eggs, the influenza viruses having been grown in hen's eggs.

Nasoflu contains live virus particles (attenuated strains) and is given by instillation into the nostrils. It is suitable in certain cases but the killed vaccines are usually preferable.

Typhoid vaccine

The vaccine generally employed to produce immunity to enteric fever contains killed typhoid bacilli together with the bacilli which cause paratyphoid A and paratyphoid B, in order that it may be effective against all the organisms of the typhoid group. It is sometimes called TAB, and usually contains (in 1 ml):

Typhoid bacilli	1000 million organisms
Paratyphoid A	500 million organisms
Paratyphoid B	500 million organisms.

A 1st dose of 0·5 ml subcutaneously is followed by a 2nd dose of 1 ml after an interval of 28 days. A 3rd dose should be given 6 to 12 months after the second. Those frequently exposed to infection should be revaccinated every 12 months.

A local reaction occurring at the site of injection, consisting of tenderness, redness and swelling after 4 hours, is common. General symptoms including pyrexia or malaise lasting 24 hours are quite common. The subject should restrict activity during this period and avoid alcohol. Reactions are less severe if an intradermal preparation of typhoid vaccine is used (dose 0·1 ml).

A preparation of the toxin of tetanus (tetanus toxoid) may be included in order to produce immunity to tetanus at the same time (TABT). The interval between doses should be 4 to 6 weeks. A 3rd dose may be given after 6 months. Typhoid vaccine may also be combined with cholera vaccine.

Other vaccines are available and used according to regional requirements. They include: cholera, yellow fever, typhus, and plague vaccines.

Yellow fever vaccine

Yellow fever vaccine is prepared from attenuated living virus. It gives sound immunity for 10 years and all visitors to tropical Africa and tropical America should be vaccinated with it.

Rabies vaccine

This is desirable for workers in quarantine kennels and when local outbreaks occur. Stocks are held by the Public Health Laboratory Service at 4 centres in Britain. Fortunately, rabies has a long (but variable) incubation period, which permits effective immunization early after exposure to the virus. The severe adverse reactions to the older vaccines are not seen after injections of the newer vaccine prepared from rabies virus cultivated in human cell cultures.

Anthrax vaccine

This is desirable for workers in tanneries and similar occupations handling raw leather and other animal products.

NB.—Details of available vaccines, their dosage and interval requirements are clearly listed in the British National Formulary and literature is also supplied by the manufacturers.

Tests of immunity

Although bacterial toxins themselves are too dangerous for therapeutic use, very dilute solutions are used in order to test the immunity of individuals to certain diseases.

If a minute dose of toxin is injected into the skin (intradermally) and the individual has antibodies to that disease circulating in the blood, the effect of the toxin will be neutralized and there will be no reaction (negative response).

On the other hand, if the blood is deficient in antibodies, the toxin will produce local inflammation (redness, swelling, etc.) and the reaction is said to be positive. In other words, it indicates that the individual is susceptible to the disease. Examples of this are:

1. The Schick test for diphtheria

A minute dose (0·2 ml) of diluted diphtheria toxin is injected directly into the skin of the forearm (intradermally). If the individual has a sufficient amount of diphtheria antitoxin circulating in the blood, the toxin is neutralized and no reaction takes place.

Such a patient is immune to diphtheria and the test is said to be negative.

On the other hand, if the patient has not sufficient antibodies to diphtheria present, an area of redness 1·5–2·5 cm (0·5–1 in) in diameter develops at the site of injection within 24 hours and persists for 2 to 3 days. This is a positive reaction.

A control injection is made into the other forearm consisting of diphtheria toxin which has been destroyed by heat. This is done in order to make sure that a positive reaction is due to the toxin and not to the protein contained in it, as some individuals are sensitive to the protein alone.

Immunization

Those patients who have been found to be susceptible to diphtheria by means of the Schick test can be rendered immune by injecting one of the diphtheria prophylactics already mentioned. The body is stimulated to produce a supply of antibodies which lasts for several years. Two or more subcutaneous injections are given and immunity develops about 6 weeks after the last injection has been made. By this means it has been possible to reduce very considerably the incidence of infection among school children and among those nursing diphtheria.

2. The Dick test for scarlet fever

This is a similar test to the above, using the toxin of the scarlet fever streptococcus in place of diphtheria toxin.

Tuberculin tests

The basis of the various tests for tuberculous infection is tuberculin. This is an extract obtained from tubercle bacilli and contains some of their toxins.

3. The Mantoux test

This consists of the intradermal injection of 0·1 ml of 1 in 10 000 dilution of Old Tuberculin into the forearm. In a positive reaction an area of redness and swelling develops at the site of inoculation within a few hours and reaches its maximum in 24 to 48 hours. If negative, subsequent tests may be carried out with stronger solutions, i.e. 1 in 1000 and 1 in 100.

This test is interpreted on a different basis from the tests for diphtheria and scarlet fever. Firstly, a distinction must be made between turberculous infection and tuberculous disease. Sooner or later tubercle bacilli gain entrance to the body of almost every individual, but it is only in a few that active clinical tuberculous disease develops.

A positive reaction means that an individual has been infected by the tubercle bacillus at some time which may or may not have produced evidence of disease. By this infection he has been rendered sensitive or allergic to the toxins of the tubercle bacillus and the positive Mantoux test is an allergic reaction in the skin to the proteins contained in these toxins.

A positive reaction in young children often indicates active tuberculous disease. Except in special circumstances, a negative reaction indicates that there has been no tuberculous infection.

4. The Heaf test

For this test tuberculin purified protein derivative (PPD) is used. A ring of superficial punctures is made in the skin with a special instrument. The punctures are made through a spread-out drop of PPD. The result is judged by the number of papules which develop.

5. The tine test

This is performed using a disposable unit with 4 prongs or 'tines', of 2 mm length, which are coated with Old Tuberculin.

6. Patch tests

These are similar in principle and consist of the application to the surface of the skin of a patch of material saturated with tuberculin. This is left in position for 24 hours. Local redness and swelling indicate a positive reaction.

Sera

The term serum used in therapeutics refers to the blood serum of an animal which has been rendered immune to a disease by means of a vaccine or toxin. Sometimes, also, serum is obtained from a human being who is convalescent from, or has previously had, a particular disease. Such sera, therefore, contain antibodies to the disease which have the power either of neutralizing the toxins or destroying the bacteria which cause the condition. They may be either:

(1) Antitoxic.
(2) Antibacterial.

Because they contain antibodies 'ready made' by another animal and the individual to whom they are given takes no part in the formation of these antibodies, they are described as producing 'passive immunity'.

Unfortunately it is not possible to produce sera which are effective against all organisms. Further, the introduction of chemotherapy and antibiotics have rendered the use of certain sera obsolete, for example, antistreptococcal serum and meningococcus antitoxin.

Among the more important sera are:

diphtheria antitoxin
tetanus antitoxin
gas gangrene antitoxin (NB. hyperbaric oxygen may be more valuable than serum
or antibiotics)
snake antisera.

Serum may be used (i) as a prophylactic agent after exposure to infection in order to prevent an attack or to minimize its severity, or (ii) in the treatment of established disease.

Immunity acquired as a result of an infection lasts for a considerable period and often for a lifetime. Active immunity produced by a vaccine may last several years, but passive immunity obtained by the injection of a serum is of short duration which rarely exceeds a few weeks.

Sera may be administered by the subcutaneous, intramuscular, intravenous, intraperitoneal or intrathecal routes. The rate of absorption is most rapid when the intravenous route is used and this method is also of advantage when large doses have to be given. Intramuscular injection produces quicker results than subcutaneous.

Serum sickness

Because serum contains protein which is foreign in character to that of the individual receiving it, allergic reactions are sometimes observed 8 to 12 days after its administration. These consist of pyrexia, joint pains, rashes such as urticaria (wheals), erythema (general redness), etc. This condition is known as serum sickness and may be relieved by injections of adrenaline (1 in 1000), 0·5 ml, and applications of calamine lotion if the rash is irritating. Antihistamine drugs are also given.

Modern methods of preparing serum have, however, reduced the amount of protein present to a minimum and reactions are not so common as formerly.

Anaphylactic shock

This is a severe type of allergic reaction. If a patient has at any time had an injection of horse serum, in any form, great care must be taken if another dose is given, as the individual is rendered over-sensitive to the proteins contained in horse serum. This over-sensitivity takes about 10 days to develop and persists for a very long time. Once it has developed a second injection of serum may cause immediate and severe collapse or even sudden death. These symptoms are known as anaphylactic shock. Asthmatic patients are often sensitive to the injection of horse serum, and for these reasons, all patients should be asked if they suffer from asthma or if they have previously had serum, before the injection is given. Most cases of anaphylactic shock follow the administration of drugs by injection. Apart from horse serum, examples are penicillin, streptomycin, and even ACTH and tetracosactrin.

Treatment consists of the intramuscular injection of adrenaline, 0·5 to 0·75 ml of a 1:1000 solution, repeated if necessary after 10 minutes and again after 30 minutes. In addition, an injection of an antihistamine is given, e.g. chlorpheniramine (Piriton) 10 mg intravenously. A corticosteroid may also be given, e.g. hydrocortisone 100 mg intravenously.

The foot of the bed should be raised. Artificial respiration may be necessary.

Persons known to be sensitive may be desensitized by giving a series of small amounts before the main dose, e.g. 0·5 ml, 1 ml, 2 ml, 5 ml at intervals of 5 minutes.

In patients with diphtheria who have previously had antitoxin, a preliminary intramuscular injection of 1 ml followed 6 hours later by the full intramuscular dose of serum has been found satisfactory.

Adrenaline should always be at hand in case of emergency.

Diphtheria antitoxin

This may be given subcutaneously, intramuscularly or intravenously. When large doses are used, the latter method is preferable. The dose is ordered in units according to the severity of the case, irrespective of the age of the patient, and may be repeated in 12 to 24 hours, e.g.:

in mild cases and nasal diphtheria	8 000 units
for moderately severe cases	16 000 units
for severe cases and laryngeal diphtheria	24 000 to
	100 000 units.

Tetanus antitoxin

Human tetanus immunoglobulin (Humotet) or antitetanic horse serum may be used prophylactically and for the treatment of the disease.

Prophylaxis

If the patient has not been adequately immunized the incidence of tetanus may be greatly reduced by giving appropriate doses of antitoxin without delay to all cases of accidental wounds, in particular those contaminated with road dirt. The minimal dose of tetanus antitoxin (antitetanic horse serum) is 1500 units. In extensive and badly contaminated wounds it is repeated in a week.

A preliminary test dose for serum sensitivity of 0·2 ml should be given first, followed by the remainder in 30 minutes if there is no reaction.

Human tetanus immunoglobulin is preferable to horse serum. The dose is 250 IU by intramuscular injection and this gives protection for 4 weeks. A dose of 500 IU is used if the wound is more than 24 hours old or if it is likely to be heavily contaminated with *Clostridium tetani*.

Treatment

Once the disease has developed, the only hope of success is to administer repeated large doses of antitoxin, e.g. human tetanus immunoglobulin 30–300 IU/kg intramuscularly or tetanus antitoxin (horse serum) as follows:

initial dose:	25 000 to 100 000 units
	intravenously
repeated daily dose:	50 000 units
total dosage:	300 000 to 400 000 units.

The symptoms of tetanus are caused by the toxins of the germ in the wound spreading up the nerves (or possibly by the blood stream) to the brain and spinal cord. Once they have reached the central nervous system, the toxins become 'fixed' in the tissues and are unaffected by antitoxin. The effect of the latter is to neutralize any more toxin manufactured in the wound and to render it harmless before it can reach the central nervous system.

At the same time, the spasms are controlled by sedatives such as pentothal, phenobarbitone, chlorpromazine, bromethol (Avertin) or paraldehyde, the last two being given per rectum. Muscle relaxants, tracheostomy and mechanical ventilation may be required.

The prevention of tetanus

In view of its high mortality the prevention of tetanus is of great importance and prophylactic measures are essential in most wounds due to trauma, especially in agricultural and garage workers. Individuals may be divided into two main groups:

1. **Immune,** i.e. those who have received 3 injections of tetanus vaccine within 5 years. A subsequent boosting dose will have given a further period of 5 years' immunity.

    Procedure:

    Such casualties only require a further 0·5 ml of tetanus vaccine intramuscularly, unless the wound is likely to be heavily infected with *Clostridium tetani*. In the latter case, 500 IU of human tetanus immunoglobulin are also given.

2. **Non-immune,** i.e. (a) those who have never received a full course of tetanus vaccine or who have not received a boosting dose within 5 years; (b) if more than a week has elapsed since a previous dose of tetanus antitoxin.

    Procedure:

    (i) Provided non-immune patients have never had any type of serum before and have no history of allergic disease, they should be given not less than 1500 units of tetanus antitoxin (horse serum) or 250 IU of human tetanus immunoglobulin at once.

    (ii) If horse serum is used and serum sensitivity is likely to be present, give test dose of 0·2 ml antitoxin subcutaneously and wait 30 minutes before the remainder of the dose is given.

    (iii) In allergic subjects for whom no human tetanus immunoglobulin is available, the test dose of antitoxin should be diluted 10 times with saline and 0·2 ml of this mixture given. If no symptoms develop give 0·2 ml undiluted toxin followed by the full dose in 30 minutes as in (ii). If allergic shock symptoms develop the patient should be kept warm, lying down and given 0·5 ml of 1 in 1000 adrenaline intramuscularly. An antihistamine may be required. If shock symptoms have developed wait until these have subsided (6–12 hours) before further doses of antitoxin are given.

(iv) Following the administration of human tetanus immunoglobulin or antitoxin the patient should be instructed to have a course of tetanus vaccine, viz.

0·5 ml of absorbed tetanus toxoid on the same day as the antitoxin but in the other arm
0·5 ml 6 weeks later
0·5 ml 6 to 12 months later with subsequent boosting doses at intervals of 5 years.

It is important that the patient should have a record card indicating the treatment which has been given.

Human tetanus immunoglobulin is obtained from the serum of healthy donors who, as the result of active immunization, have high levels of tetanus antitoxin. Horse serum would now normally be used only when the human product is not available.

Snake antivenoms

These are used in the treatment of snake-bite. Monospecific and polyvalent antivenoms are available, the former neutralizing the venom of one specific snake (e.g. Russel's viper) and the latter containing the antidotes to the venoms of several snakes. The antivenoms are supplied in a freeze-dried or liquid form and the solutions are administered intravenously. In the UK, stocks of antivenoms for the treatment of bites from foreign snakes are held at the National Poisons Information Centre, London, and at Walton Hospital, Liverpool.

Human immunoglobulin (gamma globulin)

Normal human immunoglobulin (gamma globulin) is prepared from the pooled serum obtained from a large number of healthy adults which necessarily contains antibodies to some common diseases from which most of them have suffered in childhood or against which they have been immunized.

Under special circumstances serum from adults convalescent

from a particular disease or who have been recently immunized will have an even higher content of antibodies to that particular condition. This fact may be used in the treatment of vaccinia and in previously unvaccinated smallpox contacts and in women who have been exposed to rubella during the first 4 months of pregnancy. The importance of its use in early pregnancy is the well-known fact that rubella at this stage of pregnancy is very liable to produce congenital deformities in the fetus. It may also be used in children who are exposed to measles for the first time, especially if they are suffering from some intercurrent disease or are likely to cause an epidemic in a hospital ward or institution when they are in contact with other non-immunes. It is also useful in contacts of infective hepatitis and, possibly, poliomyelitis.

Human immunoglobulins give potential victims of a disease a partial short-term passive immunity. This applies to measles, infective hepatitis and possibly poliomyelitis in high-risk persons and conditions.

To prevent infective hepatitis, travellers to remote areas are given an intramuscular injection of immunoglobulin in a dose depending on body weight and likely degree of risk of hepatitis. Adults are given 500–750 mg intramuscularly and this dose is repeated every 6 months during a visit to a developing country.

Other biological products

Fibrinogen is available for the treatment of bleeding due to deficiency of this protein (afibrinogenaemia).

Anti-haemophilic globulin (AHG) is available, in short supply, for use in haemophilia.

20 Radioactive isotopes

Although not many doctors and nurses will handle these substances personally their increasing use in medicine justifies a brief reference to the subject which, however, cannot be fully understood without extensive knowledge of atomic physics. Nevertheless some of the more simple aspects can be generally appreciated.

(1) Basically, matter consists of a number of individual elements alone or in combination.

(2) Elements consist of atoms.

(3) An atom consists of a central nucleus with a number of electrons revolving round it.

(4) The nucleus of an atom consists of two types of particles, (a) protons, (b) neutrons.

(5) The number of protons in the nucleus of an atom equals the number of electrons which revolve round it.

(6) The chemical properties and characteristics of each element are determined by the number of electrons in its atom.

(7) Under certain circumstances the number of neutrons in the atom of an element may be varied. Although the element will then have the same general chemical characteristics its atom will be unstable and it will emit radiation of particles and rays, i.e. it becomes a radioactive isotope of the element.

(8) Certain elements, e.g. uranium and radium, occur in a natural state as a mixture of normal atoms and their radioactive isotopes. Radioactive isotopes of other elements can be produced by subjecting the normal atom of that element to the action of a nuclear reactor.

(9) In some instances the isotopes are very unstable and have a short life, that is, after emitting their radiation at a rapid rate the atoms soon return to normal. In others, this process may take days, weeks or many years before the radioactivity ceases, although in fact it is diminishing at a steady rate all the time. This loss of activity is described in terms of 'half-life'. For example radioactive iodine (^{131}I) has a 'half-life' of 8 days which means that at the end of each 8-day period only half of the radioactivity present at the commencement of that period remains.

(10) Radioactivity can be detected and measured by special apparatus, (*a*) Geiger counter, (*b*) scintillation counter.

(11) Living cells cannot distinguish between the normal element and the radioactive isotope. If, therefore, a tissue takes up the isotope its presence can be detected and measured by a 'counter'.

These facts are applied to medicine in the following ways: (1) research and diagnosis, (2) therapy.

A great deal of information has been obtained by isotope research on the metabolism and distribution of various substances throughout the body, e.g. the absorption of iodine, its concentration in the thyroid gland and use in the formation of thyroxine. Subsequently, the release and distribution of radioactive thyroxine into the blood stream has been demonstrated.

Although deep x-rays and radium remain the most useful and generally employed methods of radiation therapy for appropriate conditions, radioactive isotopes may be used in certain circumstances, e.g. malignant tumours of the tongue and bladder which were formerly treated by implanting radium needles may now be dealt with by using smaller needles or wires containing isotopes which are more easily handled. Liquid solutions can also be used, e.g. radioactive gold (^{198}Au) solution may be introduced into the pleural cavity in certain cases of malignant pleural effusion or into the peritoneal cavity in some cases of malignant ascites.

Other radioactive isotopes in use are:

(*a*) ^{131}I which given orally in appropriate dosage is an effective method of treating some cases of thyrotoxicosis and a small number of cases of thyroid carcinoma.

Possible risks of ^{131}I therapy in patients with thyrotoxicosis are the induction of thyroid carcinoma or leukaemia. Fortunately these risks appear to be entirely theoretical but, nevertheless, it is recommended that the treatment is reserved for patients over 40 years of age. Even then, for fear of genetic effects, it is withheld from women who are or might become pregnant.

A considerable proportion of patients treated with ^{131}I develop hypothyroidism. This requires treatment with thyroxine, usually 0·2 mg daily, which imposes no hardship.

(*b*) Radioactive phosphorus (^{32}P) is used in the treatment of polycythaemia vera, a condition in which there is an excess of red blood corpuscles. This substance acts by depressing the overactive bone marrow.

(c) ^{131}I and ^{32}P may be used for the treatment of malignant metastases in lymph nodes. The radioactive element, in an oily medium, is introduced into one of the lymphatic vessels which drain into the affected lymph nodes.

The use of isotopes in hospital

All forms of radioactivity, except in the most carefully controlled and minute doses, may affect health adversely. An individual who has been given a radioactive isotope will continue to excrete this

Table 20.1. Isotopes used in medicine

Isotope		Principal clinical uses
Chromium-51	^{51}Cr	Labelling of red cells for measurement of their life-span in haemolytic anaemias, or of their loss by gastro-intestinal haemorrhage.
Indium-111	^{111}In	Complexed with bleomycin for localization of primary and secondary tumours
Indium-113	^{113}In	Brain scanning to detect tumours, etc. Placental localization and liver and kidney scanning
Iodine-131	^{131}I	Diagnosis and treatment of thyrotoxicosis
Iodine-125	^{125}I	As ^{125}I-fibrinogen for the detection of venous thrombosis
Selenium-75	^{75}Se	As Se-75 selenomethionine iodide in pancreatic scanning for pancreatic carcinoma and chronic pancreatitis and as a Se-75-labelled agent for adrenal imaging
Strontium-87m	^{87}Sr	Bone scanning for the detection of tumour metastases in bone
Technetium-99m	^{99}Tc	Detection and localization of brain tumours (brain scan) Liver scanning (with sulphur colloid) Bone scanning (with Technetium (MDP) Agent) Lung scanning (with Technetium (MAA) Agent)
Thallium-201	^{201}Tl	Myocardial imaging: assessment of myocardial infarct
Xenon-133	^{133}Xe	Measurement of blood flow in brain, muscle, skin and other organs Lung function tests
Yttrium-90	^{90}Y	Implantation into pituitary tumours

in the urine and faeces for some time. The radiation from these excreta might be dangerous to others, especially children and pregnant women, who come in contact with them. Special precautions are, therefore, necessary. A specially screened storage room is essential. All urine, etc., must be collected and stored for several days or even weeks until the radioactivity has decayed sufficiently for it to be disposed of in the normal sewage system. Similar precautions are necessary for any contaminated bedding or clothing.

A hospital unit handling these substances will have special rules and provided they are strictly followed by the staff and patients, the administration of these substances is quite simple and will probably play an increasingly important part in the therapy of the future.

21   Cancer therapy

'We can speak of the cure of a disease when, perhaps a decade or so after the treatment, there remains a group of disease-free survivors whose annual death rate is similar to that of a normal population group of the same sex and age-distribution.'

This definition of cure was given by the late Marion Russell of Manchester in 1958. Today it can increasingly be applied to cancer. Some cancers which were incurable 10–15 years ago are now yielding to treatment and among them are chorioncarcinoma, Burkitt's lymphoma, Wilm's tumour, medulloblastoma and lymphoblastic leukaemia in children.

Cancer therapy may include surgery, radiotherapy, hyperbaric oxygen and neutron bombardment, chemotherapy, hormonal therapy and immunotherapy. One of these alone may be adequate or two or more may be used in combination or in sequence.

Radiotherapy uses x-rays, the 'cobalt bomb', linear accelerators and radioactive isotopes—e.g. ^{131}I in the treatment of thyroid carcinoma.

Cancer chemotherapy

Cancer chemotherapy involves the use of **cytotoxic drugs,** individually and in combination with each other. Combination therapy is particularly successful in acute lymphoblastic leukaemia. Chemotherapy has increased the median survival in this type of leukaemia from 3·5 months to 36 months.

Cytotoxic drugs may conveniently be grouped as follows:

alkylating agents
antimetabolites
plant products
antibiotics
miscellaneous.

Of the alkylating agents, **busulphan** (Myleran) is well known in the treatment of chronic myeloid leukaemia and Treosulfan is used to treat ovarian cancer. The antimetabolites are divided into folic acid antagonists (e.g. **methotrexate,** which is used in the treatment of acute leukaemia), antipurines (e.g. **6-mercapto-purine,** which is also used in acute leukaemia) and antipyrimidines (e.g. **5-fluorouracil,** which may be used in certain cases of carcinoma of the bowel and breast).

Plant products include the Vinca alkaloids extracted from the periwinkle (*Vinca rosea*). Of these, **vinblastine** (Velbe) is used to treat Hodgkin's disease and **vincristine** (Oncovin) is used in acute leukaemia.

Among the antibiotics which have antineoplastic activity are **actinomycin D,** which is useful in the management of Wilm's tumour, **daunorubicin** (Cerubidin) which is active against acute leukaemia and **doxorubicin** (Adriamycin) which is used against certain leukaemias and solid tumours. **Bleomycin** is an antibiotic which is highly effective against many malignant diseases, including certain metastatic tumours of the testes. The most important adverse effect of the drug is interstitial pneumonia, progressing to chronic pulmonary fibrosis.

The miscellaneous drugs, which cannot be classified under the above groupings, include **procarbazine** (Natulan), which is used in Hodgkin's disease and a variety of other malignant conditions, and **decarbazine** (DTIC) which is used against malignant melanoma, sarcoma and Hodgkin's disease. **Cytarabine** ('Cytosar') is used in the treatment of acute myeloblastic leukaemia. Colaspase, (L-asparaginase, Crasnitin) is used in cases of acute lymphoblastic leukaemia. It is an enzyme which is used to take advantage of a specific metabolic defect of certain malignant cells.

Hormonal therapy

Oestrogens (e.g. stilboestrol) are used for the treatment of disseminated prostatic carcinoma and **androgens** (e.g. testosterone) are used in the treatment of inoperable carcinoma of the breast in post-menopausal women. Oestrogens cause hypertrophy of the male breast (gynecomastia), and androgens have a virilizing effect on the female, causing the growth of facial hair, but the benefit to those who respond is often great.

Immunotherapy

The cell membranes of cancer cells differ from those of normal cells. The abnormal constituents may act as antigens which excite the production of antibodies. In other words, the body has an immunological defence mechanism against cancer cells, as it has against bacteria. Malignant tumours 'escape' this mechanism. Attempts are therefore being made to treat cancer by boosting the patient's immunity, a process called **active immunotherapy.** For example, the reticulo-endothelial (RE) system may be stimulated non-specifically by BCG vaccine in the hope of increasing the patient's immune reaction to cancer cells. Injections of BCG vaccine (attenuated tubercle bacilli) are being used experimentally for this purpose. Combinations of immunological stimulants and chemotherapeutic agents seem to offer hope for the future in cancer therapy.

22 Weights, measures, prescriptions and miscellaneous tables

The English systems of weights and measures are complicated. In addition to the Imperial or avoirdupois measures used in everyday life, there is a system of Apothecaries' weights which was employed exclusively in dispensing but is no longer lawful.

The metric system

The Metric System is the only system by which drugs may legally be dispensed in Britain. All drugs are prescribed in micrograms (mcg), milligrams (mg), grams (g) or millilitres (ml). Laboratory workers abbreviate microgram to μg, but this abbreviation is best avoided on prescriptions to prevent confusion with mg.

Metric weight

The unit of weight is one gram, which is the weight of one millilitre of water.

1 microgram	=1 millionth part of 1 gram	
1000 micrograms	=1 milligram=$\frac{1}{60}$ grain	
10 milligrams	=1 centigram=$\frac{1}{6}$ grain	
10 centigrams	=1 decigram=1·5 grains	
10 decigrams	=1 gram=1000 milligrams=15 grains	
1000 grains	=1 kilogram=2·2 (2$\frac{1}{4}$) pounds.	

Metric volume

1 millilitre (ml)=1 cubic centimetre (cc) or 15 minims approx.
1000 millilitres =1 litre=1·75 (1$\frac{3}{4}$) pints=35 fluid ounces.

Metric length

The standard measure of length is the metre (about 39 inches).

1 centimetre=$\frac{1}{100}$ part of a metre (0·01 metre)
1 millimetre=$\frac{1}{10}$ part of a centimetre (0·001 metre).

Measures of length, area and volume

1 inch=2·54 cm
12 inches, 1 foot =0·3 metre
36 inches, 1 yard=0·91 metre
16·5 feet=5·0 metres

1 sq inch $= 6\cdot45$ cm²
1 sq foot $= 0\cdot09$ metre²
1 cu inch $= 1\cdot64$ cm³
1 cu foot $= 0\cdot03$ metre³.

Approximate equivalents

The following are the approximate equivalents used in dispensing.
(BP 1963)

Grains	Milligrams	Grains	Milligrams
15	1000 (1 g)	1/10	6
12	800	1/12	5
10	600	1/25	2·5
5	300	1/60	1
1	60	1/120	0·5 = 500 micrograms
1/2	30	1/150	0·4 = 400 micrograms
1/3	20	1/200	0·3 = 300 micrograms
1/4	15	1/300	0·2 = 200 micrograms
1/6	10	1/600	0·1 = 100 micrograms

Minims	Millilitres	Fluid ounces	Millilitres
5	0·3	1/2	15
15	1	1	30
60	4	20 (1 pint)	600

Conversion of metric and imperial weights, etc.

The most important approximate figures are: To convert:

Weight

grains to grams   × 0·065
grams to grains   × 15
grams to ounces   × 0·03
kilograms to pounds × 2·2.

Fluid

millilitres (cc) to minims × 15
minims to millilitres   × 0·06
pints to litres   × 0·57.

Domestic measures

1 teaspoonful is just over 60 minims or 4 to 5 ml
1 dessertspoonful is about 120 minims or 8 ml
1 tablespoonful is about half a fluid ounce or 15 ml
1 tumblerful is just under half a pint or 260 ml.

These measures are very inaccurate and should not normally be used.

NB.—A standard 5 ml spoon is now issued to patients and the unit dose of paediatric mixtures has been adjusted to this. Adult mixture doses are 10 ml.

USA Liquid Measure

The minim, fluid drachm and fluid ounce of the British (Imperial) measure are slightly smaller than the corresponding measures in the US Apothecaries' Measure, but 16 ounces = 1 pint in US measure instead of 20 ounces = 1 pint in Imperial, and therefore the British (Imperial) pint, quart and gallon are considerably larger than the corresponding US measures.

To convert US minims, fluid drachms or fluid ounces into British (Imperial) measure, multiply by 1·0406. To convert the British measure into US measure, multiply by 0·9609.

To convert US pints, quarts or gallons into British (Imperial) measure, multiply by 0·8325. To convert the British measure into US measure, multiply by 1·2011.

Weights and measures

Apothecaries weight

(Formerly used in dispensing)

```
20 grains   = 1 scruple (℈)
 3 scruples = 1 drachm (ʒi) =   60 grains
 8 drachms = 1 ounce  (℥i) =  480 grains
12 ounces  = 1 pound       = 5760 grains.
```

Care must be taken to distinguish these from the domestic avoirdupois weights and from fluid measures.

Avoirdupois weight

```
16 drachms = 1 ounce (oz) =  437 grains = 28·35 g
16 ounces  = 1 pound      = 7000 grains = 0·45 kg
14 pounds  = 1 stone      = 6·5 kilograms.
```

Apothecaries fluid measure

```
60 minims        = 1 fluid drachm =  4 ml (approx.)
 8 fluid drachms = 1 fluid ounce  = 30 ml (approx.)
20 fluid ounces  = 1 pint         =  0·57 litre
 2 pints         = 1 quart        =  1·13 litre
 4 quarts        = 1 gallon       =  4·54 litres.
```

Thermometric equivalents

°C	°F	°C	°F	°C	°F
0·0	32·0	36·2	97·16	39·4	102·92
1·0	33·8	36·4	97·52	39·6	103·28
5·0	41·0	36·6	97·88	39·8	103·64
10·0	50·0	36·8	98·24	40·0	104·0
15·5	60·0	37·0	98·60	40·2	104·36
18·5	65·0	37·2	98·96	40·4	104·72
20·0	68·0	37·4	99·32	40·6	105·08
25·0	77·0	37·6	99·68	40·8	105·44
30·0	86·0	37·8	100·04	41·0	105·80
31·0	87·8	38·0	100·40	42·0	107·60
32·0	89·6	38·2	100·76	43·0	109·40
33·0	91·4	38·4	101·12	44·0	111·20
34·0	93·2	38·8	101·84	49·0	120·0
35·0	95·0	39·0	102·20	100·0	212·0
36·0	96·80	39·2	102·56		

To convert °C to °F multiply by $\frac{9}{5}$ and add 32.
Thus $37\,°C \times \frac{9}{5} = 66·6 + 32 = 98·6\,°F$.
To convert °F to °C subtract 32 and multiply by $\frac{5}{9}$.
Thus $100\,°F - 32 = 68 \times \frac{5}{9} = 37·7\,°C$.
NB. A change of 1 °C = a change of 1·8 °F.

Solutions

The nurse may be called upon to make up solutions of a certain strength from other stronger solutions or solid drugs. This practice involves various mathematical calculations in which accuracy is obviously of great importance.

Solutions may be:
(1) Hypertonic, isotonic, hypotonic (p. 119).
(2) Expressed as a percentage.
(3) Expressed in the Metric System, i.e. grams in 100 ml.
(4) Saturated solutions.

Saturated solutions

A saturated solution is one which contains as much solid as it is capable of dissolving; any additional amount of solid remains undissolved as a sediment.

It will be clear from experience that some substances (e.g.

sodium chloride, common salt) are very soluble and will dissolve
in a small amount of water. Others are less soluble, dissolve slowly
and require a much greater quantity of water; while some are insoluble.

Further, the rate and degree of solubility is usually increased
when the temperature of the water is raised.

Percentage solutions

A percentage solution expresses the number of parts of a drug in
one hundred parts of the final solution. The abbreviations 'per
cent' or '%' are used to denote this. For example:

A 5 per cent solution of dextrose contains:
5 parts of dextrose in 100 parts of the solution
1 part ,,   ,,   ,, 20   ,,   ,,   ,,
5 grams   ,,   ,, 100 ml   ,,   ,,

Dilution of solutions

The strengths of various solutions may be expressed either as a
percentage or as 1 part of the substance in a definite volume of
the solution, e.g.

1 in   5 solution = 20 per cent
1 in   10   ,,   = 10 per cent
1 in   40   ,,   = 2·5 per cent (2½ per cent)
1 in   80   ,,   = 1·25 per cent
1 in   100   ,,   = 1 per cent
1 in   500   ,,   = 0·2 per cent
1 in   1000   ,,   = 0·1 per cent.

The prescription

A prescription is a formula stating the ingredients of a remedy with directions
for its preparation and administration. (The term is derived from the Latin,
prae = before; *scribo* = I write.)

The modern prescription, although usually based on the original form illu-
strated below, should be written in English using ordinary numerals. The doses
are expressed in the Metric System and each mixture made up to a 10 ml
dose for adults and 5 ml for children. Metric quantities have been substituted
for the Apothecaries' measures originally used in the sample prescription below.
The classical prescription consists of a number of parts:

The name of the patient
the superscription
the inscription

the subscription
the signature
the name of the prescriber and the date of the prescription.

These terms can best be explained by examining a typical prescription.

William Smith, Esq.
    R. Potassii chloratis   .   .   .   .   . 600 micrograms
        Liquoris ferri perchloridi   .   .   . 1 ml
        Glycerini   .   .   .   .   . 2 ml
        Aquam. .   .   .   .   . ad 10 ml
             Fiat mistura.   Mitte 300 ml
        Signetur 10 ml, ter die sumenda, post cibos.

29th February, 1900   John Jones, M.D.

Using abbreviations this would also be correctly written as:

William Smith, Esq.
    R. Pot. chlor.   .   .   .   .   . 600 micrograms
        Liq. ferri perchlor. .   .   .   . 1 ml
        Glycer. .   .   .   .   . 2 ml
        Aq.   .   .   .   .   . ad 10 ml
             F.M.   M. 300 ml
            Sign. 10 ml, t.d.s., p.c.

29/2/00   John Jones, M.D.

The complete English translation of the above prescription would therefore be:

William Smith, Esq.
    Take thou (a direction to the Pharmacist)
        of potassium chlorate .   .   . .600 micrograms
        of solution of iron perchloride   .   . 1 ml
        of glycerin .   .   .   .   . 2 ml
        Put (or add) water up to 10 ml
        Let a mixture be made.   Send 300 ml.
Let it be labelled two 5ml spoonsful to be taken three times a day, after meals.

29th February, 1900.   John Jones, M.D.

The above prescription can be analysed in the following way.

Name of patient. This is obvious. The address may also be included. It is also permissible to put the patient's name at the end of the prescription.

Superscription. This is a sort of heading in the form of an instruction to the pharmacist. The symbol R is used and is an abbreviation of the Latin, *recipe* = take (thou).

The inscription. This is the prescription proper and is a list of the various ingredients, together with the amount of each. When written in Latin, it is expressed grammatically in the genitive case because it qualifies the amount 600 micrograms, i.e. 600 micrograms of potassium chlorate.

The subscription. This is an instruction to the pharmacist. It states the form which the preparation is to take and the amount to be dispensed.
Fiat mistura (F.M.) means 'Let a mixture be made'.

Mitte 300 ml means 'Send 300 ml'.
Fiat pilula would mean 'Let a pill be made'.
Fiat lotio would mean 'Let a lotion be made'.

The signature. This does not mean the signature of the prescriber but refers to the directions to be given to the patient. Signetur or Sign. means 'Let it be labelled' and the subsequent instructions to the pharmacist may be written in Latin, in abbreviated form or in English.

The prescription is completed by the addition of the doctor's name or initials and the date. When drugs controlled by the Misuse of Drugs Act are included, the total amount of the drugs to be supplied must be stated both in figures and in writing.

In modern Medicine, however, the prescription usually consists of a single, recognized ingredient (e.g. a tablet). In the case of established mixtures, the composition is usually stated in one of the recognized pharmacopoeas or in the BNF.

The letters NP (Nomen Proprium) are printed at the top right-hand corner of the NHS prescription form FP10. They instruct the pharmacist to write the proper names of drugs on their containers. This he or she will usually do unless the prescriber deletes the letters NP. For drugs subject to the Misuse of Drugs Act, the doctor in England and Wales must add his initials in the space alongside 'NP' if he wants the containers labelled. In Scotland, this is not required and no space is provided.

Latin phrases and abbreviations sometimes used in prescribing

Ana	āā.	of each
Ante cibum (cibos)	a.c.	before food (meals)
Ad libitum	ad lib.	to the amount desired
Aequales	aeq.	equal
Alternis diebus	alt. die.	alternate days (every other day)
Alternis noctibus	alt. noct.	alternate nights
Aqua	aq.	water
Bis die	b.d. ⎱	twice a day
Bis in die	b.i.d. ⎰	
Cras mane	c.m.	tomorrow morning
Cras nocte	c.n.	tomorrow night
Cum	c.	with
Ex aqua	ex. aq.	in water
Hac nocte	h.n.	this night
Mitte	m.	send
Nocte et mane	n. et m. (nmque)	night and morning
Omni mane	o.m.	every morning
Omni nocte	o.n.	every night

Parti affectae	p.a.	to the affected part
Post cibum (cibos)	p.c.	after food (meals)
Pro oculis	p.o.c.	for the eyes
Pro re nata	p.r.n.	as the occasion rises (to be repeated when required)
Quater in die	q.i.d.	four times a day
Quantum sufficiat	q.s.	a sufficient quantity
Repetatur	rep.	let it be repeated
Semissis	ss. or fs.	half
Si opus sit	s.o.s.	if necessary (a single dose)
Statim	stat.	at once
Ter die sumendum	t.d.s.	to be taken three times a day
Ter in die	t.i.d.	three times a day

Latin terminology

The fact that Latin is used, not only in connection with the official terminology of drugs but also in Anatomy and other branches of Medical Science, often adds to the difficulties of the student who has no knowledge of the language or its pronunciation. The following notes on the pronunciation usually employed and the grammar involved may be useful.

Pronunciation

Among the main rules for the pronunciation of technical Latin and of English words derived from Latin are:

ae is pronounced 'ee' as in spirochaete, mammae (breasts).

oe is pronounced 'ee' as in oedema (a very common mistake is to call this 'odema'), oesophagus, oestrin.

-i (at the end of a word) is pronounced 'i' long as in like, e.g. ferri (of iron).

-ii (at the end of a word), first 'i' short as in tin, second 'i' long as in like, as in calcii (of calcium), sodii (of sodium).

c is soft (i.e. like 's') before 'e' and 'i', as in cerebrum, cimetidine.

c is hard (i.e. like 'k') before 'a', 'o' and 'u', as in calomel, codeina, cum (with).

g is soft (i.e. like 'j') before 'e', and 'i', as in Progestin, genital, gingivitis.

g is hard (as in 'go') before 'a', 'o', and 'u', as in gastric, goitre, gumma.

Grammar

The types of word commonly encountered are:

Nouns: names of persons, places or things. In the nominative case (see below) many Latin nouns have the following endings:

-a	e.g. aqua	-as	e.g. benzoas
-us	spiritus	-is	cannabis.
-um	acidum		

Adjectives: words which express qualities of nouns:

aqua calida   = hot water
aqua destillata = distilled water.

Frequently the Latin adjective has the same ending as the noun as in the examples above, but this is not always so, e.g. injectio hypodermica.

Verbs: words which express an action or state. In the prescription the following are all verbs:

fiat (mistura) = let (a mixture) be made
mitte   = send
recipe   = take (thou).

Prepositions: words denoting the relation of nouns to other words in the sentence:

per urethram = through or by the urethra.

Conjunctions: words connecting nouns or phrases:

et = and (e.g. *Ferri et ammonii citras*—iron and ammonium citrate)
cum = with (e.g. *Hydrargyrum cum creta*, mercury with chalk).

Nouns undergo certain changes in form: Thus there is usually a different ending to denote singular (one person or thing) and plural (more than one)

aqua, water	aquae, waters
acidum, acid	acida, acids
pessus, a pessary	pessi, pessaries
vapor, an inhalation	vapores, inhalations.

There is, however, no single rule which can be given to indicate all the various changes which may occur.

The endings of nouns also change according to the case. The case of a noun depends on its relation to other words in the phrase or sentence, but the only two of importance in the present connection are the nominative and genitive cases. The former is the subject of the sentence, the latter answers the question 'of what or whom'. For example, in the description of a drug:

sodii sulphas = sulphate (nominative) of sodium (genitive).

It will be recalled that a prescription commences with the symbol R (*recipe*— take thou), the rest of the prescription is therefore written in the genitive case, i.e.

R   sodii sulphatis
take thou of sulphate of sodium (both words being in the genitive case, the genitive of sulphas being sulphatis).

Alternative names of some common drugs

Unofficial or Trade name	Approved name
Achromycin 275	tetracycline
Albucid 249	sulphacetamide
Aldomet 103	methyldopa
Amytal 155	amylobarbitone
Antepar 85	piperazine
Anthisan 106	mepyramine
Apresoline 104	hydrallazine
Aramine 99	metaraminol
Artane 177	benzhexol
Aureomycin 275	chlortetracycline
Aventyl 171	nortriptyline
Avomine 69	promethazine (chlorotheophyllinate)
Bactrim 285	cotrimoxazole
Benadryl 106	diphenhydramine
Benemid 223	probenecid
Benzedrine 174	amphetamine
Biogastrone 70	carbenoxolone
Brufen 256	ibuprofen
Butazolidin 257	phenylbutazone
Catapres 102, 179	clonidine
Cetavlon 59	cetrimide
Chloromycetin 275	chloramphenicol
Choledyl 135	choline theophyllinate
Cidomycin 277	gentamicin
Cytamen 110	cyanocobalamin (Vit. B_{12})
Dettol 45	chloroxylenol
Dexedrine 174	dexamphetamine
Diamox 141	acetazolamide
Dindevan 122	phenindione
Disprin 159	soluble aspirin
Distaquaine 269	procaine benzyl penicillin
Doriden 157	glutethimide
Dramamine 69	dimenhydrinate
Dulcolax 78, 80	bisacodyl
Edecrin 141	ethacrynic acid
Endoxana 114	cyclophosphamide
Epanutin 175	phenytoin
Equanil 169	meprobamate
Esbatal 103	bethanidine

Unofficial or Trade name	**Approved name**
Eserine 191, 248	physostigmine
Eumydrin 71	atropine methonitrate
Femergin 178	ergotamine tartrate
Fersolate 110	ferrous sulphate compound
Flaxedil 205	gallamine
Floxapen 272	flucloxacillin
Fucidin 278	sodium fusidate
Furadantin 146	nitrofurantoin
Gantrisin 285	sulphafurazole
Genticin 277	gentamicin
Glucophage 222	metformin
Hexopal 105	inositol
Hibitane 45	chlorhexidine
Hygroton 102, 143	chlorthalidone
INAH 281	isoniazid
Inderal 103, 190	propranolol
Indocid 257	indomethacin
Ismelin 103	guanethidine
Lanoxin 94	digoxin
Largactil 169	chlorpromazine
Lasix 141, 143	frusemide
Librium 169	chlordiazepoxide
Lipiodol 136	iodized oil
Luminal 156, 174	phenobarbitone
Marzine 69	cyclizine
Megimide 126	bemegride
Mesontoin 175	methoin
Miltown 169	meprobamate
Myanesin 206	mephenesin
Myleran 114	busulphan
Myocrisin 258	aurothiomalate
Mysoline 175	primidone
Nardil 170	phenelzine
Nembutal 155	pentobarbitone
Neo-mercazole 227	carbimazole
Oblivon-C 159	methylpentynol
Omnopon 165	papaveretum
Paludrine 253	proguanil
Pentothal 203	thiopentone sodium

Unofficial or Trade name	Approved name
Phanodorm 155	cyclobarbitone
Phenergan 106	promethazine
Physeptone 152	methadone (amidone)
Pitocin 237	oxytocin
Priscol 105	tolazoline
Prominal 174	methyl phenobarbitone
Pronestyl 96	procainamide
Prostigmin 174	neostigimine
Pyopen 273	carbenicillin
Rimifon 281	isoniazid
Rogitine 105	phentolamine
Salazopyrin 284	sulphasalazine
Seconal 155	quinalbarbitone
Septrin 285	cotrimoxazole
Serpasil 103	reserpine
Soneryl 155	butobarbitone
Stelazine 169	trifluoperazine
Sulfasuxidine 284	succinylsulphathiazole
Sulphamezathine 284	sulphadimidine
Sulphatriad 285	trisulphonamide
Tegretol 175, 180	carbamazepine
Terramycin 275	oxytetracycline
Tetracyn 275	tetracycline
Thalazole 284	phthalylsulphathiazole
Thephorin 106	phenindamine
Tofranil 171	imipramine
Tridione 176	troxidone
Trilene 200	trichlorethylene
Urolucosil 146	sulphamethizole
Valium 169	diazepam
Vascardin 101	sorbide nitrate
Welldorm 157	dichloralphenazone
Xylocaine 181	lignocaine
Yomesan 86	niclosamide
Zyloric 224	allopurinol

NB.—Fuller lists are given in The British National Formulary and unofficial publications such as MIMS.

Table of some adult doses

(See also Text)

NB. I.V. = Intravenous.　　I.M. = Intramuscular.
Subcut. = Subcutaneous or hypodermic.

	METRIC up to	IMPERIAL
acetazolamide (Diamox)	500 mg	gr. 2 to 4
acetomenaphthone (vitamin K) . .	10 mg	gr. $\frac{1}{8}$
adrenocorticotrophic hormone (ACTH) (I.M.)	100 mg	gr. $\frac{5}{12}$ to $\frac{2}{3}$
allopurinol (Zyloric).	100 mg	——
aminophylline (I.V.)	250 mg	——
amitriptyline	25 mg	——
amylobarbitone (Amytal) . . .	300 mg	gr. $1\frac{1}{2}$ to 5
„　　　　sodium (Sod. Amytal) .	600 mg	gr. 3 to 10
„　　　　„　　(I.V.) .	1 g	gr. 5 to 15
ammonium chloride.	4 g	gr. 5 to 60
amphetamine sulph (Benzedrine) . .	10 mg	gr. $\frac{1}{12}$ to $\frac{1}{6}$
„　　　　„　(Injection) . .	10 mg	gr. $\frac{1}{24}$ to $\frac{1}{6}$
ampicillin	250 mg	——
amyl nitrite (Inhalation) . . .	0·2 ml	m. 2 to 5
aneurine hydrochloride (vitamin B$_1$). .	50 mg	gr. $\frac{1}{50}$ to $\frac{3}{4}$
apomorphine hydrochloride . . .	8 mg	gr. $\frac{1}{32}$ to $\frac{1}{8}$
aqua chloroformi (chloroform water) .	30 ml	fl. oz. $\frac{1}{2}$ to 1
ascorbic acid (Vitamin C) . . .	250 mg	gr. $1\frac{1}{2}$ to 4
folic acid	5 mg	gr. $\frac{1}{8}$ to $\frac{1}{3}$
hydrochloric acid (dilute) . .	4 ml	m. 5 to 60
mandelic acid	4 g	gr. 30 to 60
nicotinic acid	100 mg	gr. $\frac{3}{4}$ to $1\frac{1}{2}$
aspirin (acetylsalicylic acid) . .	1 g	gr. 5 to 15
atropine: atropine sulphate . .	1 mg	gr. $\frac{1}{240}$ to $\frac{1}{60}$
atropine methonitrate (Eumydrin) . .	2 mg	gr. $\frac{1}{60}$ to $\frac{1}{30}$
bendrofluazide.	2·5 mg	
benzhexol (Artane)	(daily) increased from 2 mg to 20 mg	
bismuth carbonate	2 g	gr. 10 to 30
busulphan	2 mg	
butobarbitone (Soneryl) . . .	120 mg	gr. 1 to 2
caffeine	300 mg	gr. 2 to 5
calciferol (Vitamin D)	1·25 mg	(50 000 units)
calcium gluconate injection (I.M. or I.V) .	10 ml	gr. 30 to 60
„　　　lactate	4 g	gr. 15 to 60
carbimazole (therapeutic daily) . .	20 to 45 mg	——
„　　　(maintenance daily) . .	5 to 15 mg	——
carbon tetrachloride.	4 ml	m. 30 to 60
chloral hydrate	2 g	gr. 5 to 30
chlorambucil (Leukeran) . . .	5 mg	——
chlorothiazide	500 mg	——
chlorpromazine (oral daily) . . .	up to 800 mg	——

	METRIC up to	IMPERIAL
chlorpromazine (I.M.)	50 mg	——
chlorpropamide (Diabenese)	250 mg	——
choline theophyllinate (Choledyl)	200 mg	——
codeine: codeine phosphate	60 mg	gr. $\frac{1}{6}$ to 1
colchicine	1 mg	gr. $\frac{1}{120}$ to $\frac{1}{60}$
cortisone acetate (*oral or* I.M.)	25 mg	gr. 1 to 5
cyanocobalamin (vitamin B$_{12}$)	1000 mcg	——
cyclizine (Marzine)	50 mg	gr. $\frac{2}{5}$ to $\frac{3}{4}$
cyclophosphamide	100 mg	——
deoxycortone acetate (I.M.)	10 mg	gr. $\frac{1}{30}$ to $\frac{1}{6}$
diamorphine hydrochloride (heroin)	5 mg	gr. $\frac{1}{12}$–$\frac{1}{8}$
digoxin (Lanoxin) (*oral, initial dose*)	1·5 mg	gr. $\frac{1}{60}$ to $\frac{1}{40}$
,, ,, (*oral, maintenance*)	0·25 mg	gr. $\frac{1}{240}$
,, ,, (I.V.)	1 mg	gr. $\frac{1}{240}$ to $\frac{1}{60}$
dimenhydrinate (Dramamine)	50 mg	gr. $\frac{2}{5}$ to $\frac{3}{4}$
diphenhydramine (Benadryl)	100 mg	gr. $\frac{3}{4}$ to $1\frac{1}{2}$
elixir cascarae sagradae	4 ml	m. 30 to 60
emetine et bismuth iodide	200 mg	gr. 1 to 3
,, hydrochloride (*emetic*)	10 mg	gr. $\frac{1}{12}$ to $\frac{1}{6}$
,, ,, (*Subcut. or* I.M.)	60 mg	gr. $\frac{1}{2}$ to 1
ephedrine hydrochloride	100 mg	gr. $\frac{1}{4}$ to $1\frac{1}{2}$
ergometrine (I.M.)	1 mg	gr. $\frac{1}{240}$ to $\frac{1}{60}$
ergometrine (I.V.)	0·5 mg	gr. $\frac{1}{480}$ to $\frac{1}{240}$
ergotamine tartrate (*Subcut. or* I.M.)	0·5 mg	gr. $\frac{1}{240}$ to $\frac{1}{120}$
eserine (*see* physostigmine)		
ethinyloestradiol (*daily*)	0·02 to 0·1 mg	——
ferri et ammonii citras	2 g	gr. 5 to 30
ferrous sulphate	200 mg	gr. 1 to 5
glycerin	8 ml	dr. 1 to 2
glyceryl trinitrate (*Sublingual*)	0·5 mg	gr. $\frac{1}{120}$
guanethidine	10 mg	
heparin (I.V.)	5000 to 15 000 units	
homatropine hydrobromide	2 mg	gr. $\frac{1}{24}$ to $\frac{1}{32}$
hyoscine hydrobromide	0·6 mg	gr. $\frac{1}{200}$ to $\frac{1}{100}$
imipramine (Tofranil)	25 mg	——
indigocarmine (*subcutaneous*)	100 mg	gr. $\frac{3}{4}$ to $1\frac{1}{2}$
,, (I.V.)	16 mg	gr. $\frac{1}{8}$ to $\frac{1}{4}$
injection of adrenaline (1 in 1000)	0·5 ml	m. 2 to 15
,, ,, calcium gluconate (I.V. or I.M.)	1·0 g	m. 150 to 300
,, ,, mersalyl	2 ml	m. 8 to 30
,, ,, nikethamide (Coramine)	4 ml	m. 15 to 60
insulin		8 to 100 units
iophendylate (Myodil)	5 ml	——
iopanoic acid (Telepaque) *oral*	3 g	——
isoniazid (daily)	200 to 400 mg	——
isoprenaline (*sublingual*)	30 mg	gr. $\frac{1}{6}$ to $\frac{1}{2}$
kaolin (light)	60 g	oz. $\frac{1}{2}$ to 2
magnesium carbonate (light, heavy)	4 g	gr. 10 to 60
,, sulphate	16 g	gr. 30 to 240

	METRIC up to	IMPERIAL
magnesium trisilicate	2 g	gr. 5 to 30
meglumine iodipamide 50% (Biligrafin) I.V.	20 ml	——
mepacrine hydrochloride (Atebrin)	100 mg	gr. $\frac{3}{4}$ to $1\frac{1}{2}$
meprobamate	400 mg	gr. 6
methadone hydrochloride (Physeptone)	10 mg	gr. $\frac{1}{12}$ to $\frac{1}{6}$
methylamphetamine (Methedrine)	10 mg	gr. $\frac{1}{24}$ to $\frac{1}{6}$
,, (I.M. or I.V.)	10 mg	gr. $\frac{1}{6}$ to $\frac{1}{2}$
methyldopa	250 mg	——
methyltestosterone (daily)	50 mg	——
methylthiouracil	20 mg	gr. $\frac{3}{4}$ to 3
morphine sulphate	20 mg	gr. $\frac{1}{8}$ to $\frac{1}{3}$
nalidixic acid (*Negram*)	500 mg	——
nalorphine hydrochloride (I.V.)	40 mg	gr. $\frac{1}{6}$ to $\frac{2}{3}$
neostigmine (*Subcut. or* I.M.)	2 mg	gr. $\frac{1}{120}$ to $\frac{1}{30}$
nicotinamide	50 mg	gr. $\frac{1}{4}$ to 4
nikethamide (Coramine) (I.V.)	2 to 8 ml	——
nitrazepam (*Mogadon*)	5 mg	——
nitrofurantoin (Furadantin)	50 to 150 mg	——
oestradiol benzoate (1000 to 50 000 units)	5 mg	gr. $\frac{1}{600}$ to $\frac{1}{12}$
oestrone (1000 to 100 000 units	10 mg	gr. $\frac{1}{600}$ to $\frac{1}{6}$
paraffin (liquid)	30 ml	fl. oz. $\frac{1}{4}$ to 1
paraldehyde	8 ml	dr. $\frac{1}{2}$ to 2
penicillin (200 000 to 2 000 000 units)		——
penicillin V	250 mg	
pentobarbitone soluble (Nembutal)	200 mg	gr. $1\frac{1}{2}$ to 3
pethidine hydrochloride	100 mg	gr. $\frac{1}{2}$ to $1\frac{1}{2}$
phenformin	50 mg	——
phenobarbitone (Luminal)	120 mg	gr. $\frac{1}{2}$ to 2
phenobarbitone sodium (I.M. or I.V.)	200 mg	gr. 1 to 3
phenolphthalein	300 mg	gr. 1 to 5
phenylbutazone (Butazolidine) *daily*	200 to 400 mg	
phenytoin sodium (Epanutin)	100 mg	gr. $\frac{3}{4}$ to $1\frac{1}{2}$
physeptone (Amidone)	10 mg	gr. $\frac{1}{12}$ to $\frac{1}{6}$
physostigmine sulphate	1·2 mg	gr. $\frac{1}{100}$ to $\frac{1}{50}$
pilocarpine nitrate	12 mg	gr. $\frac{1}{20}$ to $\frac{1}{5}$
potassium bicarbonate	2 g	gr. 15 to 30
,, bromide	2 g	gr. 5 to 30
,, citrate	4 g	gr. 15 to 60
,, iodide	2 g	gr. 5 to 30
prednisone	5 mg	——
primaquine (base)	15 mg	——
primidone	250 mg	——
procaine hydrochloride	120 mg	gr. $\frac{1}{2}$ to 2
,, ,, (*subcutaneously*)	1 g	up to gr. 15
,, ,, (*intrathecally*)	150 mg	up to gr. $2\frac{1}{2}$
progesterone (1 to 5 units)	5 mg	gr. $\frac{1}{60}$ to $\frac{1}{12}$
proguanil (Paludrine) daily	400 mg	gr. $1\frac{1}{2}$ to 6
propantheline (Probanthine)	15–30 mg	——
propyliodone (Dionosil) for bronchoscopy	16 ml	——

	METRIC up to	IMPERIAL
propylthiouracil	50 mg	——
riboflavine	10 mg	gr. $\frac{1}{60}$ to $\frac{1}{6}$
quinalbarbitone sodium (Seconal sod.) .	200 mg	gr. $\frac{3}{4}$ to 3
quinidine sulphate	200 mg	gr. 1 to 5
quinine sulphate	600 mg	gr. 1 to 10
saccharin soluble	120 mg	gr. $\frac{1}{2}$ to 2
santonin	200 mg	gr. 1 to 3
scopolamine (*see* hyoscine) . .		
sodium bicarbonate	4 g	gr. 15 to 60
,, citrate	4 g	gr. 15 to 60
,, diatrizoate 45% (Hypaque) I.V. .	30 ml	——
,, iodide	2 g	gr. 5 to 30
,, ipodate (Biloptin) oral . . .	3 g	——
,, phosphate	16 g	gr. 30 to 240
,, ,, (acid) . . .	4 g	gr. 30 to 60
,, salicylate	2 g	gr. 10 to 30
,, sulphate	16 g	gr. 30 to 240
,, thiosulphate (I.V.) . .	25 g	gr. 5 to 15
spironolactone	25 mg	——
stibophen (Fouadin) I.V.	300 mg	gr. 1$\frac{1}{2}$ to 5
stilboestrol	2 mg	gr. $\frac{1}{120}$ to $\frac{1}{30}$
strophanthin (I.M. or I.V.) . . .	1 mg	gr. $\frac{1}{240}$ to $\frac{1}{60}$
,, G (ouabain) . . .	0·5 mg	gr. $\frac{1}{500}$ to $\frac{1}{120}$
sulphadiazine	2 g	gr. 8 to 30
sulphaguanidine	2 g	gr. 8 to 30
sulphathiazole	2 g	gr. 8 to 30
tetracycline	250 mg	——
thyroxine	0·2 mg	——
tolazoline (Priscol)	50 mg	gr. $\frac{2}{3}$ to $\frac{3}{4}$
troxidone (Tridione)	300 mg	gr. 1$\frac{1}{2}$ to 6
tryparsamide (*subcutaneously*, I.M.) . .	2 g	gr. 15 to 30
urea	16 g	gr. 15 to 240
urethane	2 g	gr. 15 to 30

Index

Index